Jim Fairlie was born in Perth and educated at Perth Academy. After graduating from Dundee University with a degree in Politics/Economics he taught for 13 years, and then became a financial adviser in 1983. He married Kay in 1961. Together they have two daughters, three sons, nine grandchildren and three great grandchildren. Jim was a member of the SNP for 35 years and held the post of Deputy Leader from 1980 until 1984. He left SNP in 1990 as a result of the party's support for EU, and is a known campaigner against euro-federalism.

UNBREAKABLE BONDS

(THEY KNOW ABOUT YOU, DAD)

JIM FAIRLIE

UNBREAKABLE BONDS

(THEY KNOW ABOUT YOU, DAD)

AUSTIN & MACAULEY

Copyright © Jim Fairlie

The right of Jim Fairlie to be identified as author of this work has been asserted by him in accordance with sections 77 and 78 of the Copyright, Designs and Patents Act 1988.

All rights reserved. No part of this publication may be reproduced, stored in a retrieval system, or transmitted in any form or by any means, electronic, mechanical, photocopying, recording, or otherwise, without the prior permission of the publishers.

Any person who commits any unauthorized act in relation to this publication may be liable to criminal prosecution and civil claims for damages.

A CIP catalogue record for this title is
available from the British Library.

ISBN 978 1 84963 034 4

www.austinmacauley.com

First Published (2010)
Austin & Macauley Publishers Ltd.
25 Canada Square
Canary Wharf
London
E14 5LB

Printed & Bound in Great Britain

DEDICATION

To my wife Kay,
for all the love and support.

ACKNOWLEDGEMENTS

I would like to achnowledge the Perthshire Advertiser for their tremendous support, and thank them for providing us with the photograph on the front cover, which featured their article, also titled 'Unbreakable Bonds'.

INTRODUCTION

This is a book which should never have been written. It is also a book which had to be written. It tells the story of a young woman, my youngest daughter Katrina, driven to the point of suicide and tormented by false images of murder, of ritual and serial rape, of being abused by her father and others, from the age of two for a period spanning over twenty years.

It tells the story of a family, my family, driven to the verge of destruction, forced to confront their parents with accusations of unspeakable crimes against their younger sister, of their pact to speak and act as one, so that each could draw strength from the others, as they fought to come to terms with the picture painted for them, of a violent and dangerous man they had always known as a loving father.

It is the story of my wife Kay, the woman who has shared my life for fifty years and who was prepared to sacrifice everything, including contact with the children and grandchildren she adored, in order to give me the love and support I so desperately needed. Her outrage and fury on my behalf has frequently been greater than my own.

Most of all, it is the story of a belief in a system gone wrong, of professionals, bureaucrats and their legal back-up teams financed by public money, all of whom were prepared to deliberately destroy an entire family rather than admit that a mistake had been made.

Recovered Memory or False Memory Syndrome has torn apart thousands of families both in this country and in the United States, where the "memory wars" so called, have been raging for more than two decades. This is not a direct contribution to the professional debate, which has so bitterly divided the psychiatric and psychology professions, because I am not qualified to comment professionally.

But I am better able than most to question a theory, the practical consequences of which has created so much heartache and misery and which has been so roundly condemned in every country in which it has been practised.

I am better able than most to challenge this theory because if I had not fought back, I would have been one of its many victims and my family would have been destroyed.

Cooperating with my Dad in the writing of this book has not been easy. When I discharged myself from Murray Royal Hospital in Perth, in March 1996 against medical advice and after having been an inpatient for fifteen months, I was determined never to go back. Unfortunately I was not well enough to be able to keep that vow. For the next year I had several short stays in the hospital, while attending the Cullen Centre in Edinburgh as an outpatient.

In February 1997 I was admitted as a voluntary patient to the Priory in Roehampton, diagnosed as suffering from anorexia nervosa, among other things, and spent the next ten months as an inpatient, subjected to much the same therapy I had been receiving since first being admitted to Murray Royal Hospital in November 1994. When I walked out of the Priory in November 1997, again against medical advice, I was determined that this time, I would stay out. Despite a few relapses, when I was admitted to Liff Hospital in Dundee for short periods, I have managed to regain my independence and have avoided any further contact with psychiatrists and their so-called profession.

I had no intention of taking part in the writing of this book because I wanted only to forget the most frightening period of my life. Those who have been subjected to Recovered Memory Therapy (RMT) will know that you tend to continue to have the images which were created, long after the therapy has ceased. I was repeatedly told that I was so ill that I might never get well enough to function as a normal person. Had I been prepared to listen and continue to allow the psychiatrists to keep me in therapy, I am convinced I would not have survived. During my time under their care in Murray Royal in Perth, a period of fifteen months, there were 66 incidents when I self-harmed or attempted suicide. At least four of those attempts almost succeeded. Since discharging myself from their tender mercies, there has not been a single instance of either self-harming or attempted suicide.

Why then, would I want to revive the memories of the most harrowing period of my life, by participating in the writing of this book with my Dad? Why would I want to relive the horror of the nightmares, nightmares induced by the drugs the psychiatric team prescribed? There is no simple or straightforward answer to that question. Perhaps the best answer is to say it is the same reason I would give to victims of rape for why they should speak out. Silence on the part of the victims, is the best and most potent weapon those who are guilty of rape have. Similarly silence is the best protection practitioners of Recovered Memory Therapy have. When they refuse to give answers to questions they have to be challenged. They also have to be stopped.

I feel an enormous sense of betrayal, by the health service, the legal profession and the justice system. Perhaps the most appropriate question that should be asked of me, is why would I not speak out?

Katrina

CHAPTER ONE

October 16th 1995

The unexpectedness, rather than the sound, of the telephone startled me because I had given instructions that I wanted no calls. Snatching at the telephone, the irritation in my voice was evident when I answered. "I am sorry," said the receptionist, "but it is your son Andrew on the 'phone and he says it is urgent."

"Alright, put him through."

"I need to speak to you Dad, can you come up to Philip's house?"

"Can it not wait? I'm pretty tied up just now."

"Sorry Dad, I need to see you right away."

"It must be serious if you want me to come up right now. What is it?"

"Sorry, I can't tell you on the 'phone."

After a moment's hesitation I said, "My car is in the garage being serviced and I can't get it back until after 5pm, but I will be up as soon as I can get a taxi."

The car journey to Philip's house took no more than ten minutes and the taxi driver chattered throughout, making it difficult for me to give much thought to what this was all about. It was only when we arrived that I discovered I did not have enough money to pay the driver. Andrew met me at the door and I asked him to pay the taxi while I went into the house. One look at the faces of my wife and the other three of our five children left me in no doubt that whatever was wrong, it was serious. My first question was, "Has something happened to Katrina?"

"You had better sit down Dad," said Sharon our eldest child.

"Has something happened to Katrina?" I repeated, looking from face to face, wondering why no one would look at me directly.

"The hospital knows about you Dad," said Sharon quietly, looking straight at me for the first time.

"Knows what about me?" I asked.

"They know you have been abusing Katrina for years."

"What? What are you talking about?"

There was silence as I looked from one to the other.

"What are you talking about? Is this some kind of wind up, because I don't think it is very funny."

"Katrina has made a statement to the police and they are making enquiries. So is the Child Protection Unit of the Social Work Department," said Sharon, whose pinched white face convinced me very quickly that this was no joke. I looked from her to the rest of the family. Philip and Andrew could not look at me but seemed to find the carpet fascinating.

Jim, our youngest son, was rocking back and forward in his seat, looking straight at the wall on the other side of the room. My wife Kay, sat rigid by the fire, her gaze had not wavered from the same spot somewhere in the middle distance.

"What statement could Katrina make to the police?" What am I supposed to have done?"

My voice was beginning to rise.

"We can't tell you because of the police enquiry," said Sharon.

"We're not telling you anything you don't already know," said Jim, speaking for the first time.

"What am I supposed to know? If there is a police enquiry, what are they looking for? Are you going to tell me what the hell is going on?" Anger was beginning to take over and I was rapidly losing patience. The questions were being spat out.

"The police are checking up on the paedophile ring you have been running in Perth and Dundee," said Sharon.

"Paedophile ring?" I shouted. "What bloody paedophile ring? Have you all taken leave of your senses?" Turning to Kay, "What have you got to say? Do you believe any of this?"

Kay's gaze was still fixed somewhere in space. "They say they have a lot of evidence," she mumbled.

"What evidence? Who says they have a lot of evidence? Evidence of what? What am I supposed to have done?"

"We're not telling you anything you don't already know," repeated Jim, still rocking back and forward in his seat.

"You will know there has been a SNP Councillor making enquiries to the police, asking if you were under investigation," said Sharon.

"What SNP Councillor? Making enquiries about what? I don't know what you are talking about!" I was beginning to sound as frantic as I felt. I had arrived expecting to be told something had happened to Katrina. Instead, I was being accused of being a paedophile, of abusing my youngest daughter. And I was being accused by my wife and the rest of my family.

By now I was standing in the middle of the room but the only person who actually looked at me was Sharon. Kay was sitting as if in a trance. Jim kept rocking back and forward in his seat, sometimes hugging himself, sometimes sitting on his hands. His response to every question was the same, "We are not telling you anything you don't already know." Philip and Andrew both stood with heads bowed, looking at the floor and saying nothing. I kept looking at each one in turn. This was my family who were condemning me as a paedophile and yet refusing to tell me what I was supposed to have done, other than to say that I had abused Katrina and was now being investigated by the police.

Kay and I had been at the school together, we were only seventeen when we had our first date and we had just celebrated our thirty third wedding anniversary the previous month.

And yet she seemed ready to believe that I could have done these things. I had always believed that I had a good relationship with my sons and Sharon, as the eldest in the family, had always been as close to me as any daughter could have been to a father. I would have given my life for any one of the five people who were in that room with me and yet they seemed like strangers. I have never felt so alone, so isolated. The hostility was almost tangible.

The impact of what had just been said to me finally penetrated. Speaking slowly and quietly, although seething inside, I said, "Don't think for a minute I am going to leave it like this. You can either tell me now what I am supposed to have done, or you will tell me in court." I had no idea of what I was going to do beyond getting out of that room and court was actually a long way from my mind. But what I did know was that I had been accused and convicted of something I had not done, albeit I had only the vaguest idea of what it was. Someone had made an accusation, someone had claimed to have evidence and I had no intention of hanging around waiting for the police to come looking for me. I decided to go to them first.

"Is it too much to ask for a lift into town as I don't have a car?"

There was no response and I stood for a moment or two, waiting. Finally I turned without another word and made for the door, at which point Sharon said, "I'll give you a lift. Where do you want to go?"

"I'll come with you," said Jim.

"The police station," I said, walking out into the hall without a backward glance.

We left the house in silence. Philip and Andrew still had not spoken and Kay had said no more than half a dozen words. In less than fifteen minutes, my entire world had collapsed around me. Not having the car annoyed me because I didn't want to be near any of them. I didn't want to have to speak to any of them until I could find out what was going on. Hesitating as we walked towards Sharon's car, I was on the verge of telling her and Jim that I would find my own way to the police station but impatience to get there and to speak to someone who could give me some information, overcame the need to get away from the family.

The journey seemed to take forever although it lasted only a few minutes, but silent hostility makes an uncomfortable travelling companion. I felt sick. My insides and my mind were churning. By the time we reached the police station I was desperate to get out of the car and had the door open before we had stopped. I had one foot on the ground when Sharon said, "You will need to speak to Rhona Anderson, she is the police constable who took Katrina's statement."

Without looking at either her or Jim I closed the car door and walked into the police station, passing a sergeant I had known for several years. We passed a few pleasantries, asking how each other's families were, while I wondered if he knew about the allegations. There was no obvious reaction from him when I said the family were doing well.

Crossing to the office counter, it didn't help to discover that of the two officers on duty, one was an ex-pupil of mine and the other was someone with whom I had played five-a-side football on a regular basis until only a short time previously. Both greeted me heartily, giving no indication that their attitude to me had changed in any way. But I still felt deeply uncomfortable and dreaded having to ask to speak to constable Anderson who worked in Child Protection.

Neither of them asked why I wanted to speak to Constable Anderson and continued to chat amiably while waiting for her to appear. On her arrival at the front office I was shown into a small interview room and discovered that although I had never actually taught her, Constable Anderson had been a pupil at the school at which I had taught economics for close on a decade.

She obviously knew who I was but there was no smile of recognition. The expression on her face did not convey hostility, just a professional neutrality. There was no greeting, no comment whatsoever – she just stood and waited.

"You'll know why I'm here. I've just been told I am under police investigation for running a paedophile ring and abusing my youngest daughter. What's it all about?"

"I'm sorry, I can't talk to you. Investigations are ongoing and we will contact you when we want to interview you. We are not ready to do that yet."

"You have to be able to tell me something," I protested. "My family have just told me that my youngest daughter has accused me of abusing her. What am I supposed to have done? And when?"

"I am sorry. There is nothing I can tell you at the moment. When we complete our enquiries we will call you in for questioning," said Constable Anderson.

"How long will that be? When can I expect to hear?"

"All I can say is that enquiries are ongoing and I don't know how long they will take." I was getting the official script. It had always amused me when, as a young probationary police constable, we learned to write official reports. Policemen never walked, they proceeded. A report of an incident would start off, "I was proceeding in a westerly direction on the south side of High Street, when…"

Constable Anderson was "proceeding" as the book demanded. It was obvious I was going to learn nothing, either about what I was supposed to have done, or about what was going on. It may have been my imagination but the look on the young policewoman's face seemed to register disgust.

It seemed pointless to ask any more questions and there was nothing else I could think of to say, despite feeling increasingly angry at this wall of silence. At the same time I was determined I was not going to be simply dismissed, to be treated as if I had already been tried and convicted of being a pervert, although given the attitude of my wife and family, and now this policewoman who had spoken to Katrina, that is exactly how they saw me.

"I'll expect to hear from you shortly because there is nothing to investigate." This was thrown over my shoulder as I made for the door, but I could not resist looking to see the reaction on Constable Anderson's face. It had not changed and she made no reply.

There were several messages waiting for me when I returned to the office but there was only one thing on my mind – to speak to the psychiatrist who had been treating Katrina. The telephone rang several times before there was any response at the other end. I spent those few moments going over in my mind what I was going to ask him, the questions literally tumbling over one another. "What did

Katrina say about me? When did she start making the accusations? What is wrong with her?" The same questions – over and over.

"Murray Royal." The clipped tones of the receptionist interrupted the mental rehearsal and for the moment I forgot why or who I was calling, until she repeated, "Murray Royal."

"I'd like to speak to Dr Yellowlees please."

"Yes, can I say who is calling please?"

"It is Mr Fairlie, Katrina Fairlie's father."

The silence went on for so long I began to wonder if I had been cut off and was about to redial when the reply came, "I'm sorry, Dr Yellowlees is not available at the moment."

"Can you say when he will be available? It is rather important that I speak to him."

"I'm sorry, I can't but if you care to leave a contact number, Dr Yellowlees will return your call."

"Can I speak to Nurse Hogg then?" Senior Charge Nurse Jenny Hogg was Katrina's main carer. We knew Katrina had spent a great deal of time with her therefore I assumed she would know what was going on.

More minutes passed and when Jenny Hogg finally came on the line, I found it difficult to frame the questions I needed to have answered.

"Maybe it is not appropriate for me to be speaking to you at all, but you will know why I am calling."

"No, I'm sorry I don't."

"But you are bound to know about Katrina's allegations."

"I'm sorry, I don't know anything about that."

The rest of the conversation went nowhere.

It was the same wall of silence. Jenny Hogg was to write in her notes of that day that she had found me, "calm, polite and pleasant" and that she "had responded likewise." It was no more than one hour after having been confronted by the family and Nurse Hogg's assessment of my manner so soon after, was in stark contrast to the way in which Dr Yellowlees was to claim I had spoken to him a full three and a half months later.

I sat and stared at the telephone, trying to think of someone else I could call, who could tell me what was going on. It was unreal. I could not believe what was happening. The telephone rang and I ignored it. It rang several times more and I ignored it each time. I just sat there, replaying the scene in Philip's house again and again. The same words kept coming back. "You have been abusing Katrina for years! Can't tell you! They have a lot of evidence! Ongoing enquiries! Can't tell you! Pervert! Paedophile ring! Can't tell you!"

"Bastards!" The word exploded from me as I threw my self up from the chair. It was almost five o'clock and I had still to collect the car. I left the office without speaking to anyone, collected the car and made for the first off-licence I could find. Armed with a bottle of The Famous Grouse, my first thought was to drive somewhere and get drunk. There was no way I was going home. I wasn't even sure I still had a home to go to.

Feeling drained, I was driving aimlessly, my stomach turning somersaults, the same thoughts cascading through my mind endlessly. The initial anger had begun to subside, leaving a numbness I had never experienced before, and was never to experience again. But the anger which had been driving me since the confrontation, was nothing compared to the sheer fury I was to feel later, when we started to piece together the full story of what had been done to our family, in the name of psychiatry.

It wasn't a conscious decision to look for somewhere to stay the night, it just happened. Driving north on Dunkeld Road, one of the main arteries out of Perth and a road which had a long string of houses offering Bed & Breakfast, I suddenly stopped and booked into one of them for the night. Although I had eaten nothing since morning, the last thing I felt like doing was eating. Drinking seemed a much better idea. It also helped me to think because it calmed me down.

Never one to sleep more than five hours, even on a good night, I knew I had a long stretch ahead of me. The other problems I faced now began to impact on my mind. What was I going to tell the Partners in the legal firm which employed me? If there was a police enquiry, it was bound to hit the press. What was I going to tell the editor of the local paper, for which I wrote two columns every week? How do you tell other people your family think you are a pervert?

As it happened, that turned out to be a lot less difficult than I had expected but there was no way I could know that as I lay on top of the bed, slowly demolishing the bottle of Grouse. At least it seemed to be slowly, but it soon became obvious that the night was going to last a great deal longer than the bottle. By that time I was too drunk to care. While the confrontation with the family had been brutal, I was more confused and angry than hurt, but getting drunk was still the best thing that had happened to me all day. I passed out rather than fell asleep.

CHAPTER TWO

I was not the only one who had been devastated by the events of that day. My wife Kay, was hurrying to get ready for a hair appointment when the telephone rang about 8.30am. The voice at the other end of the line was Sharon.

"Mum, what are you doing this morning?"

"I have a hair appointment at 9 o'clock and I'm just getting ready to leave."

"Can you cancel it and come into Perth?"

Kay's heart immediately missed a beat.

"Why, what is wrong, has something happened?"

"I can't tell you on the 'phone. I will tell you when you come in. I will pick you up at the bus stop."

"Why can't you tell me now? What is wrong? Has something happened to Katrina?"

Kay's first thoughts were exactly the same as mine, as were her concerns.

"Sorry Mum, I can't tell you anything on the 'phone. Please just come into Perth and I will tell you then."

Kay agreed reluctantly, cancelled her hair appointment but she had an hour to wait before the next bus to Perth was due. It was a very long hour as she turned over and over in her mind, what the problem was likely to be. Never for an instant did she get anywhere near to thinking what the actual problem was, her thoughts were for Katrina and that something had happened to her. The journey to Perth from our home in Crieff takes about forty minutes but it could have taken twice as long, or half as long, for all the difference it made to Kay. The time meant nothing to her as her mind was in such a turmoil.

Sharon was standing at the bus stop, on her own and there was not the usual warm greeting as Kay stepped down from the bus. Both she and Kay walked across the road in silence to Sharon's car, where Kay asked Sharon again,

"What is wrong, what has happened?"

Sharon's tone was quiet, her words clipped.

"Wait until we get to the house Mum, you'll find out then."

The journey from bus to house was no more than a few minutes but those were the last words Sharon spoke. She kept clearing her throat as if there was something stuck there. But it was a nervous cough and she kept glancing at Kay as if to say something, then changing her mind. Kay could feel her tension as well as her own, with the result that Kay became convinced that something had happened to Katrina, confirmed in her own mind when she saw our sons' cars parked in front of Sharon's house.

Kay was prepared for the worst as she saw Philip and Andrew sitting on chairs, while Jim paced back and forward, none of them prepared to meet her eyes. The tension built up even further as Sharon closed the sitting room door quite deliberately and quietly before turning to Kay to say,

"You better sit down Mum. Look Mum it is vital you believe what I am going to tell you because Katrina's life depends on it. It doesn't matter what the rest of us believe, but you have to believe it."

That immediately threw Kay into confusion. If what she was about to be told meant life or death to Katrina, she must still be alive. She looked in utter confusion from one to the other of the children but none of the boys said a word. Sharon looked to be struggling to say whatever it was she was trying to tell Kay and there were a few moments of silence before Sharon finally blurted,

"Dad has been abusing Katrina for years."

Kay was absolutely stunned. She had entered the room utterly convinced Katrina was dead. Now she was being told her husband was a serial abuser. She looked frantically at each of our four children. The boys avoided her gaze and Sharon looked quite distraught. Before any of them could say any more, Kay said, with an involuntary and nervous laugh,

"Don't be ridiculous. What are you talking about?"

It was if a dam had finally broken. Kay was given a litany of alleged abuse that I was accused of committing. She tried to interrupt frequently but was told,

"They have evidence."

"Who is they and what evidence?"

"We can't tell you just now."

Other names were mentioned, all of them known to Kay, as she was bombarded with details of alleged abuse. Each time she raised a question, or was about to raise a question, she was interrupted by the same mantra,

"They have evidence but we can't tell you yet."

Finally Kay exploded,

"Who is this man you are talking about? It certainly is not your father."

There was a pause, as if the children suddenly realised they had gone too far. Kay had stopped smoking three months previously, after almost thirty years of addiction to the weed, but she suddenly reached for someone else's cigarettes and took a long and very deep drag.

"Mum, I am going to get Katrina and it is vital you tell her you will support her."

It was Sharon, speaking very slowly, as she readied herself to go back out. Katrina was at the Murray Royal Hospital and it would take Sharon at least three quarters of an hour to get there and back. Kay looked at her and said very slowly,

"I will always support Katrina."

After Sharon left there was an awkward silence as none of the boys seemed to want to pursue the discussion. Kay sat quietly for a few moments and now that she had started to smoke, she was lighting one cigarette after the other. Suddenly Andrew asked,

"Would you like to go for a walk Mum?"

To Kay, this was the opportunity she had been looking for. When she had first entered the room and was being bombarded with the details of my alleged abuse, she had looked to either Andrew, our eldest son, or Philip to call a halt. Jim, our youngest son, was very upset and seemed to be quite overwhelmed with what was going on. Kay was now convinced Andrew would put a different slant on what she had been told, albeit he had contributed to the accusations that had been levelled at me, without any qualification.

"Andrew, this cannot be true. Surely you don't believe what is being said about your Dad?"

"I'm sorry Mum, but they have a lot of evidence."

"What evidence?"

"We can't tell you yet but you are just going to have to accept that it is true."

"But this is not the man you know. How can you believe this?"

Whatever Kay's expectations had been, that I might be exonerated, that Andrew had a different opinion about my alleged abuse, she was to be bitterly disappointed. Despite her pleading, Andrew was as adamant now as he had been in the house, with everyone present. He believed, just as they all did, that I had abused Katrina and had been doing so for years.

When Katrina arrived with Sharon, she looked dreadful. Her hair was a mass of curls when she was a child, something that had continued into adulthood and when Katrina allowed it to grow naturally it just looked unkempt. She looked as if she had not had a comb near her hair for weeks. She was obviously very heavily medicated and shambled into the room. As soon as she saw Kay she burst into tears and said,

"I'm sorry Mum."

As Kay hugged Katrina, she said,

"No, I'm sorry you have had to go through this."

As Katrina was embraced by her brothers, there was very little conversation, beyond asking Katrina how she was. It was obvious she was in no state to be involved in detailed accounts of what had happened to her and after a short time, Sharon took her back to the hospital. On Sharon's return to the house, it was decided they should all go to Philip and Alison's house, to which I would be summoned. Philip's wife Alison and Andrew's wife Ashley had arrived at Sharon's house by this time, while Jim's wife Anne, looked after the children at their place. I was to learn much later that neither Alison nor Ashley believed any of the allegations that had been made and were very much opposed to my being confronted.

While waiting for me to arrive at Philip's house, Kay's mind was still in turmoil. She felt physically sick, haunted by the very thought of the allegations that had been made about me, unable to come to terms with the fact that the children were so adamant that there was "proof" of what I was supposed to have done, even although they had provided none. She now felt certain that when I arrived, I would be given details of this "proof" and together, she and I would be able to convince the family that the whole thing was an absolute nonsense. Unfortunately, again her expectations were to be completely dashed.

When I arrived and was subjected to the same allegations, the same claims of the hospital, police, social work department all having "evidence", but with none provided, she simply froze. She had been told that I would probably deny it and that she should be prepared for that. She was also assured that when I finally admitted to the allegations, "they" – the family – would "get me help". The significance of these remarks were not really to sink in until days later when Kay and I had had time to go over for the umpteenth time, the events of that hellish day. It is one of the reasons her outrage on my behalf has been so enormous and why she took a long time to forgive the family.

When I turned to her and asked what she had to say about the allegations, her response of, "They say they have a lot of evidence," was no more than the line she had been fed all day. By that time, her state of mind was such that she was incapable of rational thought. She desperately wanted to scream, "It is not true. It is not true." but to her deep shame, she was incapable of saying anything that made any sense or added anything to my defence. She desperately wanted to get up and leave with me but she found she was physically incapable of getting up from the chair. When Sharon and Jim returned to the house after dropping me off at the police station, Kay said she wanted to go home to Crieff but Sharon objected.

"I don't think that is a good idea Mum. Why don't you stay with Neil and me tonight?"

"No, I want to go home."

"But what if Dad comes home?"

"What do you mean?"

"Will you be safe enough with Dad on your own? He is going to be very angry."

It was now being hinted that I was capable of abusing my wife, that I could be violent to Kay, despite the fact that the very idea of that happening, never entered anyone's imagination in all the years we had been together. The children had never, ever seen me even threaten to raise my hands to Kay. Kay's response was immediate and brooked no further discussion or argument. On the journey back to Crieff, accompanied by Sharon and Andrew, there was very little conversation other than a "warning" to Kay that she should not contact Jane (this is not her real name but she and her husband were our closest friends). Sharon's actual words were,

"If you are going to telephone anyone Mum, don't 'phone Jane because Bill is one of the other men involved."

"The last thing I will be doing is broadcasting this on the telephone to Jane or to anyone else."

That conversation went no further.

On arrival at Crieff, Sharon and Andrew refused tea or coffee and a fair measure of Kay's state of mind can be gauged when she said,

"Do you like the new curtains?"

We had just re-decorated the sitting room and Sharon's and Andrew's reaction to the question was bemusement, expressed in further concern that Kay would be OK if left on her own.

When they left shortly after, Kay sat in a large chair near to the window, staring into space and with the same thoughts churning relentlessly through her mind. It was approximately 4.30pm and quite dark but Kay sat without lights. She sat there until 10pm, when she finally called our own doctor, David Mitchell, who had been tremendous in the support he had given us throughout the early problems with Katrina and would continue to give us unstinting support in the years to come.

Within minutes he arrived at the house and was given the details of what had happened. His first question to Kay was what her own thoughts and feelings were. Did she think I had done it? When she said under no circumstances, he said he agreed and while he had not known us for very long, he felt he knew me well enough as a patient to say he did not believe I could have been guilty of the abuse of which I was accused. He was concerned however, that I was safe. He asked Kay if she thought I would do anything to harm myself. Kay assured him that it would be totally out of character for me to do anything like that but she did concede I was very angry when I had left Philip's house.

David Mitchell impressed on Kay that no matter what time it was when I returned home, she should call him. Kay had hoped that he could give her an explanation for Katrina's accusations but of course he couldn't. He was not a psychiatrist and the only explanation he could offer was the possibility that Katrina had transferred the guilt for the abuse from my father to me. It did not help much but his support was very important and the fact he did not believe I was guilty of the abuse, meant a great deal to Kay at the time. It was the first voice of reason she had heard all day.

The doctor sat with Kay until 11pm and she spent the rest of the night sitting in the chair, turning the day's events over and over in her mind. Philip had called twice in the early evening and Sharon had called once, both of them expressing concern for Kay and asking if she had heard anything from me. They were told Kay would call as soon as she had heard from me.

Kay spent the night turning over and over in her mind, the events of the day and the allegations of abuse. By 8am, she had decided what she was going to do. She was worried sick about what had happened to me and deeply ashamed that she had allowed me to walk out of the door at Philip's house on my own. She was equally concerned about Katrina and the claims she had made, while at the same time she was ecstatic that her original fears were unfounded. She called each of the family in turn and told them that no matter what "proof" or "evidence" they claimed they had, the allegations of abuse of Katrina were false. It did not happen.

She then called Katrina and assured her that she would always have her support. Kay told her that she would visit her in hospital but the abuse I was supposed to have committed did not happen. She also told Katrina that if she did visit her in hospital, she, Kay, was not prepared to listen to Katrina accusing me of abuse. The next telephone conversation Kay had was with me. It was short and curt. I told her I was on my way home to pick up my things and then hung up.

In the space of 24 hours Kay had watched her world fall apart. She had been summoned to her daughter's house and she had gone in fully expecting to be told her youngest daughter had died. Instead, she was told her husband of 34 years and the man with whom she had shared her life since the age of seventeen, had been abusing her youngest daughter for years. She had just told her family that she did not believe the allegations and was prepared to run the risk of losing them. Finally, her husband had just telephoned to tell her he was coming home to collect his things, obviously in order to move out. It was hard to imagine a more terrible or hellish set of experiences in a single 24 hour period. Nevertheless, there were many days to follow that offered strong competition.

CHAPTER THREE

October 16th 1995

I had never wanted my Dad confronted. I had never wanted anyone to know that my Dad had abused me but that decision was taken from me, just as so much else was taken from me. At first I did not believe that Dad had abused me. I had always been a Daddy's girl, the youngest of five, with an older sister and three older brothers, I knew I had been spoiled. Dad had never once lifted his hands to me, a disapproving look was enough but Dad didn't lift his hands to any of us. He just shouted a lot – and we laughed and giggled, although not to his face.

I knew I was ill, and had been for months, tormented by nightmares, flashbacks and hallucinations of what seemed like endless abuse at the hands of my Dad and his friends. My first "memory" of being abused by my Dad came in the form of a nightmare. I was told by the duty nurse that my Dad had been in the nightmare and that I was "acting out" sexual intercourse.

"Do you know your Dad was in that nightmare?" I was asked.

"You are lying," I shouted, "my Dad would never do that to me."

"I am sorry but your father was in that nightmare," she said.

"He wasn't, you're making a mistake. He wouldn't do that," I insisted.

The very idea horrified me, made me feel sick, but as the weeks wore on and the nightmares and flashbacks became more horrific and intense, Dad became the central figure among a group of men who seemed to abuse me constantly. My medication was increased as I grew worse and the more medication I was given, the worse I became. The man I remembered taking us to the swimming baths after long runs up Kinnoull Hill every Sunday, teaching us all judo at the club where he coached, taking me to school every morning because I attended the same school where he taught, going horseback riding when I got older, had disappeared. His stock phrase had been,

"You can do it Katrina," as he encouraged me at whatever I was doing. Judo is a hard sport and injuries are common but he was never rough and never encouraged the juniors to be rough with each other. He couldn't stand bullying and bullies.

"Practise the technique, get the technique right and the rest will come," he would say. When riding it was always,

"Keep your hands soft, be gentle on his mouth."

I barely remembered how much I used to love curling up on the couch where he was sitting, loving it when he gave me a cuddle for no reason, as he also did with Sharon, receiving approval without having to look for it. The fun we had decorating my first flat was typical of the type of fun we had all had, growing up in a family that did so much together.

In his place was a monster who beat me, raped me, murdered a young friend with an iron bar, to teach me to be nice to the group of men who abused me. The great difficulty I had was that this monster only appeared in my nightmares and flashbacks. I had no clear memories of my Dad ever abusing me, although I said he did because I believed he did. I was encouraged in those beliefs by the staff who looked after me because I was always given support and told I would always be given their support. The more support I got, the needier I became and it developed into a vicious circle of medication, nightmares and flashbacks, more medication and appeals for support, more nightmares, more medication and so on.

That was why I did not want anyone to know Dad had abused me. The consultant psychiatrist Dr Yellowlees insisted I tell Sharon, my oldest sister when I said I wanted to go to my brother Jim's wedding. My Dad had been stopped visiting me months before and Dr Yellowlees did not want me to be in his, Dad's, company unless someone else who knew about the abuse, was there to "protect me".

"Your father appears constantly in your flashbacks Katrina," he said, "and it is necessary for me to know you will be looked after if you are in his company. I would be very concerned if you went there without anyone else who was with you, knowing about the abuse. I am also concerned about your sister Sharon's two boys and the other grandchildren. Your parents see them regularly I believe?"

"Yes, Mum and Dad babysit with the grandchildren almost every weekend." I answered, "but Dad wouldn't touch them," I argued.

"You don't know that and I can no longer take that chance," Dr Yellowlees replied. "If you insist on going to your brother's wedding, against my advice, I have to insist you tell Sharon about the abuse."

The day I told Sharon, I was very uncertain and said at one point that I wasn't sure if the abuse had taken place. Long before Dad appeared in my nightmares, my main carer, Jenny Hogg had asked if my father ever abused me. I was upset and very angry, and said,

"No, he didn't."

When I told Mum she was equally angry because she said they were making suggestions to me and that was wrong.

When finally faced with having to tell Sharon I had been abused by Dad, it did not feel right and I hesitated. Dr Yellowlees became quite sharp and said,

"Come on now Katrina, after all we have been through are you now going to say you're not sure?"

Not wanting to get his disapproval, I told Sharon,

"Yes, Dad did abuse me."

Having to tell my brothers was worse. Several weeks had gone by after I had told Sharon and my mental health deteriorated. The nightmares and flashbacks became progressively worse and I seemed to be terrified most of the time. Sharon insisted she could not go on being the only one to know and in any case, she felt the boys had a right to know because of their own children. Mum and Dad were still visiting the family every week, seeing the grandchildren and Dr Yellowlees had frightened her by telling her how concerned he was for their safety. Sharon was also finding it very difficult to keep up the pretence with Mum and Dad. The pressure seemed to get worse and I saved my medication over a period of two weeks and then took an overdose. As I was on a cocktail of 12 different pills every day, a two week supply amounted to a large number of pills. The result was a stomach pump, several days locked up in a secure unit and no visitors.

The boys had grilled me and became impatient when I could not supply many of the answers they were looking for. I was convinced they did not believe me and told Jenny Hogg I was terrified of losing their support. Jim worshipped Dad and was the most upset of the boys, running out of the building at one point, until Andrew ran after him and brought him back. Philip was not at that meeting because he was working in Edinburgh that day but Andrew kept asking me about details that were impossible to give him.

"How do you know it is true, if you have no actual memories and you only know about the abuse because of your nightmares?" Andrew asked angrily.

"Because I've been told the flashbacks are memories I have repressed," I answered, still not even sure myself if what I was saying was true.

"I don't know Andrew, speak to Jenny Hogg or Yellowlees."

"But it is so hard to believe that Dad would do anything like that," he insisted.

"If you could witness her flashbacks, you would have no doubt," interrupted Jenny Hogg.

The questions had gone on and on until I could take no more and asked to go back to the ward. After they had gone, I had to be medicated to calm me down but it took several days before I felt able to speak to Sharon again. They were days filled with fear of losing my family and more flashbacks and nightmares. They just never seemed to stop. The staff assured me of their support and said no one could get at me as long as I was in their care. It did not stop the nightmares.

As the pressure increased, to continue to tell more and more of what had happened to me, as the nightmares and flashbacks became more vivid and frightening, it was decided to involve the police and Social Work Department. I was encouraged to make a police statement and told Sharon would also make one. Now that I had spoken to Sharon and the boys, some of the original reluctance to speak about what Dad had done, had gone. I knew that speaking to the police meant that Dad would now be questioned but I was told it also meant I would be protected. There was no way the police would allow any of the men who had abused me, some of them important in politics, the opportunity to harm me any more. Jenny Hogg sat with me as I gave my statement to a young police woman. She encouraged me to tell as much as I remembered, to name as many of the other men involved, to give as much detail as possible.

"I realise how difficult this must be for you but just take your time and tell us as much as you can," she said. When I hesitated, she reassured me.

"I just find it difficult to tell you some of the things that were done to me, some of the things that happened," I said.

"You have done nothing wrong," she said, "you have nothing to be ashamed of and nothing you tell us will shock us in any way because we will have heard it before."

It was not easy but I was not bullied or pressured, just encouraged. Jenny Hogg was asked to confirm the details of what I was saying and after it was over, I felt relieved. I was more relaxed, it was as if the assurances that I was now going to be safe were beginning to sink in.

When Sharon told me they were going to confront Dad, I was terrified. She told me that she and the boys could not carry on pretending that nothing had happened. They were finding it more and more difficult to face Mum and Dad, avoiding contact with them as much as possible and dealing with the social workers. I was sure something would happen to me. I wanted to speak to Mum, I needed to speak to her, to make sure it was all right with her. I didn't want Dad punished. I didn't know what I wanted. I just wanted it all to end. Sharon came to the hospital to tell them I wanted to speak to Mum because if Dad was to be confronted, I had to be sure she would support me. Jenny Hogg, as the main carer, was not keen to let me go, saying they were afraid for my safety. This did not help my own fears but I still wanted to see Mum and after some persuasion, Jenny Hogg agreed I could go – but just for one hour, then I had to return to the hospital.

Now that the day of the confrontation had arrived, I was very frightened. I was scared of what my Dad would do. I was scared of what my Mum would say, which is why I needed to see her; but at the same time I was scared she would not believe me and I would lose her. The build up to the day had been terrible. I could not eat, I had not showered for a couple of days. I could not sleep and when I did, I had more nightmares. The medication seemed to do little to calm me down and I was given it virtually on demand.

Sharon had been very concerned about whether or not I could cope, after the confrontation, reminding me that after it was done, there was no going back. There would be no place for me to hide and I couldn't pretend it hadn't happened.

"Are you sure you are ready for this?" she asked, "This is not going to be pleasant Katrina and Mum might be difficult to convince."

"I know it is going to be bad," I said, "and I am terrified at the thought of it."

"You don't have to come, we can speak to Mum," Sharon said.

"No, that would not be fair and I have to do this for my own peace of mind," I replied.

At the same time she did not try to stop me seeing Mum and assured me that the boys and her supported me and would continue to support me, whatever happened. As I waited for Sharon to come and collect me, I just wanted it to be all over. Sharon had telephoned the hospital to tell them she would be coming to collect me over two hours before, and I was worried something had happened. A member of staff sat with me while I waited, trying to reassure me that everything would be all right, trying to keep me calm.

When I walked into the room at Sharon's house and saw Mum and the boys, I could not help it, I just burst into tears. I had been so sure that if only I could speak to Mum, I could explain it all. I could convince her of what had happened to me. I had played out all the scenes in my head over and over again. I would just tell Mum what had happened and clarify things, so that she would see I had to do this. Instead, all I could do was hold on to her and cry, as she hugged me. I remember saying to her,

"I am sorry Mum."

"No," she said, "I am sorry you have had to go through this."

Any thought of giving an explanation disappeared because I found I had nothing I could say. I could not find the words. I just cried. All the plans, all the words I had prepared to say to Mum, were no longer there. The reason we were all meeting was my Dad's abuse of me but nobody mentioned it, nobody said anything about what had happened. The boys seemed to want to avoid looking at me and I sat with my head down. Everybody just sat and said very little. I was convinced Mum didn't believe me but I was afraid to ask her because she might have given me the answer I dreaded.

As I had been given only an hour's pass from the hospital, the time with Mum just seemed to fly past.

"Katrina," It was Sharon. As I lifted my head, I could sense rather than see the boys and Mum looking at me.

"We are going to have to leave to get back to the hospital and we still have to call Dad. We are going down to Philip's house to meet him there. Are you going to be all right?"

"Yes," I muttered, "I'll be fine" although I felt anything but. Mum came towards me and held out her arms. As she hugged me she said,

"Katrina, you know I love you and you know I will support you."

Somehow I didn't believe her but I held on to her as if I knew I would never see her again.

The boys hugged me in turn but they had said little or nothing and the time I had spent with them and Mum seemed to be a complete waste of time. I had been so certain I could explain everything to Mum and then it would be OK but I had just sat there and cried. The journey back to the hospital was miserable. Sharon kept glancing over to me,

"Will you be all right?" she asked for the umpteenth time.

"Mum didn't believe me Sharon," I said, "I knew she wouldn't. She will take Dad's side."

"She has had a hell of a shock Katrina," said Sharon, " but she told you she would support you."

"I wanted her to believe me," I replied, "and she didn't."

Nothing Sharon said made me feel any better.

When we arrived back at the hospital, Jenny Hogg met us at the door and asked what had happened. I said,

"My Mum didn't believe me."

She looked at me, a knowing look crossing her face as she replied,

"Your mother has a lot to lose, but it is good it is now out in the open."

"But I wanted her to believe me, not just get it into the open. I knew we should never have agreed to confront Dad," I said.

"He had to be confronted Katrina, for the sake of the grandchildren, and to make him pay for what he did to you," said Jenny, as she turned towards Sharon.

They spoke for a short time before Sharon left to return to the house. I don't know what was said but I was immediately sectioned, which meant I was not allowed out of the hospital. Jenny Hogg spoke to me for a while about what had happened but there was little I could tell her.

"I could not find anything to say to Mum, I just cried the whole time," I said. "The boys hardly opened their mouths to me and I just feel it was a waste of time."

"Sharon is going to telephone the hospital as soon as the confrontation with your Dad has happened. It will soon all be over," Jenny said.

How little she knew. The confrontation with Dad was just the start.

The telephone call came later. I have no idea how long after Sharon had left but she telephoned to say that Dad had been confronted and had been furious. She told Jenny that Dad had taken off and gone to the police, but that she had no idea what he was going to do then and no one had heard from him since. I was panic stricken.

"What if he comes here?" I asked Jenny, "What will you do?"

"There is nothing he can do because he won't be able to get in," she assured me. Nevertheless she organised the staff to have me locked in the secure unit.

"Your Dad is not going to get anywhere near you in here Katrina. You will have to relax." she said.

I was heavily medicated but it was a bad night. I was the only one in the unit and hallucinated several times during the night, absolutely terrified that something would happen to me.

The night had been very disturbed and I slept very little. The staff told me I had hallucinated but I have very little memory of any of what had taken place. When I was told my Mum was on the telephone and wanted to speak to me, I knew what was going to happen. I just knew. The telephone call lasted only a short time.

"Katrina," Mum's voice was quiet but strong, "you know I will support you and give you as much help as I can, but I have been thinking about the accusations you made about your Dad all night. I haven't slept and have done nothing but think about what you said. I know you believe it happened, but I am telling you it didn't."

Although I had expected this, I was immediately angry and very upset and tried to interrupt Mum, but she continued as if I hadn't spoken.

"I will come and visit you if you want me to but I am not going to allow you to say those things about your Dad. I am going to find out what has happened but I know your Dad did not abuse you."

Whatever else was said did not matter. I had known Mum did not believe me when I saw her at Sharon's house. Now she had confirmed it and I was going to lose her support, whatever she said. I became hysterical and tried to run away from the ward where the telephone was. The staff immediately overpowered me and I was injected with something to calm me down. I was screaming and trying to get free but the drugs soon took effect and I was taken back to the secure unit, where I was to spend the next few days.

The confrontation with Dad was supposed to make things better. Dr Yellowlees had convinced Sharon and I that my Dad would deny it at first but that he would soon realise he had been found out and admit it. They would then be able to get help for him but in any case, it would be out in the open and I would be safe. It was supposed to force him to admit he and his friends had abused me. Instead, I had lost not only my Dad but my Mum as well as the rest of my family. I knew the boys had not believed me, although they said they would support me. The only place I knew I had real support was in hospital because they did believe me. It would be a long time before I was forced to realise that the kind of support they offered was destroying me as a person and would almost destroy my entire family.

CHAPTER FOUR

THE FIRST MISTAKE
July 1994 – December 1994

"There's a postcard from Katrina. She says she will be home on Saturday, so we will see her on Sunday."

Kay had just brought in the mail from the front door and was reading from a postcard from Katrina who had just spent two weeks in North Wales with her friend. They had gone there because they could get in some good horse riding.

"Hmm, she says she has had a pretty miserable few days with stomach pains, I hope it didn't spoil the holiday. She says she will be glad to get home." said Kay.

"If she and Eileen have been able to get some good hacking in, I doubt she will have let a sore stomach spoil things for her," I laughed.

However, when we saw Katrina on the Sunday, it was obvious she was not well. She looked quite drawn and pale and also looked as if she had lost a little weight. She told us the pain had been so severe at times, it had actually made her vomit. Both she and Eileen were due to start work the following day but if Katrina was no better, it looked unlikely she was going to be going anywhere. I promised to call in the next day on my way to the office.

Katrina and Eileen shared a flat no more than three hundred yards from my office, in a very desirable part of Perth, both worked in the Post Office on irregular shifts and sometimes saw very little of each other from day to day. When her work allowed, Katrina and I frequently went for something to eat at lunchtime. I called in the next day on the way to the office just before 9am, and noting that she was no better, I suggested she come out to Crieff to stay with Kay and I.

"Katrina, why don't you come out to Crieff? Your Mum and me are worried about you being here all day by yourself."

"No Dad, it's OK. Eileen comes home by 7 o'clock and she is here in the evening and at night, when I'm usually at my worst. Anyway, I think I'm a bit better than I was and I don't want to have too much time off my work. You know what they can be like if you lose too much time."

"OK, but if you are no better tomorrow, you are getting no choice. You're going to be coming out to Crieff."

She refused to budge the next day, Tuesday, arguing that she would probably be fine within the next day or so. She was no better on the Tuesday evening when I called in on the way home and when she looked slightly worse on the Wednesday, this time, she was given no choice about coming out to Crieff.

By the Friday of that week, with no improvement in Katrina's condition, Kay was concerned enough to call our own GP, whose first thoughts were that Katrina might have appendicitis. He had her admitted to Perth Royal Infirmary (PRI) that same day and she was operated on that night, when her appendix was removed. We visited her the next morning and arrived in the ward just in time to meet the surgeon who had operated on Katrina. He was in the process of telling her that there had been nothing wrong with her appendix.

Naturally we were concerned to know why, if there was nothing wrong with her appendix, the surgeon had removed it. He explained that it was considered better to remove the healthy appendix, because if at some time in the future, Katrina was to suffer from an inflamed or diseased appendix, any doctor examining her could be misled by the abdominal scar into thinking it had already been removed. And that could prove to be potentially dangerous.

The explanation seemed to be reasonable to us at the time and, as our main concern was that the doctors should find the real cause of Katrina's pain, if it was not her appendix, we did not pursue the issue. We asked the doctor if they knew what the problem was and were told that at that precise time they did not have a clue, nor were they prepared to offer any possibilities until they had conducted further tests.. The operation had taken place on the 22nd of July and Katrina was discharged on the 2nd of August, with still no answer to what was causing the pain.

For the next week our GPs called in on a regular basis, both to administer pain relief to Katrina and to monitor her condition, which continued to cause them concern. As a consequence of that concern, Katrina was re-admitted to PRI on the 12th August and without giving either her or Kay and I any explanation, the medical team decided to remove her gall bladder on the 16th August. The following day, we asked to speak to the surgeon and much to our dismay, we were told that her gall bladder was also clear, there was absolutely nothing wrong with it. When we spoke to Katrina, she was very upset and quite depressed, having been given no explanation as to why the gall bladder had been removed.

By now not only were we worried sick about what was wrong with Katrina, we were also rapidly losing faith in the doctors who were treating her. She had had two abdominal operations in the space of three weeks, neither of which had been necessary, by the hospital's own admission. Not only that, but she had had two perfectly healthy organs removed and no one was able to give us any kind of explanation that made any sense.

Kay had been a nurse before we were married; her ability to ask the right questions, and more importantly, to know when she was being given the right answers, was obviously resented by some of the staff and one of the doctors in particular, who dubbed us "the parents from hell". It was an attitude we were to encounter time and again throughout the nightmare that was to follow. It was as if we had no right to be concerned parents. We were a nuisance, timewasters, who should just be fobbed off with whatever answer it was thought we would accept, as they attempted to intimidate us with the use of medical terms that no lay person could possibly understand.

The medical staff were to learn very quickly we did not take kindly to being fobbed off, nor were we going to be intimidated by the use of medical language we did not understand. All we asked for was a bit of courtesy and patience. We were prepared to show the same courtesy, unless we were given non-answers or "explanations" that were an insult to our intelligence. During much of this time and throughout the majority of the discussions which took place with the medical team, I was a mere bystander, having little or no medical knowledge and being quite content to follow Kay's lead.

Three days after her second operation, on the 19th August, Katrina was released into her mother's care. The Discharge Sheet noted "Good Family Support". She was released with a wound so badly infected, it required to be dressed several times each day and daily visits from a nurse, to administer pain relief. Those visits were to continue for almost three weeks at the end of which Kay took responsibility for dressing Katrina's wound. During this later period there were also regular visits from our GP to continue with administering pain relief, which initially took the form of injections into Katrina's hips. As a consequence of the weight loss associated with her operations and lengthy period of convalescence, the regular injections caused Katrina further pain and discomfort. To alleviate this, the pain relief was soon being administered orally.

Weeks went by with the doctors at a loss to understand the cause of the original pain. Both appendix and gall bladder had been shown to be clear of infection after they had been removed but there was no doubt at the time – Katrina had been experiencing severe abdominal pain. It was also very obvious, given that the wound from the gall bladder operation had been badly infected, that the post-operative pain was equally severe. What was not so obvious was that Katrina had become addicted to the Pethidine which had been prescribed to alleviate her pain. The switch to oral medication made it easier to feed that addiction.

Towards the end of September, Kay and I decided to take a quick break, spending a week in Brittany. We found a small hotel in St Cast, about twenty kilometres west of St Malo, ideally situated in an area renowned for its beaches. We were to make good use of them, passing the days like a couple of beach bums. Armed with a plastic bag containing a freshly roasted chicken, a baguette and a bottle of wine (or two), we just lay there soaking up the late September sun. The evenings were spent as evenings should be spent while in France, eating good food and drinking French wine.

While we were in France, Katrina stayed with her sister Sharon and her husband Neil, moving back in with us on our return. By that time our GP was expressing increasing concern at her apparent inability to be without pain relief. There was still no solution being offered for her original pain and he pressed to have her re-admitted to PRI for further tests, and more importantly, to have her weaned off Pethidine.

Kay and I had returned from France greatly refreshed and looking forward to Katrina showing signs of recovery. To our dismay, her recovery seemed to be as far off as ever and we were to look back later and reflect on how that short holiday was to be the last time for several years, we could be truly relaxed. The doctors had made their first mistake, a mistake that was to have horrendous consequences for both Katrina and her entire family. It was to be compounded several times over with what was to follow.

Under pressure from our GP, Katrina was re-admitted to PRI in early November in order to have her condition re-assessed and her addiction to Pethidine addressed. "Cold turkey" was just an expression we had heard. We knew it referred to coming off hard drugs with no back-up, but having had no experience of having witnessed its effects, we had no real idea of what it actually meant. But it is a reasonable description of what Katrina went through during the first few days after her re-admission to PRI, when she was immediately taken off of all medication.

She suffered the sweats, the nightmares, the shakes, the crawling sensations under her skin, while we were constantly assured that things were progressing as planned. We were to learn later that although we had been assured by the medical staff that they had taken advice on how to deal with Katrina's addiction, it was not until she had been in hospital for almost a week, that contact had been made with Dr Yellowlees, Consultant Psychiatrist at Murray Royal Hospital, to ask about appropriate back-up. We were also to learn that although they were given advice on the proper required dosage of Diazapam, it was administered for too short a period and in too small dosage to be effective in allowing Katrina to be "brought down" slowly. The adverse effects of withdrawal from Pethidine continued, as Katrina became more depressed, Kay and I became more anxious and the medical staff became more impatient.

Our anxiety increased tenfold when, on the Sunday afternoon of the beginning of the third week of Katrina's stay in hospital, she collapsed on the way back to the ward and was to remain unconscious for over an hour and a half. To relieve the monotony of hospital routine, she had been given permission to go to the hospital cafeteria with us during one of our visits. She had undergone more tests, all of them negative and none of them taking her any nearer to solving the riddle of the causes of her pain. As we were making our way back to the ward, she suddenly pitched forward on to her face.

Katrina struck her head as she fell to the floor and Kay was concerned that the long period of unconsciousness was as a consequence of a possible serious head injury, rather than as a consequence of the withdrawal of Pethidine. Despite our concern, there was a strong reluctance on the part of the medical staff to investigate further the possibility of a head injury by taking an x-ray, leading to a stand up fight between Kay and the duty doctor. Kay persisted and the x-ray was taken, showing there was no injury but the episode was another example of the deteriorating relationship between us and the medical team.

Although there was no evidence of a head injury, the periods of prolonged unconsciousness were to continue over the next few weeks, with Katrina collapsing at regular intervals; in the middle of the ward, in the shower and even when sitting up in bed. There was a visit from at least one member of the family every day and each day there seemed to be another bruise or scrape on Katrina's arms or face, where she had struck the floor or some piece of furniture when she lost consciousness. The staff found it impossible to rouse her, even when they stuck her with pins.

By late November the medical staff had decided that they needed further assistance and Dr Yellowlees, who was the Consultant Psychotherapist as well as the Consultant Psychiatrist at Murray Royal Hospital, was asked if he would see Katrina. His report to the PRI, dated 24th November gave his diagnosis of Katrina's condition as:-

1) Drug addiction
2) Abnormal behaviour and reaction to illness

"I think that most of her current complaints and behaviour can be seen in terms of drug withdrawal symptoms... Her "collapses" are more likely to be abnormal illness behaviour, designed to persuade the staff that she requires more medication". He went on to suggest that as she was still experiencing considerable craving for Pethidine, if the hospital had completed their physical investigations, he would consider transfer to Murray Royal for completion of drug withdrawal "if she is willing to come".

As we were given only a verbal report of Dr Yellowlees's diagnosis of Katrina's condition and were not to see the written medical reports until some two and a half years later, we were not aware that even at this early stage in her dealings with the psychiatric team that would cause so much damage, there was a certain bias against Katrina. This was noted and underlined by Dr Janet Boakes, who would later provide expert testimony on behalf of Katrina. Dr Boakes noted that in his initial diagnosis, Dr Yellowlees had failed to note that the drug addiction was iatrogenic. In other words it was under medical supervision and on prescription. She also noted that it could hardly be concluded that Katrina was suffering from abnormal reaction to illness when Dr Yellowlees had not examined her medical records nor had he spoken to either Kay or me in order to determine if Katrina's recent reactions were out of the ordinary.

Not only was Katrina not willing to go to Murray Royal, there was no way she was going to be persuaded. Despite Kay's and my best efforts, she discharged herself and returned to her own flat. Sharon called in to see her during her lunch hour the next day, only to find her lying unconscious on the floor, one side of her face very badly bruised where she had struck the fireplace as she fell. The PRI refused to re-admit her, stating there was nothing more they could do and with Katrina still unwilling to go to Murray Royal, Sharon finally persuaded her to move in with her and Neil, at least for a few days. Katrina was never to move back into her flat.

The next couple of weeks were very difficult for all of us, but particularly so for Sharon and Neil. Katrina still complained of abdominal pain and was obviously in very low spirits. Sharon had two lively boys as well as a fulltime job and Neil worked long and irregular hours as a AA patrol man. Kay visited as often as possible and a great deal of time was spent discussing the possibility of Katrina's going into Murray Royal. Finally, after a few days of feeling very low, and after further discussion with her own GP, Katrina decided to go in to Murray Royal on a voluntary basis, which meant she could leave whenever she wanted to. It was December 15th 1994. She would not leave until March 1996, and against medical advice.

CHAPTER FIVE

December 1994

The very thought of going into a psychiatric hospital horrified Katrina, who objected very strongly to the suggestion that the pain she had been suffering had no physical cause and that it was psychosomatic. On the day she went in, she was very subdued and when I passed the bedroom where her mother and her were packing her case, I could hear her quietly crying. Kay told me later they had been discussing the prospect of her having to be in hospital for some weeks and that terrified her. The experience in the PRI and the attitude of the staff there had done little to encourage her to believe she would be treated sympathetically.

Kay and I took her to Gilgal House, an annex of Murray Royal, where the drug rehabilitation section was situated, on the evening of December 15th. We were all in tears; Katrina sobbed as she clung to her mother but was eventually persuaded by the sympathetic treatment of the staff to leave us and be admitted to the ward. Kay and I were asked to give some background information for the admission sheet, to Charge Nurse Wilson. Kay was still very tearful and the initial details were left to me and as I began to relate the circumstances which had led up to this meeting, the two unnecessary abdominal operations, the drug addiction, the lapses into unconsciousness, the anger at what had happened began to surface.

There were no histrionics, there was no ranting and raving, there was not even a raised voice, but it must have been obvious from the intensity with which I detailed events how I felt. Charge Nurse Wilson certainly was able to tell because she commented on my obvious anger and tried to re-assure us that while the system had apparently fallen down in its treatment of Katrina so far, they would do their best to rectify that as soon as possible.

"I am afraid Kay and I are going to take some convincing of that," I said. "We simply cannot understand why two operations were carried out, two organs removed and yet, there was nothing wrong with either of them,"

"They did several tests so there must have been something shown in the second tests for them to remove the gall bladder," Kay said. "But they insist there was nothing wrong with the gall bladder either. If the tests were done properly, and they did a scan," looking at me for confirmation, "the fact there was nothing wrong should have shown up." She continued, "So, please, we don't have much faith in any assurances we might get now. Our concern is that Katrina is looked after and you get her off the Pethidine."

"Did you discuss this with the doctors at PRI?" Nurse Wilson asked.

"Of course we discussed it," I answered, "but we could not get any answers. They just kept saying there was "no pathology found" which means, I take it, there was nothing wrong."

"I am afraid I can't answer for the doctors at the PRI," answered nurse Wilson, "I can only give you some reassurance that we will look after Katrina as best we can."

That is one conversation Kay and I have had cause to remember, in light of not just what happened at Murray Royal, but the way in which Katrina's care was managed for the next fifteen months. No doubt Nurse Wilson meant it at the time.

But there was something else, something which we felt it important to tell Nurse Wilson. It was something we felt could have an important bearing on Katrina's problem and something which we had discussed, it seemed endlessly, before bringing her to Gilgal.

Katrina had been abused as a child. Kay had overheard a telephone conversation between her and one of her cousins that made her stop and listen. She had had no intention of eavesdropping. Katrina was fifteen years old and a young adult, therefore she was given the privacy that any young adult of that age should feel entitled to, but a couple of words jumped out of the conversation at Kay, which was enough to make her more than just curious. It was obvious what the topic of conversation was about and that disturbed Kay, who waited until she could speak to Katrina privately before tackling her.

Despite being distressed that Kay had overheard the conversation, as there had been no intention of ever telling her, Katrina finally admitted that my father had abused her when she was a child, as he had also abused two others in our extended family. She confirmed the abuse had stopped before she had left primary school and that she felt she had dealt with it. Kay's first thought was to tell me but Katrina begged her not to, expressing her fear that I might feel she was diminished, that I might see her as being dirty. Despite Kay's assurances that I would feel nothing of the kind, that I would be incandescent with anger but not at Katrina, she was adamant that I should not be told. Seeing how distressed Katrina became at the thought of my finding out, Kay promised her that she would not tell me.

Although Kay agreed not to tell me, she convinced Katrina she, Kay, had to speak to the mother of the other girls. With great reluctance Katrina agreed. Kay contacted the mother of the other girls the next day and she in turn, confronted her daughters. They were appalled that their secret was out and also begged their mother not to tell their father for much the same reasons as had been expressed by Katrina. While all the girls admitted it had happened, they would give no details to their mothers, neither of whom pressed them beyond confirming that abuse of some description had actually taken place.

Naturally the mother of the other girls was just as sick and furious as Kay was. Not only that, she wanted something done about it, although she had agreed not to tell her husband. That was obviously going to be very difficult and Kay impressed on her that she had assured Katrina that I would not be told. She insisted that whatever the other mother did, whether or not she eventually told her husband, under no circumstances would Kay tell me and she expected the woman to honour that commitment. For that reason and that reason only, both mothers resolved to deal with the situation themselves and to make sure the girls were protected, although all had agreed the abuse had stopped.

We saw my parents on a fairly irregular basis but my father very occasionally called in to our house on his own. From the day and hour she found out about his abuse of Katrina, Kay made sure there was never a minute when he was left on his own with her. At the same time, for Katrina's sake and mine, she succeeded in acting as if nothing had happened, while at times feeling as if she wanted to kill him. As she was now fifteen years old, Katrina was not as defenceless as she had been as a young child and now that her mother knew, there was less fear that it might happen again. Of course, the three girls all claimed the abuse stopped as soon as they had left primary school and it appeared the interest in them as targets for abuse, had gone. For two years Katrina and Kay shared their secret and neither of them would ever have told me. But that decision was taken for them.

My younger brother Brian, who lived in Glasgow with his wife and family, had taken what was to prove to be some kind of virus which attacked his brain. In the early stages of his illness however, the x-rays showed only that he had a swelling which covered the whole of one side of his brain, including the stem. Brian very quickly slipped into a coma in which he had remained for about three months. The doctors at the Southern General Hospital in Glasgow confirmed that what they thought was a tumour, was inoperable. I had been travelling to the hospital three or four times a week and had been involved in all the discussions which took place between Brian's wife and the medical team responsible for his care.

While the doctors were at a loss to explain what had caused the tumour, they were certain there was no cure for Brian. At the end of a series of tests, they took his wife and I aside one afternoon and told us it was only a matter of time before Brian slipped away. It could be hours, days or weeks and the only thing about which they were certain, was that Brian was dying. I had not long returned after leaving his wife at their house in Glasgow, stopping off to tell my own parents what to expect and making sure my sister could stay with them. I was telling Kay and the family what had happened when the telephone rang.

We were in the kitchen, I was looking out of the window, my hands cupping a mug of coffee, talking about Brian, about the years when we were growing up. Kay, who had answered the telephone, returned several minutes later. It was the sound of her voice that made me turn round. She was in tears and said simply, "It is for you and you're going to be upset."

"Is it about Brian? Is he…" I could not finish the sentence.

Kay was too obviously upset to speak and just shook her head.

Expecting to be told that Brian had died, I picked up the receiver. The female voice at the other end was icily cold, berating me about abuse, my father and her daughter. I had to stop her several times so that I could make sense of what she was saying. It was the mother of the abused girls, telling me that my father had made an obscene telephone call to her daughter. She then proceeded to tell me how Kay and she had known about the earlier abuse for two years, about how they had agreed not to tell me but that this was the last straw. Her daughter had been hysterical when the mother returned from town and was so incoherent, she had taken over an hour to explain what had happened. The mother had not telephoned the police but she wanted something done about it and expected me to do it.

I was devastated and when the initial shock wore off, was very angry. Why was I not told? How could I not have known? A hundred and one emotions took over in the space of a few moments – rage at my father, guilt that I had allowed it to happen, anger at Kay for not telling me, concern for Katrina. Kay stopped me before I could return to the kitchen, where she and the family were still waiting. She had had to tell Katrina what had happened and she was now inconsolable and speaking to Sharon. Kay took me to the sitting room and told me the rest of the story, particularly about how upset Katrina was.

The next few weeks were an absolute hell. For the sake of all the girls, not just Katrina, I had to confront my father. At the same time I felt I needed to protect my mother, who, I was convinced, could not possibly have known anything about what had taken place. The women, that is the girls and their mothers, took the final decisions, as they and only they had the right to, that there should be no police involvement. That was decided for the sake of the girls but my father still had to be confronted. The repercussions were to be enormous; for me, for my parents and the rest of the family but most of all for Katrina. For a time, things were very difficult as she was almost inconsolable for much of the time but, after a few weeks, Kay and I thought she was over the worst. Until the evening she did not return home at her usual time, having gone out earlier in the evening with her boyfriend.

It was three o'clock in the morning when she returned, by which time Kay and I were frantic. It was obvious she had been drinking and she was told in no uncertain terms that we would not tolerate that kind of behaviour from a seventeen year old. We finally went upstairs to bed, leaving Katrina in the sitting room, but finding it difficult to settle and having a sixth sense that something was wrong, Kay went downstairs again to find Katrina unconscious. She had swallowed a large number of Codeine tablets.

After spending a few days in hospital, during which time she spoke for the first time to a counsellor, Katrina returned home, having agreed to see the counsellor as an out-patient.

We learned that her late night drinking had arisen because she had split with her boyfriend, that our reaction to her staying out so late, on top of the recent disclosure to me of her earlier abuse, had all been just too much for her to cope with.

It brought home to us just how deeply affected she had been and made me realise I had a long way to go before I could convince Katrina that she was not to blame, that she was just as precious to me now as she had ever been. Kay and I encouraged her to continue with the counselling, we offered to speak to the counsellor – an offer which Katrina declined – and after a period of about four months of fairly irregular sessions, she stopped. As far as we could tell, for the next seven years she enjoyed a normal and enjoyable lifestyle, with her own flat, a steady job in the Post Office and regular horse riding. There was no further contact with psychiatric services and no evidence that any was needed.

Katrina's counsellor was a psychiatric social worker called Emily Powrie. The name meant nothing to us at the time, we never met the woman and Katrina said very little about what was discussed during their sessions. The name was to crop up again seven years later, when she was to play a leading role in Yellowlees's team and in involving the Child Protection Unit of the Social Work Department, in giving my family instructions in how to screen my grandchildren for suspected abuse.

We had no idea whether any of this was of any significance but having been told by the medical team that there was nothing wrong with either Katrina's appendix or her gall bladder, that her condition was psychosomatic, the alarm bells sounded for Kay and I. Perhaps Katrina had not coped with the abuse as well as we had thought, perhaps she was in need of further counselling. We just didn't know. But we thought it better to tell the psychiatric staff and allow them to be the judges. We thought that if they knew about the earlier abuse they would at least have a starting point, a base on which to work towards finding the cause of Katrina's pain. Nurse Wilson listened sympathetically and noted it down. She did not dismiss any of what we had told her as being irrelevant but the nightmare was just about to begin.

CHAPTER SIX

THE NIGHTMARE BEGINS
December 1994 – October 1995

Katrina's hostility to being in Gilgal at all, manifested itself in her growing hostility to the staff, her determination not to cooperate and her equal determination to come home. Every visit followed the same pattern; Katrina voicing her agitation and her anger while we tried to persuade her that she should listen to what the staff had to say and to work with them. By early January of 1995 we were increasingly concerned and asked to speak to one of her doctors.

On January 6th we met Dr White, the psychologist who was at that time treating Katrina. There had been much discussion among ourselves about disclosure and whether or not it would be beneficial for Katrina. Both Kay and Sharon knew a great deal more about it than I did and their concern was that it might not be in Katrina's interest to disclose what had happened to her. At the same time, we were also concerned that the lack of disclosure could have been the cause of her recent problems, after all we had been told her pain was psychosomatic.

As was customary in the early meetings with the psychiatric staff, Kay did most of the talking. Sharon had previously met Dr White in late December and had questioned her closely about the possible effects on Katrina of disclosure. Dr White had assured Sharon that "in a safe and secure ward environment any potential problems would be minimised". Kay went further, asking if the defensive barriers which Katrina had built were to be dismantled, thereby in some respects dismantling Katrina herself, would they (the psychiatric staff) be able to put her back together again?

We were assured that all avenues were still being explored, including physical causes of the original pain, that disclosure work would be carried out only if it was thought to be appropriate. We were also assured that if Katrina's defensive barriers were to be dismantled during disclosure, the resultant psychiatric care she would receive would allow her to cope. Yes, they could rebuild her. Given the number of attempts Katrina was to make on her own life in the following months, that interview now seems laughable, but as Dr White recorded in her notes of that day, "they (Kay and I) seemed reasonably re-assured".

She could not have been more mistaken but it was simply a confirmation of the level of self delusion under which the staff laboured even at that early stage in their dealings with Katrina and her family. We were far from convinced that Katrina was improving, in fact we saw a distinct deterioration in her mood when we visited. The process which Kay was to refer to later as, "like watching Katrina disappearing down a tunnel" had begun. Her personality began to change and she complained constantly. When asked about Dr Yellowlees, the psychiatrist who was her consultant, she replied, "He's an asshole Mum! He's an asshole!! However much we were to later agree with her assessment and to wish we had listened more closely to her, at the time we saw no alternative but for her to continue to work with them.

It was about this time that her behaviour started to cause us to have serious misgivings about the course of her treatment. About the third week in January she suddenly appeared at my office in a very distressed condition, having absconded from the ward. I was on the telephone when the door suddenly opened and Katrina walked in, sat down and burst into tears.

"What is wrong? How did you get here Katrina?" I asked. It took several moments for Katrina to compose herself enough to answer me.

"I've run away Dad, I can't stand it any more. I hate that place. They keep on at me to talk about the abuse with Poppa and I don't want to," she answered.

"Will the hospital know you have gone? How long have you been away?" I wanted to know.

"I don't know but it has been a while."

"Where did you go?

"I walked down by the river and sat there for a while," she said.

On contacting the hospital, I learned she had been missing for about two hours and extensive searches of the hospital grounds and city centre had already been conducted. I took her back to the ward but was unable to speak to anyone in authority to voice my concern that I had not been told Katrina was missing. She was very upset when I took her back to the hospital and it meant she was sectioned and kept under lock and key for the next two days, until the staff felt she had calmed down enough to be allowed back into the general ward. What concerned Kay and I when we discussed it later that night was the fact she had sat by the river. We had been well aware of Katrina's mood recently, her obvious depression and we were worried she might harm herself. Her presence at the river did nothing to allay our fears.

It was a pattern of behaviour that was to be repeated often during her period in Gilgal/Murray Royal. The hospital lies on the main road leading to one of Perth's most popular beauty spots Kinnoull Hill, whose seven hundred and twenty nine foot sheer cliff face dominates the Carse of Gowrie. It is also one of the favourite suicide spots for patients at that hospital, something which is common knowledge in Perth and something which was certainly known to us.

Sharon, whose training in behavioural support and child psychology gave her a much deeper insight to the problems associated with abuse, was giving Katrina as much support as she could. She suggested that we should speak again to a member of staff and it was arranged that she and I would meet with a Dr Hull, another psychologist involved in Katrina's treatment, on February 9th. It turned out to be a complete and utter waste of time as we were told nothing.

The medical notes for that day state no more than that the interview lasted approximately one hour, "during which her sister in particular asked a number of questions which have previously been addressed by other members of staff.." None of us knew at the time that Katrina had been experiencing nightmares and "flashbacks" which were causing her great distress. Three days later she was to make her first serious suicide attempt by overdosing on her medication which she had been saving. It was only the first of many.

At the beginning of March Katrina was more determined than ever to discharge herself and agreed to a weekend pass with Sharon, which if it was successful, would help her to assess whether or not she could cope. It was a disaster. She suffered severe nightmares and "flashbacks" and Sharon was forced to return her to the hospital during the second night out. Sharon was now Katrina's main support as it was becoming more and more obvious that Katrina did not really want to see Kay and I.

We had noticed Katrina becoming more and more withdrawn and on some occasions was so heavily medicated that the visits were cut to no more than ten or fifteen minutes at a time. She appeared to have lost not only her personality but also any willpower, being incapable of saying whether or not she wanted to go back to the ward or to stay and talk to us. In any case, talking consisted of no more than monosyllabic replies to our questions and there were times we were not sure if she would remember our visits within minutes of our leaving her. As it turned out we were right, there are still considerable gaps in Katrina's memories of her time in Gilgal.

As usual Kay was the first to notice the change in mood. At the end of one of our visits, when Katrina had been reasonably bright and the conversation had been a little more animated, I put my arms around her as I always did when we arrived and when we were leaving. We had always been a tactile family and it was the most natural thing in the world for me to give my daughters a hug. It must have been the expression on her face which prompted Kay to say to her,

"You didn't really want that did you?"

The reply was short, "No." at which I became embarrassed. Kay followed that up by saying,

"If you would rather we didn't come so often, just say. In fact we will wait until you telephone us before we come the next time."

In the car I asked Kay,

"What was all that about?"

She explained she had been aware that Katrina was sometimes quite hostile to us, something which we had discussed before, and put it down to her feeling angry at us for not having protected her. It was an assumption on Kay's part but it seemed to be a reasonable assumption. There had also been at least two occasions when I arrived at the hospital to visit on my way home from the office and was told Katrina was sleeping and should not be disturbed, when in fact she had left instructions she did not want to see me. By early April the invitations to visit had stopped and I was not to see Katrina again until the day of our youngest son Jim's wedding on 4th August, although Kay had spoken to her several times on the telephone, except for one occasion on the day before we left for France at the beginning of July.

Sharon saw Katrina more often than any of the rest of the family and the boys rarely saw her at all. The deterioration in Katrina's health therefore, also became very obvious to Sharon who had some contact with the staff when she visited the hospital. Despite her concerns being expressed to the staff, she was also assured Katrina was progressing just as planned. Far from satisfied with those assurances, Sharon insisted on a meeting with Dr Yellowlees, who agreed to meet her with a friend of hers on the 7th April. Sharon asked for her friend to accompany her, with the agreement of Dr Yellowlees, because her friend was a practising psychologist and she felt she would be able to pose rather more searching questions if it was thought necessary.

In her statement to my lawyers on the 18th of December 1995, Sharon gave details of that meeting. She states, "By April 1995, I was concerned about Katrina's deteriorating mental state, and her dependence on a charge nurse in her ward. I expressed my concern about Katrina's mental state, with her dependence on Jenny (the charge nurse) and that she seemed to be institutionalised. She (Katrina) also stated that there was pressure on her to disclose, but that she did not want to. Dr Yellowlees said he was aware of her behaviour… that there was no pressure on Katrina to disclose as this would replicate the abuse, and indeed he felt that at this stage it would not be helpful for Katrina to disclose…"

Sharon came away from that meeting reasonably re-assured, particularly as her friend felt the approach being used with Katrina was appropriate. She took extensive notes of the meeting, which in light of Yellowlees's denials later, were very important. The notes include the following comment," ..the recorded statements (by Yellowlees) were made in response to Sharon telling Dr Yellowlees that Katrina was relying heavily on her at this time, and sharing her views that the staff were no good (apart from Jenny). And that she would not co-operate with clinical psychologist assigned to her."

They go on to record Yellowlees's statements as follows,

"The only reason Katrina is in hospital now, is to start work with clinical psychologist on managing flashbacks and coping mechanisms, which can continue as an outpatient, with additional support of a Community Psychiatric Nurse.

The original reason for admission – drug detox/pain relief – are now gone.

It is not good for Katrina to remain in hospital and become dependent.

The main therapeutic relationship should be with the clinical psychologist and that can be available as an outpatient

Nobody could or should force Katrina to do disclosure work, as this would replicate abuse…It would be very dubious indeed if this would be in Katrina's interest at present.

It is not a pre-requisite for getting better, or starting to get better…

The eating problem is not critical…it comes and goes."

There was much more but it is important to note that this meeting took place a full four months after Katrina was admitted to

Murray Royal and Yellowlees is stating, without qualification, that no one would force or even encourage her to disclose if she did not want to, that disclosure was not a pre-requisite to getting better and that the "eating problem" was not critical. That is in stark contrast to the reality of Katrina's treatment as recorded in the medical notes, examined by Dr Janet Boakes whose statement for the Court, in order to counter the Health Trust's Court statement, carried the following, "She began to talk about her sexual abuse as the direct consequence of the treatment plan to carry out "disclosure work", not spontaneously." He was also saying that Katrina should not really be in hospital but she would remain there for another year and discharge herself "against medical advice" – his advice.

In other words Yellowlees was lying and although Katrina had been under his care for four months, it was still in the early stages of her treatment and we have to ask why he felt it necessary to lie at this early stage. In retrospect we have been able to piece together a number of things which seemed to be totally unconnected at the time. Katrina telephoned her mother one day in March to tell her that charge nurse Hogg had asked her,

"Did your father ever abuse you?"

Katrina had been furious, as was Kay, who saw far greater significance in the question than I did. My response had been, "So what?" which was a measure of my naivety. We were to learn much later that Katrina's first allegation that I had sexually abused her was made in early April 1995 but that disclosure work had started several months before, despite Yellowlees's assurances to Sharon.

Given that Sharon seemed to be reasonably reassured after her meeting with Yellowlees and that Katrina did not seem to want to see us, Kay and I were prepared to accept that from then on our main contact with Katrina should be through Sharon. The other members of the family telephoned or visited on occasion but Katrina was leaning more and more heavily on Sharon. We also had something else to occupy our mind – our youngest son Jim was getting married on 4th August. He and his girlfriend Ann had been living together for some time and had two girls, Jean who would be two years old in June and Susan who had just been born in March. The small matter of when to take our holidays, so that they could be fitted around everything else, had also still to be settled.

We thought about waiting until after the wedding, but that would have meant being on holiday at the same time as the English and the French, when every resort would have been bursting at the seams. Neither did we want to wait until September because it was too far away. Thus by the process of elimination it was decided to go at the end of June, so that on our return we would have plenty of time to make all the last minute arrangements for the wedding. The only problem with that was the uncertainty of the weather – unless we went far enough south to be sure of getting some sun. We intended to go camping with Keycamp, in one of their mobile homes. We also intended driving there, therefore we had to find a spot which would be far enough south to give us a good chance of decent weather and at the same time, close enough to the Normandy or Brittany ports to allow us to get there in one day.

The obvious choice was the Vendee. We were able to get a last minute booking with Keycamp at their site located within the grounds of an old chateau called La Garangeoire, close to the village of St Julien des Landes. It was ideal for what we wanted, a quiet, restful holiday with nothing to do but laze in the sun, or if the mood took us, take in the sights of the lovely Vendean countryside. The mood didn't take us very often although I found a nearby stable with some excellent horses and managed to fit in several good hacks in some of the best riding country in France.

We had gone to visit Katrina, at her invitation, on the day before we left for France but she was decidedly off-hand and we left with the nagging sensation the situation was getting worse. Although the holiday did us good, the weather was superb and we did very little to exert ourselves, we were never really relaxed. We telephoned every day to get an update and had left instructions we were to be contacted immediately if anything happened.

Katrina made no attempt to contact us after our return, although Kay telephoned the hospital and spoke to her very briefly the day after we arrived back. Of more immediate concern now, was the wedding, the arrangements for which Jim and Ann had made themselves. We did not know until the very last minute whether or not Katrina would be there and any information we received came via Sharon. We were told that Yellowlees did not want her to go at all, but if she did go, it should be only for the ceremony and not to the reception.

The ceremony and the wedding meal were to be attended by only the immediate families and a few friends, although a great many more were invited to attend the evening reception. When Kay and I arrived at the registrars for the ceremony, Katrina, Sharon and some of the rest of the family were already standing outside. The transformation in Katrina's appearance was quite startling, she looked lovely. It was obvious she had made an effort to look her best, something which encouraged Kay and I but there was barely a nod in our direction and although Katrina looked lovely, she also looked very stressed. Neither Kay nor I attempted to engage her or Sharon in conversation, thinking it best to allow her to come to us if she wanted to. At the same time, it hurt to be so obviously ignored on a day when we should all have been enjoying ourselves. Kay was to be even more hurt later at the reception.

Sharon did not leave Katrina's side the whole time she was in our company. They left the registrar's in the same car to go to the reception, they were together while we waited for Jim and Ann to return from having their photographs taken and they sat together at the meal. A short time after the meal started and without having eaten a bite, Katrina had to leave the table, Kay following her and Sharon to the toilet, where Kay was told to go back to the meal, that Katrina would be all right. Neither of them returned, the message being relayed to us that Katrina had had to be taken back to the hospital by Sharon and Neil.

The reception was in full swing by the time they returned and Kay went immediately to Sharon to ask how Katrina was. She was stopped in her tracks with, "Not here Mum, this is neither the time nor the place!" as Sharon swept by her to join some of her friends. It was the second time Kay had been cut dead that afternoon. I didn't fare much better when I asked Sharon to dance, conversation being almost non-existent and the atmosphere stony. At the end of the evening we were glad to get home. We had no idea what was wrong but we deeply resented the way in which we had been treated.

Ann and Jim had arranged to go away for only a few days, as they did not want to leave the girls too long, but the babysitter had had to call off at the last moment. We received a telephone call from Ann the next day, asking if we could take the girls for a couple of days. Rather than take the girls to our house, we moved into their house as it made more sense to have their clothes and toys and anything else we would need there at hand. The girls were a delight to look after and each evening after tea, I took them for a walk through the fields beside the cottage where Ann and Jim Lived.

Jean was just two and we never walked far enough to be out of sight of the house but it gave Kay some time to herself in the evening before the girls went to bed. It also allowed me to spend some time with them, to hear Jean chatter non-stop about what had happened that day, or to sing her latest song or recite her nursery rhymes. It was to cause the psychiatric staff some concern and was noted.

The next time the family were to spend the whole day together was on the occasion of Andrew and Ashley's daughter Ilona's seventh birthday on August 15th. As they lived in Milngavie, near Glasgow, it was easier to come to Perth to celebrate than for the rest of the family to go to Milngavie. They decided therefore to have a barbeque at Quarrymill, a park and picnic area near Perth which provides those facilities and plenty of space for children to enjoy themselves. Only Katrina was missing. Sharon and Neil, their boys Euan and Craig, our middle son Philip, his wife Alison and their children Stacey, Jenna and Jamie; Ann and Jim with Jean and Susan, Kay and I joined Ashley, Andrew, Ilona and Ashley's mother Lillian in what we thought was going to be a lovely family day out.

It was a lovely day in many respects. The kids thoroughly enjoyed themselves and there were enough of us for the adults to spell each other in playing with them. But there was an atmosphere, a lack of warmth which we found strange. At one point during the day Kay and I found ourselves on our own, walking among the trees which bordered some of the footpaths, trying to figure out what was wrong. The relationship with Sharon had been strained since the wedding but we put it down to the stress we knew she was under because she spent so much time with Katrina.

That did not explain the atmosphere that seemed to exist with the rest of the family. Earlier in the day, when we were all seated having something to eat, Kay had attempted to involve Philip in a conversation which normally would have provoked a furious debate in our house. The family had never known a time when I was not involved in politics. They had been brought up in a political household where political debate was the daily conversation. I had spent thirty-five years in the Scottish National Party, contested five parliamentary elections and was deputy leader of the SNP for a number of years in the 1980s, under the leadership of Gordon Wilson, who at the time was the MP for Dundee East.

Both Sharon and Philip had contested local government seats, Philip winning a seat on the Tayside Regional council and serving four years as a SNP councillor. I resigned from the party in December 1990 because of their commitment to membership of the European Union, their support for the Maastricht Treaty and the European Single Currency. I considered the party's policy of "Independence in Europe" to be nothing more than a slogan, and a dishonest one at that. It was a contradiction in terms which I refused on principle to try to sell to the electorate.

At the time of my resignation I had been re-adopted as the prospective parliamentary candidate for Perth & Kinross, a seat I had contested in 1987, running second to the Conservative MP Sir Nicky Fairbairn. The SNP had had high hopes of taking the seat at the next election, which took place in 1992, when the candidate who replaced me, Roseanna Cunningham came an even closer second to Sir Nicky. My interest in politics did not diminish in the slightest on leaving the SNP. I had become involved with a group of dissident nationalists called Sovereignty and then another group called the "Independence Movement" and maintained a high public profile, being asked to comment frequently on political matters on radio and TV.

I was a regular contributor to the Scottish newspaper columns, taking every opportunity to try to open up the debate on the future of Europe as opposed to the European Union, and Scotland's place in the kind of Europe I hoped to see. I also wrote two weekly columns for the local newspaper, one of which usually had a heavy political content. Sovereignty had discussed the possibility of putting up parliamentary candidates and I was under pressure to stand against the SNP in Perth & Kinross. Kay was very much opposed to the idea and in broaching the subject with Philip, expected to get an animated response. There was no response at all; Philip merely shrugged and made little or no comment. Kay said later, she felt as if she had been slapped. At home that evening we discussed any number of possible reasons why we seemed to be on the outside of the family looking in. None of them came even close to what was really wrong.

Over the next few weeks the general situation changed little, except that we saw a great deal less of the family. It was not that we saw them less frequently, we just saw them for shorter periods. Kay and I usually made a trip into Perth at some time during the weekend and we would normally call in to see each of our children and their kids. I passed Ann and Jim's house twice every day on my way to and from the office and while I did not call in every evening, I called in a couple of times every week. Jim tended to work long hours as a self-employed agricultural contractor and was seldom there when I visited. It was only later I was to learn that each visit I made was purgatory for Ann, as she tried to pretend everything was normal.

There was one major change to our customary routine which we did notice. There was rarely a week went by that we were not asked to babysit, either in our family's own homes or, as often happened at weekends, the grandchildren were brought out to Crieff where we had plenty of room. The kids would have what they called "an action weekend" starting with pony rides, followed by long walks or picnics, an hour or so in the children's park and then swimming at the Crieff Hydro. Getting them to sleep was never a problem and we loved having them, as much as they enjoyed coming. During the whole of August and September we were not asked to babysit once, even when we asked if they were coming out, there was always a reason why they couldn't.

About the middle of September Katrina telephoned her mother and asked her to come in to Perth to take her out for a short time. Kay would normally have telephoned me to let me know she was coming in to Perth so that I could arrange to pick her up because she did not drive and always came in to Perth by public transport. She had been unable to contact me at the office that day and therefore it was quite a surprise to see Katrina and her walking across the Smeaton Bridge as if heading for my office. Unfortunately I was having lunch with a business colleague in a restaurant immediately across from my office and had Kay and Katrina gone in, I intended to run over and asked them to join us. In the event they walked by without even looking in.

Kay called me later to say that she was at the hospital and asked me to pick her up there. On arriving just after five o'clock, Kay was waiting at the door and there was no sign of Katrina. I asked why they had not come in to the office and why Katrina had not waited to see me just now. Kay replied that Katrina had said she just did not want to see me and that she (Kay) did not want to pressure her. But it was getting to the point where I was beginning to get more than a little annoyed. I had begun to feel like a pariah. It was only a few days later that I learned I was not only a pariah, I was the worst kind of pariah. I was a paedophile.

CHAPTER SEVEN

July 1994 – April 1995

When Eileen and I came back from Wales I was never so glad to get home. The last three days of the holiday had been spent going from the bed in the small bedroom in the hotel, to the toilet in the hall. The journey home was a nightmare as I was sick several times in the train. When Mum and Dad came to see me on the Sunday, the day after we arrived home, I felt better and hoped the worst of the sickness was over but the rest of the week showed no improvement and I was actually glad when I was admitted to PRI because I felt sure that the doctors would find out what was wrong and do something about it. The operation to remove my appendix was performed at 6pm on the Friday evening of the day I was admitted to hospital.

I felt no better on the Saturday morning, when the surgeon came to see me, but I assumed that this was the consequence of the operation and that once the immediate pain passed I would be fine. When he told me that there had been nothing wrong with my appendix, my immediate reaction was to ask why he had taken it out and what were they going to do now. More importantly, if my appendix was OK, why had I been so ill? The surgeon and the doctor were perfectly honest about what was wrong with me – they had no idea but they intended to find out before I left the hospital. I had several x-rays over the next few days as well as a scan but no one came to tell me what had been found. I was given pain killers to relieve the discomfort from the operation but I felt no better when I was discharged a few days later and went to stay with my parents in Crieff. Neither my parents nor I were given any information about the scan that had been carried out.

I was sure I would be given some information from my parents' GP who attended me, coming in every couple of days, but he insisted he had heard nothing from PRI. He expressed his concern that the pain continued but that I could not be certain whether it was the original pain or the pain from the operation to remove my appendix. I suspected it was the original pain because I was still very nauseous and the scar from the operation was not very large, although it was quite inflamed. His persistence and insistence that the PRI re-admit me, led to my being taken back to PRI on August 12th. More tests were carried out, although I was still given no information before they decided to remove my gall bladder on August 16th.

The first few weeks after the gall bladder operation were passed in a fog of pain from the infected wound. Moving back in with my parents and being nursed by my mother was certainly preferable to being in hospital but it was a pretty miserable time for all of us. When I managed to get my clothes on after the first few days and was allowed to get out of bed, I simply moved from my bed to the couch in the sitting room. The weight just seemed to fall off me and the daily injections I was getting for pain relief became so uncomfortable and painful that I asked the doctor if there was no other way to give me relief. I was given the same dosage of Pethidine in tablet form and when the pain became too severe, I was able to take more than the prescribed dose, which contributed to my rapid addiction to the drug.

I was totally opposed to being re-admitted to PRI but my parents' GP was too concerned that the pain had continued, to allow the situation to go on. Although I was just as concerned, I dreaded having to go back for more tests, to be treated by doctors who did not seem to have a clue what they were doing. I was in constant pain, frightened to go back to hospital and frightened not to go. The dosage of Pethidine had been increased and I was taking more than I was prescribed, therefore when I had relief from the pain, I hardly knew what time of day it was. If the further tests told the doctors anything, they did not tell either me or my parents and the fact we were getting no information made things worse because it allowed my imagination to play havoc with my emotions. I felt very depressed for much of the time and swung from periods of being agitated to the point of climbing the walls, to deep despair when I just sat and cried.

The first time I collapsed in hospital, in the corridor going back to the ward with my parents, I got absolutely no warning. I did not feel dizzy or unsteady on my feet. One minute I was walking along the corridor very slowly, speaking to my Mum, the next I was coming round in the ward. I had no recollection of what had happened and was amazed when I was told I had been unconscious for an hour and a half. My parents had refused to leave until I was x-rayed and I was told there had been a fight with the duty doctor. It was perfectly obvious the staff were furious with me but I had no idea why. They had no patience with me and I invariably had to ask for anything I needed such as water for the bedside cabinet. There was no conversation with staff, other than the normal ward rounds when they would discuss my condition as if I was not there and was not even an interested bystander. Rarely was I asked how I felt or if I needed anything. My mood tended to be very low most of the time and the attitude of the staff did nothing to improve it.

Over the next two or three weeks the periods of unconsciousness became worse and totally unpredictable. On one occasion I was sitting up in bed drinking a cup of tea and the next I was coming to on the floor beside the bed. Another time I collapsed in the shower and pulled down the curtain as I fell. Several times the falls were so severe that I suffered extensive bruising to my face, my arms and on a couple of occasions, my head. Obviously this was of concern to my parents who grilled the doctors relentlessly about my treatment. The regular confrontations between my Mum and some of the staff did nothing to help their attitude to me

My recollection of some of the time I spent in PRI is hazy to say the least. I was taken off Pethidine and suffered nightmares, inability to sleep and sweats. When I fell into unconsciousness the staff attempted to waken me by sticking pins in my hands and feet and I later learned they thought I was doing it deliberately, which is why they always seemed to be annoyed with me. How they thought it was possible to feign unconsciousness when being stuck with pins is beyond me. When they eventually admitted they did not know what else to do, they called in Dr Yellowlees, a psychiatrist. I was not prepared to speak to him because of the counselling sessions I had had ten years before, after the abuse by my grandfather was discovered, but was assured it was to do no more than discuss the addiction to Pethidine and treating the withdrawal from it.

There was very little discussion with Dr Yellowlees about what had happened. He confirmed that I had had both appendix and gall bladder removed but gave no opinion about the fact that nothing had been found wrong with either. He discussed the drugs I had been taking and told me I had become addicted to Pethidine and the first thing he would have to do, would be to reduce my dependency gradually by replacing the Pethidine with Diazapam. When I told him that I had been taken off all medication when I came back to PRI, he said he thought that would help to explain the lapses into unconsciousness, although in his opinion, they sounded as if they were too severe to be caused by the withdrawal of Pethidine alone. I explained that eventually I had been given some other drugs but had no idea what they were. His response was that the dosages had obviously been incorrect or, that the drugs themselves were not the right drugs to "bring me down".

When he suggested I go into Gilgal so that he could better monitor the drug intake, so that the withdrawl from Pethidine could be completed in a properly controlled environment, I refused without even considering it. I knew Gilgal was a psychiatric hospital and the thought terrified me. Probably in an effort to persuade me that it was important, he suggested my pain may not be physical at all but psychosomatic and that a short stay in Gilgal would allow him to evaluate my condition that much better. The suggestion that I was imagining the pain, that there might be nothing physically wrong with me at all, infuriated me and convinced me that the last place I would go was Gilgal. On his final visit he told me that his report to the hospital would be that I was addicted to Pethidine and that my reaction to illness was not normal. He also said he would recommend my admission to Gilgal on a voluntary basis but only if I agreed.

As far as I was concerned it was not going to happen but my first day at home in my own flat was a disaster. When Sharon found me lying unconscious on the floor in front of the fire, with a large bruise on the side of my face where I had struck the fireplace as I fell, and PRI refused to re-admit me on the grounds there was no more they could do, it became obvious to me that eventually, I was not going to be given any alternative. That did not mean I was going to give in without a fight and initially insisted I would not go in but allowed myself to be persuaded to go and stay with Sharon and Neil, in the hope that things would work themselves out. How they were going to do that, I had no idea but I was desperate to avoid going into a psychiatric hospital.

I loved the flat I shared with Eileen. It had a large sitting room which faced on to the North Inch, one of the two large parks for which Perth is well known. The flats along the street had all been converted from large town houses and all the rooms had high ceilings with attractive cornices. We got on very well, we both worked in the Post Office where I had been since I was seventeen; we both loved horses and we spent every spare minute we had at the stables on the outskirts of Perth, working with them if not actually riding. My Dad and I had had great fun decorating it when I first took over the tenancy and the day Mum and Dad helped me to move in with Sharon and Neil and I did a last minute tidy up before leaving, the last thing on my mind was that it would be the last time I ever set foot in the place.

The next two weeks spent with Sharon and Neil put great strain on their family life. Sharon taught at the local primary school quite close to where she stayed but Euan and Craig, their two young sons, were only nine and seven respectively. It was still only early December and the school holidays had not yet started. Neil worked awkward shifts as a AA Patrolman, therefore there was really no one to look after me and be with me as much as I needed, as I was still having spells of unconsciousness. Mum visited almost on a daily basis and she and I spent the days talking about what I should do. Both Dad and her were concerned for me but they were also concerned for Sharon and her family.

The day before I finally agreed to go into Gilgal, the three of us, Mum, Dad and me, sat for hours discussing what should be done.

"I really don't want to go Mum because I am frightened I'll never come out again," I said.

"Why should you not come out again?" Dad laughed. "That's just daft, you are going in only to get you off the drugs and, as you are going in on a voluntary basis, you can leave anytime you like."

"I don't know and it's maybe daft to you, but I'm just scared." Dad gave me a hug and laughed again,

"It is not even the part of the hospital where the really disturbed psychiatric patients are. The people you will be with are recovering alcoholics, and people who have had nervous breakdowns."

"You really don't have much choice Katrina," said Mum. The strain is beginning to tell on Sharon and Neil and you are not getting the treatment and care you should be getting."

"I know Mum, I'm being selfish, but I'm just scared stiff."

I hated Gilgal as soon as I stepped in the front door. It had been a large country house, converted into an annex to the main hospital called Murray Royal. There was a large open foyer with a wide staircase leading to the upper floor. Corridors led right and left of the foyer, giving access to private rooms as well as the main wards at either end of the corridors, for male and female patients. Although it was early evening it was dark on the approach paths to the main door, with overhead lights giving a dim reflection through overhanging trees on both sides of the path. The dark, traditional wooden doors, together with subdued interior lighting, gave the whole place a dark and forbidding atmosphere, which made my already low mood even worse. I was given only a short time to say goodbye to Mum and Dad, before being led to the room in which I would spend the first few days, while being assessed.

"It is better if you don't stay too long saying cheerio to your parents," said the nurse who took me to my room. She was very pleasant and smiled a lot, giving the impression she was a very warm person. That was in stark contrast to the staff at PRI and made me feel slightly less apprehensive. As she helped me to unpack she said,

"We hear you have had a pretty rough time at the PRI. It must be terrible to have both your appendix and your gall bladder taken out only to be told there was nothing wrong with either of them."

"It certainly wasn't pleasant and I'm scared there is something seriously wrong that they haven't found yet." I answered.

"I know it is easy for me to say, but you should try not to worry. The staff here are pretty good and we'll soon have you home and well again." This was said as she was walking towards the door. I saw that nurse only another couple of times before she was transferred and I wonder if she ever thinks back to that conversation, in light of the outcome of my stay in Gilgal?

My first night was very disturbed and despite being given a sedative, I slept very little, being aware of not only the surroundings but the presence of patients moving about the wards. It was frightening because I had no experience of being this close to mental illness, nor did I have any knowledge of how patients might behave. Gilgal was not the ward for the very seriously disturbed but the noises I heard coming from various parts of the building suggested that some of the other patients were far from being well. Sheer exhaustion and the fact I had hardly stopped crying for hours, finally caused me to fall into a very fitful sleep.

The introduction to the nursing staff was friendly and they made an obvious effort to relax me and put me at my ease. Nevertheless, the fact I resented being there at all, made it difficult for the nursing staff to make any impression. Given the state of utter confusion which I was in for much of the time I spent in Gilgal, the initial entries in my nursing notes for the first few days, are worth noting. The diagnosis of my illness was written up as, "*Prescribed* drug addiction and abnormal illness behaviour." Where it asked if "Patient has understanding of reasons for admission", the named nurse had written, "None initially. Thinks that everyone thinks her illness is in her head".

Those entries are worth noting because it underlines the fact that the drugs to which I became addicted had been prescribed, as this was to cause controversy later when the experts had a major disagreement over how I had become addicted. At the end of the first two weeks on the 27th December, the "Goals" were still being written up as, "To establish the cause of Katrina's pain and prevent further abuse of pain relief." However, the "Evaluation" contained the following assessment, "Katrina has been receiving her pain relief on average 3 times per day for past two weeks. Observations have been recorded but no definite pattern has developed as yet. Continue with present regime."

Of much greater importance however, was the following, "Cause of pain could be due to experiences she went through in the past. SCN Hogg to investigate Katrina's physical feelings with her *when she is doing disclosure work with Katrina to try to establish any links and common factors or issues, which could identify further causes.*" Jenny Hogg became my main carer from the outset and within a very short time, I became totally dependent on her, which merely underlined the rapid deterioration in my health. The reference to disclosure work within 12 days of going in to Gilgal completely contradicts the assurances I had been given before I went in and which my parents received that none was being done, when they expressed their concerns about my health.

When Dr Yellowlees first suggested to me in PRI that the cause of my pain could be psychosomatic and made a tentative reference to looking into anything in my past that might have caused distress, I told him immediately that I had no intention of discussing anything in my past. My first reaction was that he meant the abuse I had suffered at the hands of my grandfather, although he did not mention it specifically. I had dealt with it when it happened ten years previously and had no intention of talking about it. It was brought up again within the first two or three days of my stay in

Gilgal by Jenny Hogg and I told her the same – I did not want to discuss it.

When I was introduced to Jenny Hogg, I was told she would be my charge nurse and that if I wanted to discuss anything, I should go initially to her. She introduced the topic when she said, "Well, we are going to have to find the cause of this pain Katrina, so you and I have some work to do."

"What do you mean?" I asked, "I thought I was here to get me off the addiction to Pethidine."

"Yes, you are but getting you off Pethidine is not going to get rid of the pain, at least not just getting you off the Pethidine."

That made me angry because she was obviously suggesting the cause of the pain was psychosomatic.

"Why will nobody believe I have a physical pain, that it's not psychosomatic? I asked.

"The pain you are feeling Katrina is real enough and it feels as if there is a physical cause, but we have to look at the possibility there might be another cause."

"How are you going to do that?"

"We can just talk about anything that is bothering you," she answered. "You were abused by your grandfather, weren't you?"

"I told Dr Yellowlees I was not going to speak about that and I was promised I wouldn't have to, if I didn't want to," I stormed

Jenny Hogg immediately backed off and let it lie for the rest of that first meeting.

Despite my determination not to do disclosure work, the pressure to disclose was constant and I became angry and totally uncooperative. Perhaps it would have been better if I had not been so aware of my surroundings in Gilgal because they added to my feelings of depression. Within days, I was introduced to anti-depressants both morning and evening, with a different drug administered during the day to "lift my mood". I was very soon being given the medication on demand and as my mood plummeted, largely because of the constant pressure to disclose, the "demands" became more frequent and I was quickly back on the treadmill of addiction to prescribed drugs.

Three or four days after being admitted to Gilgal I was introduced to the main ward and several young girls who were to become my constant companions and in at least two cases, my friends, over the following months. At least three of them claimed to have been sexually abused as children, a claim vehemently denied by the mother of one of the girls with whom I became particularly friendly. With constant pressure to disclose and talk about the abuse by my grandfather coming from the staff, and increasing discussion of abuse among the girls in the ward, it seemed, in a short period of time, that my sole topic of conversation with both staff and patients, was sexual abuse.

Within the first few days, I was given a book called Courage to Heal by Ellen Bass and Laura Davis, subtitled – A guide for Women Survivors of Child Sexual Abuse – and sometimes described as one of the most pernicious self-help books ever written. Every girl in the ward who claimed to have been abused read that book. No, that is wrong – we devoured the book and were encouraged to discuss its contents. Under a section entitled, "But I Don't Have any Memories", it says, "*If you don't remember your abuse, you are not alone. Many women don't have memories, and some never get memories. This doesn't mean they weren't abused.*" It then continues, "If you don't have any memory of it, it can be hard to believe the abuse really happened. You may....want proof of your abuse. This is a very natural desire, but *it is not one that can always be met.*"

An example is given of one "survivor", "One thirty-eight -year-old survivor described her relationship with her father as "emotionally incestuous". She has never had specific memories of any physical contact between them, and for a long time she was haunted by the fact that she couldn't come up with solid data. Over time, she's come to terms with her lack of memories. Her story is a good model if you don't have specific pictures to draw from." This woman was initially concerned that she might be accusing her father of something he had not done but she attended "Incest Survivor

Groups" and found she "empathised" with everything they said and took comfort from the fact that no one ever said to her, "You do not belong here".

This woman suffered feelings of anxiety and in her need to know why, she decided to play the "All right, let's act as if" game. She did not know why she felt anxious therefore decided to invent a reason – and that reason was sexual abuse by her father. Despite having no memories of actual abuse, she decided it had happened anyway because it gave her a reason for her anxiety. She convinced herself that this process was healing her and when she went to the incest groups and said, "I don't have any pictures" she simply "talked all about her father". The fact she was not told that she did not belong there helped to convince her the abuse took place.

Another "survivor" described her memories thus, "*The more I worked on the abuse, the more I remembered.* First I remembered my brother, and then my grandfather. About six months after that I remembered my father and then, about a year later, I remembered my mother. I remembered the "easiest"first and the "hardest" last. Even though it was traumatic for me to realise that everyone in my family abused me, there was something reassuring about it. Remembering the rest of the abuse was actually one of the most grounding things to happen. My life suddenly made sense."

There is a chapter in the book entitled "EFFECTS: RECOGNISING THE DAMAGE". Despite the title, the introduction to the chapter goes on, "The long-term effects of child sexual abuse can be so pervasive that it's sometimes hard to pinpoint exactly how the abuse affected you. It permeates everything: your sense of self, your intimate relationships, your sexuality, your parenting, your work life, even your sanity." Then follows a series of subheadings and lists of "affects" that can be "identifiers" of having been sexually abused. That some of them are contradictory seems to have gone unnoticed, or perhaps it is simply a case of nothing being left to chance, every personality trait or behaviour pattern can be used as an "identifier of sexual abuse" if the therapist so wishes.

In the section on self-esteem and personal power, it asks,

Are you afraid to succeed?
*Can you accomplish things you set out to do?

On sexuality it states;
* Are you able to stay present when making love?
* Do you go through sex numb or in a panic?
* Do you experience sexual pleasure?
* Do you think pleasure is bad?

On parenting:
* Have you ever been abusive, or feared you might be?
* Are you overprotective?
* Do you have a hard time feeling close to your children?
* Are you comfortable being affectionate with them?

The environment created by the use of this book, together with the constant discussion of abuse and the pressure to disclose previous abuse, was very unhealthy. Add to the environment the fact that I was on increasing medication and I soon became as obsessed with abuse as everyone else, including the staff. Sleep was disturbed by nightmares where I was being abused but the nursing staff told me the nightmares were "flashbacks", where I was re-living actual events. When the flashbacks became too severe, the nurses would waken me and "reorient" me. I was given the names of people I saw and called out to during the flashbacks and was encouraged to write the details down, as they were given to me by the nurses. I was soon having the flashbacks during the day, if I fell asleep and was told they were frequently quite violent. I was also told I simulated having sexual intercourse during the course of the flashbacks, which was extremely embarrassing and the thought of doing this in the open ward, in front of other patients horrified me.

As the intensity of the flashbacks increased, I was encouraged to disclose more about the abuse with my grandfather but I continued to be hostile to any attempt to get me to talk during the sessions I had with Jenny Hogg. My feelings of guilt about the abuse and the fact I was in Gilgal, began to make me feel increasingly dirty. I began to experience the kind of feelings I was afraid I would feel if my Dad found out. I spent long periods in the shower trying to wash the dirt away and the more I scrubbed myself, the more obsessed I felt about getting clean. The one thing that did improve was the abdominal pain I had been experiencing since the previous June, over eight months before had disappeared almost completely and I no longer needed regular pain relief.

In an attempt to create as much normality as possible, I was given "time-out" in Perth with members of staff. This would last approximately two hours and involved no more than a walk around the shops and perhaps a visit to a café for a cup of coffee. There was an endless supply of coffee and tea in the hospital and no restriction on how many cups per day we had, therefore any visit to the town would always involve at least two visits to a café to keep the intake at its usual level. It also seemed to allow me to talk a bit more freely to staff, although never about the abuse. I was also given the very occasional visit to Sharon's house for a few hours, providing her and Neil could guarantee they would return me to the hospital at the required time.

On one of those time-out visits to the town on my own, I experienced a flashback which caused me to collapse in the street. The police were called and fortunately the flashback was not as severe as those I normally had in hospital and I was able to tell them about my being an inpatient in Gilgal. Obviously I was very embarrassed and humiliated when the staff came to collect me and for the first time, contemplated suicide. I had reached a point where I could not see myself getting any better and the episode in the town came at the end of a period when I had been experiencing intense flashbacks, where I could recognise my grandfather and another member of the family, who had suddenly started to appear. In the second week of March 1995, after several days of feeling like this, I absconded from the ward. I got no further than a mile from the hospital before the staff picked me up and I provided little resistance to being taken back to the ward, but it was an indication that the situation was deteriorating.

As the deterioration set in, I thought more and more about ending it by committing suicide. Speaking to the staff or Jenny Hogg did nothing to lighten my moods and the future frightened me. I did not want to carry on with this kind of life indefinitely, finally resolving to do something about it. Towards the end of February, the flashbacks were more frequent and severe and over the period of seven days, I saved the bulk of my medication by only pretending to swallow it. The staff never checked to make sure I had swallowed the medication, therefore it was easy to keep it under my tongue until after they had gone. The attempt was unsuccessful because there were not enough pills and those I took made me violently sick, so that the staff were able to see what had made me vomit.

From then on, the staff paid much closer attention when I was given medication, making sure I had actually swallowed it before leaving me. Despite their attentions, I was able to make another attempt shortly after. Although my mood had obviously deteriorated and there was little sign of progress, the staff allowed me time-out on my own. My forays into town usually lasted no more than two hours and I rarely took the full two hours because there was really nothing I wanted to do or see. Sharon and Neil worked, my parents were in Crieff and the boys all lived outside Perth, so there was no one I could visit. The only person I had any possibility of seeing during the week was my Dad, but he was always busy, unless my Mum came in from Crieff. On one of the trips into Perth, I bought a packet of Ibuprofen and took them all when I returned to Gilgal. The sixteen pills again made me very sick and again, the staff discovered what I had done.

Despite the trips to Sharon and Neil's and the trips to town, the weekly Evaluation sheets for January, February and March had a distressingly familiar content, underlining the almost complete lack of progress in my mental condition. Invariable they would note, "Katrina shows little change from last valuation. She continues to experience two or three flashbacks every night but staff quickly reorientate her. Flashbacks also occur daily, sometimes several times per day. Continues to have counselling sessions with Nurse J Hogg but little progress as Katrina finds it difficult to work through her guilt. Still hostile to staff and sometimes with other patients. Has very negative outlook and fears for the future." One of the last evaluations at the beginning of April noted I was "having increasing difficulty coping with flashbacks which can sometimes be quite violent."

After a fairly severe flashback one day, the nurse who had reoriented me, said,

"Katrina, your flashbacks are getting worse and there is a lot of violence in them. Maybe if you tried to do disclosure with Jenny Hogg, you would find it relieved the pressure and you would be able to cope better."

"I'm too ashamed," I said.

"You have no need to be ashamed, you have done nothing wrong," she said quite sharply.

"But Jenny might think I am dirty," I countered.

"She will think nothing of the kind. She will be supportive and help you through it," the nurse said. "The staff are all here to help you and none of us will ever think of any abused girl as dirty. Why would you think that?"

"Because that is how I think of myself," I replied quietly.

By this time I had started regular sessions with a psychologist which I thought a complete waste of time. There were times when Jenny Hogg failed to turn up for a counselling session and this left me feeling very let down and upset, even although I resented being pushed to disclose. Although I did not realise it, I was becoming more and more reliant on her and felt rejected if she failed to keep our regular appointments. She also seemed to be able to reorient me much more quickly than some of the other staff, which made the flashbacks less severe if she was there.

At the beginning of April, as I was leaving the room where we had had one of our usual sessions, Jenny Hogg suddenly asked me,

"Did your father ever abuse you?"

"What, my father? Of course he didn't. Why are you asking?"

"I was just asking, it doesn't matter".

I was very angry and told Jenny Hogg I was but she just shrugged, as if it was of no consequence. When I later told my Mum that evening when I telephoned home, she was equally angry. She said that to suggest that to me, because that was what had been done, was dangerous because of my confused state of mind. Confused did not even begin to describe how I felt. Jenny Hogg's question had upset me a great deal.

There had never been any mention of my Dad abusing me. He had been white with fury when he found out about his own father, my grandfather, and the only reason he had not pressed to have him charged was because I could not face it becoming known. I knew he didn't abuse me, therefore the question simply did not arise. There was no need even to think about it Unfortunately the suggestion had been made and it started a chain of events that almost destroyed the entire family.

CHAPTER EIGHT

April 1995 – October 1995

When I think back fourteen years on, to that terrible time, I can hardly believe how close my mind came to completely unravelling. The months leading up to the confrontation with my Dad in October 1995, were the worst months of all the time I spent under psychiatric care, with my mind filled with horrific pictures of abuse, including witnessing the murder of a six year old "friend" by my father. I was told repeatedly that I was not mentally ill but that I displayed all the symptoms of someone who had been badly physically beaten and sexually abused over a very long period of time. Despite those assurances, I was convinced I was losing my mind.

Not only was I having flashbacks and nightmares, I was also having oral, tactile and visual hallucinations. I began to see fairies, black ones which frightened me to death and white ones which danced and made me laugh. They seemed to be so real that I spoke to them or, in the case of the black fairies, just cowered in fear. I heard voices telling me to harm myself or to take my own life. I could feel people touching me but not in a pleasant or friendly way and I accused some of the staff of being the Devil, or frequently misidentified staff completely confusing one with the other. Despite all of this, I was assured by staff constantly, that they believed whatever I told them, whatever accusations I made about the abuse I was suffering.

My medical records of this time are full of references to my mood swings, flashbacks, hostility to staff and growing inability to cope with the flashbacks. There are also references to the start of self-harming and violence, generally directed at furniture or the windows in the ward. On more than one occasion I attempted to put my fist through the window. As a consequence of this, my medication was changed and increased so that there were times I felt totally confused about my surroundings, my behaviour and even the people with whom I was in contact. I still kept company with the girls in the ward who had also been abused and our discussions were all about our experiences at the hands of our abusers.

An important part of the treatment was keeping a diary of what had taken place each day, particularly if I had had a flashback. My flashbacks were apparently getting more and more violent, where I would thrash all over the place and scream and call out. I was frequently told I was simulating vigorous sexual intercourse and on more than one occasion was told my hands had been tied behind my back while I was anally assaulted. After being reoriented by the staff, I was given details of what had happened while I was in the flashback and encouraged to write them down. The contents of this diary, or journal as it was called, was then discussed with Jenny Hogg and I was encouraged to believe that what was contained in the flashbacks were in fact memories which I had buried. On occasion I was encouraged to write with my non-dominant hand as this was supposed to ensure that what I wrote was in fact the truth.

After a particularly violent flashback and I was slowly recovering, one of the staff said to me,

"Did you know your father was in that flashback?"

My reaction was immediate and I called her a liar but another member of staff who had also been present, confirmed I had called out to my Dad while I was still in the flashback. I still did not believe them and told them so but it upset me greatly to think of my Dad appearing. I spoke to Jenny Hogg about it and she encouraged me to trust my "memories". When I told her he had appeared in a flashback and that I did not have any memories of being abused by him, she told me that flashbacks were simply things that had happened to us but which we had buried, coming to the surface. I refused to accept my Dad had abused me and although I had no problem when my grandfather appeared in the flashbacks, because I had vivid memories of his abuse, it was different for my Dad. I did not have any memories of being abused by him.

Although I had no actual memories of Dad ever abusing me, after the first time he appeared in a flashback, he began to appear regularly in a whole series of bizarre episodes which, no matter how horrendous they became, were invariably accepted by the staff as the "truth". One of the last times Dad ever saw me on his own at the hospital, was at the beginning of February and we went for a walk in the extensive grounds of Gilgal. Some time later he appeared in a flashback, walking with me at the hospital and telling me it would be better for everyone if I killed myself. I immediately related this to the staff because I was so upset and it was recorded in my diary.

The flashbacks where he abused me now began to include not just historical abuse when I was a child, but more recent and current abuse when I moved into my flat before Eileen moved in with me, and in the hospital itself. Other men began to appear also, friends and colleagues of my Dad's including some senior members of the SNP. One violent flashback showed Dad and his closest friend raping me at my flat and then my Dad accepting money. As the number of flashbacks including him continued, he appeared at my flat regularly either alone or with other men and I would invariably be beaten and raped, before money, cigarettes or drink changed hands. These assaults always happened during the day and I would go on to work after as if nothing had happened.

On another occasion I visited Sharon's house with my Mum when my Dad called in. Mum had agreed to collect Sharon's oldest son Euan from the school and when she left to walk to the school about a mile from the house, I decided to take a shower. No sooner had I stepped under the shower than my Dad came into the bathroom and raped me. Not only did he rape me but he sexually assaulted me with a hairbrush. The use of instruments had become a feature of the assaults by my Dad and he used a variety of articles on me, including on one occasion a screwdriver. He was also becoming more aggressive and willing to take chances. After one flashback I was hysterical and it had taken almost thirty minutes for the staff to reorient me. I had seen my Dad murder a six year old girl with an iron bar in order to make me more compliant for his friends. He had also raped me in the hospital grounds and forced me to give him oral sex in one of the visiting rooms at the front of Gilgal House.

Pressure was now being put on me to tell other members of the family but I was adamant that no one else should know. I was deeply embarrassed and very upset that the staff knew about Dad. Every incident in every flashback had been recorded in my diary and the act of writing it down somehow made it seem worse because it made it more "real". Yellowlees, who saw me only infrequently as my main contact was still Jenny Hogg, although I did see a psychologist from time to time, insisted I tell Sharon. He said he was worried about the grandchildren and that Dad might harm them if he was still in contact with them. I did not want to tell Sharon because I was terrified if she found out my Dad would also find out and he would harm me in some way. I believed he had asked me to kill myself and by this time, believed he or one of his friends might also kill me.

It was now the middle of June and as the flashbacks became more frequent and violent and my general condition deteriorated, Yellowlees increased the pressure on me to tell Sharon. During one of her visits I tried to tell her. As we were walking in the grounds I said, "I have remembered more abuse and there is someone else involved."

"Who is it?" asked Sharon.

Try as I might, I just could not bring myself to tell her, although she pressed me until she had to return to the school at which she taught. When I told Jenny Hogg and Yellowlees that I had been unable to tell Sharon, they were annoyed, insisting that sooner rather than later, I was going to have to tell her.

That time arrived the following week when Sharon returned. She was now on holiday and saw me almost every day and had been up to visit at least three times since I had started to tell her, but did not raise the subject again. Finally I plucked up the courage and said to her, "I have something I must tell you."

"Is it about the abuse, what you started to tell me the last time?" she asked.

"Have you ever wondered about Dad?" I said.

"Have I ever wondered what about Dad?"

"Dad is the other person who has been abusing me."

Sharon looked at me as if I had slapped her and just asked, "What?"

"Dad has been abusing me and is still abusing me now in the hospital." I said.

Sharon was so shocked she could hardly speak, said she couldn't believe it. I told her I had no memories of being abused by Dad, that all the abuse had taken place in flashbacks and that the staff had told me at first, when he had appeared. I also told her I had told them I did not believe it at first because I did not want them to know but I admitted I was now seeing him quite clearly, him and other men, some of them in the SNP. I gave Sharon no names and did not go into any detail about the nature of the abuse by Dad. Sharon said she still could not believe it and asked me if I was sure, since I had no actual memories of having been abused by Dad. I had to admit to her that I just did not know but that the staff had assured me the flashbacks I was having were real enough. She said she wanted to speak to Yellowlees, at which I told her it had been his idea that I tell her and that he would probably be only too glad to see her.

As expected, Yellowlees was keen to meet Sharon because he insisted he was extremely worried about the grandchildren and Dad having access to them. I was very nervous about the meeting because I did not know what to expect, nor did I want Sharon to know everything about the level of abuse I saw in the flashbacks. When Sharon arrived, I was taken from the ward because Yellowlees wanted me to tell Sharon in his presence. He knew I had told Sharon Dad had abused me but he wanted to give her the details. As he had no idea how much Sharon knew, he asked my permission to tell her everything but I refused. The abuse was so bad that I did not think Sharon could take it if she knew. At the same time, I was not even sure it had happened because I still had no "real" memories, only flashbacks and nightmares.

There were two incidents however, which helped me to speak to Sharon because I thought they would be able to prove the allegations were true. During one of the flashbacks when Dad was abusing me in our house in Tarvie Place in Perth, I recognised the figure of an ex-boyfriend of mine, Steven Houston. Steven came to the house on occasion and my parents knew him well and liked him and although he was present during the abuse, he seemed to do nothing to try to stop it, he just stood by and watched in horror. Before I could be certain about what happened then, I was reoriented by the staff but the flashback had been so clear I was able to tell the staff without prompting and they thought the presence of a witness to the abuse was a major breakthrough.

The second flashback where another witness was present, although this one was also a victim, involved my cousin Susan. She it was, who had been talking to me on the telephone about the abuse by our grandfather, when Mum had overheard us, bringing the original abuse to light. During another flashback, it was obviously at our house, when Susan was visiting, there was another vivid image of Dad abusing her, after he had raped and beaten me. I was sprawled where I had fallen on the floor, watching in terror as he also raped Susan. Again, the staff felt more and more confident we were finally going to be able to do something to bring this to an end.

Sharon told Yellowlees she could not believe Dad was an abuser and told him that I had said I was not sure because the abuse had happened in flashbacks. Yellowlees was obviously annoyed and turned to me quickly asking,

"Come on Katrina, after all we have been through and all we have discussed, are you having doubts, are you really saying you are not sure?"

I didn't have the courage to face up to Yellowlees and certainly did not want his disapproval. After a short pause I could only mutter a very soft,

"No, Dad did abuse me."

I then begged Sharon to tell no one else, I did not want the boys to know. She still seemed to be too shocked to take it all in and agreed, although at the time, I had no idea whether or not she would keep to the agreement.

After the meeting Yellowlees told me he felt much happier because they could now involve other people to ensure the grandchildren were looked after. That made me more nervous because it meant more people knowing and more chance that Dad and his friends would find out. The next two or three weeks seemed to be one long flashback and nightmare. Every day started with cups of coffee and several cigarettes. My moods fluctuated wildly and I would have a flashback before lunch, be reoriented and almost immediately have another. Despite the dissociation, where I had no idea where I was and the psychotic episodes, where I saw things and other people who were not there, I still insisted I wanted to go to Jim and Anne's wedding.

Neither Yellowlees nor Jenny Hogg were keen because they did not want me to be in my father's company and told me they were afraid for my safety. By this time, the very thought of my father petrified me. He appeared in all my flashbacks and the violence of the abuse was an ever present, helping to convince me I would be harmed if either he or his friends ever were given the opportunity. But Jim and I had been very close when we were growing up. We were the closest in age and we were the last two left in primary school together, after Sharon, Andrew and Philip had all gone to secondary school. Dad had encouraged us to take riding lessons and we did that together, as well as judo and swimming with the rest of the family.

When Jim and Anne first set up home together, Jean, their oldest daughter was just a toddler and they were always short of money, spending nights at my flat with Eileen and me. I couldn't bear to think of not going to the wedding, however scared I was of my Dad. Sharon agreed to take me to the ceremony and stay by my side the whole time. Yellowlees would not agree under any circumstances to my presence at the reception and finally agreed to allow me to go to the ceremony only on condition that I give a solemn promise to return to the hospital as soon as the ceremony was over. Sharon had also to agree.

As the two weeks before the wedding had been very difficult for the staff, coping with my flashbacks and the need for almost constant supervision, they were not sure I was going to be able to make the wedding at all. On the morning before, I had a particularly violent and lengthy flashback, which my medical notes record in detail. The staff have written, "Katrina went into flashback and thrashed continuously for over thirty minutes. She kept repeating the same name, shouting, " Please don't hurt me. That is sore. Please you're hurting me." When she came round, she was totally exhausted and felt sick. She had to be helped to bed. Her father appeared in the flashback with several other men."

The next day, I was much calmer but went into a mild flashback which lasted no more than ten minutes, about 7am. My normal medication was supplemented with more anti-depressants so that by the time, Sharon called for me, I was very subdued. She had agreed to call well before we were due at the ceremony at 11am to help with my makeup and make sure my hair was OK. She was very nervous and admitted she was not looking forward to the wedding because she did not know how to face our parents. She had not seen them since being told about Dad's abuse and had no idea how she would react. Sharon had seen me almost every day since that meeting with Yellowlees when she found out and she was well aware of how bad things had been for me and how many times I had been psychotic, or had flashbacks.

Neil called to collect us about thirty minutes before we were due at the ceremony and gave me a hug. Obviously Sharon had had to tell him. First of all he complimented me on how I looked than asked,

"How are you feeling and are you going to be all right? Are you sure you want to go through with this?"

"Yes, I'm all right and No, I'm not sure I want to go through with this but I'm going to anyway," I replied.

"If anything happens or you want to come back to the hospital, just tell us and we can leave right away," said Neil

"Nothing is going to happen," said Sharon, "because Dad doesn't know we know."

Unfortunately that wasn't to be the case.

As soon as I saw Mum and Dad outside the Registry Office where the wedding ceremony was to take place, I froze. They had just arrived and were standing on the edge of a crowd which included Philip, Alison and Andrew and, although we were separated by several yards and at least a dozen other people, I was immediately gripped by fear and concern.

"I don't want to speak to them," I said to Sharon.

"It is OK, you won't have to. We can go straight into the Registry before anyone else if you want to," she answered. We did that and accompanied by Neil, we went in and sat down until the rest of the guests arrived, followed soon after by Anne and Jim. The ceremony was soon over and as soon as Anne and jim had signed the Register, we went outside to arrange to go to the reception. I still had not spoken to my parents.

Sharon did not leave my side for a second and made sure we were no where near Mum and Dad. She was just as nervous as I was and was glad of having to look after me so that she could also avoid contact with our parents. We were seated almost directly opposite Mum and Dad and although I tried hard to avoid looking in their direction it was impossible to keep that up throughout the meal. Twice or three times both Mum and Dad tried to make eye contact and Mum signed to me, asking if I was OK. I just nodded and saw Dad speaking to her, convinced they were discussing me. Catching his eye unsettled me and I said to Sharon,

"I don't think I am going to be able to stay here. I hate being opposite Dad and I am sure he knows." I said.

"What can he know and anyway, he can't do anything here," she replied.

A few moments later, I was certain I was going to have a flashback and panicked.

"Sharon, we are going to have to get out of here. I am going to faint."

Sharon immediately spoke to Neil and without saying anything to anyone else at the table, we rose and left.

The car was parked a matter of a few yards from the door and the time it took Neil to bring it over can have been no more than a few minutes, but by that time, a combination of panic at the thought I might have to speak to Dad and fear, I was about to have a flashback, made me almost hysterical. I was no sooner in the car than I went into flashback. It was the first time Neil had witnessed this and immediately stopped the car but Sharon had told him to get us to the hospital as quickly as possible because she did not know if she could cope. When they left me at the hospital, I was very distressed. I had been desperate to go to the wedding and it had turned out to be a disaster, with no chance to speak to Anne and Jim and fear of my Dad making it impossible for me to stay for any length of time. It would have been better if I had not gone.

"I must be pregnant."

The words just burst out and Jenny Hogg looked startled and then slightly amused.

"What makes you think you're pregnant?" she asked.

"I've missed a period. I must be," I replied.

"You've been very ill for some time now and that can often lead to missed periods," Jenny Hogg said. "Are there any other signs?"

"What kind of signs?"

"Do you feel sick or is there any tenderness of your breasts?" she asked.

"I often feel sick but I just know I am. Dad raped me didn't he?"

Jenny just looked at me for a moment then said, "I will speak to Dr Yellowlees and discuss a pregnancy test."

The test was carried out within a few days with the results showing negative.

After the first meeting with Yellowlees, when I had confirmed to Sharon Dad's abuse, she had interviews with the Social Work

Department, who discussed at length, the protection of the grandchildren. Sharon felt under enormous pressure at this time and pleaded with me to allow her to tell the boys. I kept refusing because I did not want them to know. I was afraid they would find out because it meant there were other people involved and there would be a greater chance my Dad and his friends would find out. But there was a more important reason I did not want Sharon to tell the boys; they had started to appear in my flashbacks as having abused me.

The flashbacks had continued throughout August and September, with my father and several other men appearing regularly. I recognised all of them as neighbours, a couple of relatives and a number of well known SNP members. When Dad was the parliamentary candidate in Dundee, he went down to Dundee most Saturdays to campaign and speak in the City Square. As Mum worked, Jim and I went with him most days and either sat in the car with him or, if he had a meeting, we would sometimes be left with his election agent's wife at their home. At other times we spent time at the SNP offices which were always filled with SNP members.

The first one of my brothers to appear in the flashbacks was Andrew, whose name I had called out and was told by the nursing staff as they reoriented me. Soon after, both Philip and Jim appeared and all three participated in the abuse. They were always there with Dad and seemed to be forced to participate because they looked to be no more then ten or eleven years old. After those flashbacks I became very depressed at the thought that my brothers had also been involved in the abuse and Sharon's constant efforts to make me tell them only made me worse and more afraid. If they had taken part in the abuse, would they side with Dad, even although he had forced them?

During the first two weeks of September a new figure appeared in the flashbacks that depressed me to such an extent that I made two attempts to commit suicide. The brutality of the abuse did not seem to surprise the staff who, no matter what they were told, continued to tell me they supported me, that they believed me and that it was better to get it out into the open. On occasion, some discussion had centered around the part played by my mother. What had she been doing while I was abused? The obvious answer was that she did not know but Jenny had suggested that Mum might also be a victim of Dad's brutality and was too afraid to do anything.

When the staff told me she had appeared in a flashback, I told them I did not believe them, just as I had done with Dad. They assured me it was true and I sobbed my heart out that night at the very thought of Mum being involved. As the number of times she appeared increased, I began to see her more clearly. When Dad first appeared in the flashbacks, the abuse was straightforward, if such a term can be used to describe abuse of any kind, but it was non-violent. As it progressed however, it became more brutal with the introduction of instruments. It was during one such episode that Mum appeared more clearly than she had ever appeared before, as she passed Dad something which he used to assault me. I could not see what it was but she had had to go into the kitchen to get it and bring it to him.

"I can't believe Mum was involved," I told Jenny Hogg after I was reoriented.

"Perhaps she wasn't as innocent as we thought," she commented.

I looked at her, tears welling in my eyes and said, "She must have been forced, she would not do that on her own."

"Forced or not, she was definitely involved and you will have to accept it." she said. "Things are now getting too serious to be left as they are Katrina, you should speak to the police."

"I can't do that," I said quickly, "then Dad and his friends would definitely find out. I am too frightened."

Later that evening, I tried to hang myself with the cord from my dressing gown, as a consequence of which I was locked in the secure unit on suicide watch for the next four days.

Jenny Hogg was right, as much as I hated the thought, I finally agreed to tell the boys.

Sharon arranged to bring them to the hospital and Andrew, Jim, Sharon and I met in one of the visiting rooms. Jenny Hogg had brought me from the ward and as it was only a few days since I had tried to hang myself, I was accompanied everywhere. Before she left us alone, she asked Sharon to come and get her so that she could take me back to the ward. Sharon had not told the boys what they were going to hear before they arrived and when I told them they were absolutely stunned. Jim sprung to his feet looked wildly around him and suddenly smashed his head into the large bay window and shot out of the room. Andrew ran after him and Sharon and I could see the two of them run across the fields adjacent to the hospital.

It took about ten minutes for Andrew to get Jim, calm him down and bring him back. It was obvious he had been crying and he was quite distraught. Andrew was the first to speak,

"Are you sure?" he asked

"Yes," I said, "I wish I wasn't."

Sharon went on to explain about how I had appeared in the flashbacks, how she had questioned Yellowlees and how he had assured her there was no doubt.

"Where did it happen and were there any others involved?" Andrew asked.

"It happened in our house and a flat in Perth and another flat in Dundee when Jim and I went there with Dad," I answered. "I can't tell you who else was involved because I'm terrified Dad will find out and they will harm me."

"Were there any cameras, were photographs taken?" asked Andrew, who was becoming very agitated.

"Yes," I said, "But I don't want to speak about it anymore," at which point I started to cry bitterly. Throughout this, Jim had sat with his head in his hands and said nothing, while Sharon sat beside me, encouraging and helping me when I stumbled over words.

I said I wanted to go back to my room so Sharon went to look for Jenny Hogg, who, when she turned up, asked Jim to take me back while she waited to speak to Sharon and Andrew.

"Are you absolutely certain Katrina?" Jim asked. "I just can't believe Dad did it."

"I have no memories of Dad doing anything, except in flashbacks," I said. "It's not the same as with Poppa, I can remember his abuse and can tell you when it happened, whether it is at night or during the day. I can remember all of that. I don't have any memories of Dad like that. I am always in flashback. I don't know when it happened or what time of year it was or anything like that but Yellowlees and Jenny Hogg, as well as the rest of the staff keep telling me that flashbacks are memories we have locked away and that I should trust my memories."

"I am so sorry Jim, I know how much you think of Dad but I couldn't keep it to myself any longer."

By this time we had reached the door of my room, where a nurse was waiting for me. Jim gave me a quick hug and the tears were streaming down his face as he turned and walked back to find Sharon and Andrew. That night I again tried to hang myself, using the legs of the bottom of my pyjamas. Mum and Dad were told it was not a serious attempt.

Now that the boys were involved, there were several meetings between Yellowlees and them, as they and Sharon tried to come to terms with what they had been told. I was told they were also being put under pressure by the Social Work Department. Over the next two or three weeks the pressure became relentless. I was still having flashbacks several times a day, as well as during the night and finally, I was persuaded to give a statement to the police. I had refused several times because I did not think they could protect me but was told Sharon would make one too and finally, I agreed.

It was arranged that Jenny Hogg would accompany me. Two police women came to the hospital to take my statement and immediately tried to put me at my ease by assuring me they would not put me under any pressure and that I should take my time and just tell them as much as I wanted to tell them at that stage. It was extremely difficult to get started but under their encouragement, it became progressively easier. They told me they were part of a special unit in the police that did work with women who had been raped or otherwise sexually assaulted, as well as child protection.

"Nothing you tell us will come as any surprise, nor will we be shocked in any way," the senior officer said. "Try to relax and tell us in your own time and words."

I started by telling them about the earlier abuse, when no violence was involved, explaining how that had changed, the more I remembered. They prompted me from time to time, asking about where it took place and when. I explained about the difficulty of remembering when the abuse took place but was able to tell them about the rape in the shower in Sharon's house, and how I reported that as soon as I returned to the hospital, as well as the rape and assaults that had taken place in the hospital itself. They asked Jenny Hogg about the assaults in the hospital in particular, together with the rape in the shower because that had been reported so soon after it had happened. Jenny Hogg confirmed that those assaults had taken place and been reported as I had claimed.

When they pushed me about the others that were involved, I gave them a list of men some of whom were friends, relatives and neighbours but their main interest was in some of the leading members of the SNP, including two of their MPs. There were seventeen men in total and one name would take on a special significance because of later developments. That name was Jim Sillars, who had been the MP for Glasgow Govan and was one of the most high profile and best known political figures in Scotland. At the end of the statement, the police assured me I would be kept safe and for the first time, I began to think they might be telling the truth. By the end of that week, Sharon and the boys had confronted Dad.

CHAPTER NINE

A FAMILY TORN APART
July 1995 – October 1995

Sharon's early and almost total involvement with Katrina throughout her illness made it inevitable that she would be the first one of the family to be told. Yellowlees had also met her, knew she had two young boys and that Kay and I saw the grandchildren often. His concern for the grandchildren was obviously understandable, if he believed I was guilty of the abuse of Katrina. Sharon found the meeting with Katrina and Yellowlees difficult, partly because he was evidently under instructions from Katrina, to hold back some of the information Sharon would need if she was going to accept that I was an abuser. She was being asked to accept that I had violated her sister, on trust, on the word of a psychiatrist with whom she had had only a handful of contacts and she was going to need a great deal more than that.

After the initial confirmation by Katrina that I had abused her, albeit under a degree of pressure from Yellowlees, Katrina went back to her room upset and in tears but Sharon wanted and needed to pursue this with Yellowlees, therefore she hung back until Katrina had gone before questioning Yellowlees much more closely Sharon had been teaching for ten years, for eight of them as a behavioural support teacher, dealing with children who had been abused physically, sexually and emotionally by parents and relatives and sometimes by people who had no blood relationship at all. In other words her experience of child abuse and its ramifications was extensive.

"How can you be certain my Dad abused Katrina if she has no clear memories of the abuse and everything she has reported has been by way of flashbacks and nightmares?" she asked Yellowlees. "Is there not a possibility those flashbacks could be confused?

Yellowlees answered,

"Yes, they could be confused but I have no reason to think they are in this case. I have no reason to doubt what Katrina is saying."

"But Katrina isn't "saying" anything, she is having flashbacks and nightmares."

Yellowlees went on to describe and explain flashbacks, which were memories that had been buried and that could be activated by a change in circumstances or environment. For example if Katrina felt it was safe for her to speak about her abuse, and was encouraged and supported by people who were obviously willing to help her.

"I find it very difficult to believe my father is an abuser," Sharon said, "From my own experience of Dad, he is not aggressive, he is not violent in any way. He shows no disrespect for women and is not a bully. He has never lifted his hand to the girls at all and yet Katrina's description is all about violence and aggression. From my experience of child abuse, Dad does not fit the profile of an abuser."

Yellowlees countered by saying that Katrina's perception of me was entirely different from Sharon's. He went on,

"When I met your parents, I have to say I found him to be intimidating and imposing. He was also very unhappy about disclosure work being done with Katrina and did not want to have you involved at all. Personally, I find that very suspicious."

"My parents were concerned about my health because of the nature of my work, which has its own pressures, and because of the time I spent running after Katrina, which was obviously putting pressure on me," Sharon said.

"I have only good experiences of Dad and I was the only girl in the house for eight years before Katrina was born. I know I was not abused, so how do you explain that?" she asked.

Yellowlees looked directly at Sharon and said, "Perhaps you were abused and blocked it out, like Katrina did."

When Sharon shook her head and started to say something else, he quickly interrupted her,

"Perhaps he sought out only certain members of the family or maybe he just didn't fancy you. I am very concerned about the younger members of the family, the grandchildren, particularly as your father abused Katrina here in the hospital grounds. I feel strongly the rest of the family should be told but Katrina is not yet ready for that but Jenny Hogg will be working with her, to try to persuade her to tell your brothers as soon as possible. There is other evidence that I can't tell you about because of patient confidentiality and if you could only see her flashbacks, you would have no doubt it is true."

"What am I supposed to do until then?" Sharon asked.

"It is vital you do not tell your brothers until Katrina is ready but it is equally important for her mental state that you give her as much support as you can." Yellowlees answered. "I also think you should speak to the hospital social worker, with regard to the protection of the grandchildren and I will make an appointment for you to see her as soon as possible."

A few days later, Sharon received a telephone call from the Social Worker, Emily Powrie, asking to set up a meeting as soon as possible. The meeting was arranged to be held in the hospital a couple of days later. After introducing herself to Sharon, as the ward Social Worker who had sat in on several of the ward meetings where Katrina's situation was discussed at length, Powrie said,

"Katrina is very frightened because of the men involved and for her protection, I think the next stage should involve the police. There is obviously a very skilful paedophile ring involved. Katrina has no intention of making a police statement but you should make one."

The way in which this was said made Sharon think Powrie was implying I had also abused her.

"I was not abused by my father, what would I make a statement about?" asked Sharon.

Powrie seemed to accept this and went on to talk about the safety of the grandchildren.

"Now that you know about your father, you have a duty, the same as I do, to make sure the grandchildren are kept safe," she said

"I will have to wait until my brothers can be told but if any of the family need a babysitter, I will do it so that my parents are not asked."

Suddenly, Powrie turned to Sharon and asked her,

"Do you think your father would ask Katrina to kill herself?"

"Is that what has happened?" Sharon asked, once again so shocked she could barely get the words out.

"I have had a lot of experience of dealing with damaged girls and abusers can be very devious and threatening. It would not be unusual for abusers to do that," Powrie said, not really answering the question but giving the impression that that was exactly what had happened.

She then went on to tell Sharon she, Powrie, had to satisfy herself that the measures Sharon had suggested to protect the grandchildren would be sufficient and to do this, she would have to involve the Child Care Manager, Rhod Napier.

The meeting with Powrie had intimidated Sharon to such an extent she took her husband Neil with her, when she was asked to meet both Powrie and the Child Care Manager, Rhod Napier, the following week. Napier made it clear he was not prepared to accept any half measures when it came to protecting the children. He insisted that I was to have no unsupervised access to the children, therefore there was to be no babysitting, no visits that were not under the strict control of the parents.. As the boys had not yet been told about the abuse, Sharon asked how she was going to be able to fulfill that commitment. Napier told her that was for her to work out but if he became aware of anything which might cause him concern, he would have no hesitation in taking further measures.

He then dropped the real bombshell of that particular meeting. He told Sharon and Neil he saw his main role as that of Sharon's adviser in how to keep the children safe. He did not want to meet the boys, nor to have anything to do with them as, having been brought up in a "culture of abuse" they could very likely be abusers themselves. Sharon and Neil were left stunned because the contradictions were so obvious. If the Social Work Department thought the boys "could likely be abusers" having been brought up "in a culture of abuse" how on earth could Sharon be responsible for the safety of the children? That question was never answered and until that point, had obviously not even been addressed. The Social Work Department had just increased the pressure on Sharon and Neil tenfold.

Sharon had spent hours thinking about the allegations made about me. Unable to take the whole responsibility by herself, she had told Philip about the allegations and she and him had discussed all the possibilities but neither could come up with any explanation. Philip was sworn to secrecy but he found the pressure difficult to take, although he kept his promise to say nothing to either Andrew or Jim. Now, Sharon had just been told that Philip could also be an abuser. Another factor had come to mind when she thought back to their childhood and the allegation I had been abusing Katrina while they were all still children and living in the family home. Try as she might, she had no memories of anything which would have given a clue, even in hindsight, that Katrina was being brutally abused on a regular basis.

But Sharon, along with the rest of the family, knew I had spoken to the Social Work Department shortly after finding out about my father's abuse. After confronting my father I never spoke to him again but concern for my mother made it impossible to tell the rest of my family why. My mother was a woman I had never in my life ever heard swear. She did not push her religious views down anyone else's throat but she did practise it herself and was a staunch Catholic, who attended to the duties of her church. It was inconceivable to me that she would have had any idea of what had gone on, although Katrina had claimed she was abused in my parents' home from time to time. She had also been abused right under our noses in our own home and neither Kay nor I had suspected anything, therefore as far as I was concerned, it was perfectly possible for it to have happened without my mother's knowledge.

My visits to my parents' home became less and less frequent until they had all but stopped altogether. About nine months after I found out about my father, I received a call from a Social Worker who asked to come and speak to me at my office, without saying what it was about. I agreed and about half an hour later, two Social Workers turned up, a male and a female. After introducing themselves, the female by way of telling me why they were there, said, "Why have you not visited your mother in hospital?"

As it happened, I had no idea my mother was in hospital but her tone and the abruptness of the question immediately annoyed me.

"It has got bugger all to do with you," I said.

She was about to say something else and I was about to tell them to take a hike, when the man quickly put a restraining hand on her arm.

"We have just come from the hospital and the doctor is worried about your mother," he said. As I sat and just looked at him without making any attempt to answer, he continued,

"She took a heart attack about twelve days ago and although she has got over the attack, her mood has been very low, as a consequence of which we were called in. The doctor was able to get her to talk a little and she has told him that she had not had a visit from you, nor had she heard from you in some time. We were asked to contact you, which is why we are here."

After some hesitation, I explained about finding out about my father, about my confronting him and about how I had wanted to protect my mother by keeping it from her, at the expense of cutting myself off from them completely. It was not the best solution and I had paid a heavy price for taking it because I had been cut off from the rest of my family. The consequence of that was that no one had told me my mother was ill. I explained when I confronted my father, he had denied it but I had been given enough information to trip him up and there was no doubt in my mind he had done it.

"In any case," I said, "I believed my daughter."

Throughout the meeting, after my first reaction to her question, the female had sat with a face like thunder but at that last statement, she almost smiled and mouthed a single word, "Yes."

We briefly discussed what might happen to my father but they were of the opinion that his age would preclude any action being taken, particularly since he was not in any contact with any young children. I visited the hospital the next day, to be told my mother had been sent home that morning. About six months later, I was climbing the stairs to the upper floor in my office building when I bumped into my secretary, just as she was in the process of saying to the senior partner in the firm,

"Jim will probably not be in this morning."

As she suddenly saw me, she caught her breath and after a pause said,

"I'm very sorry to hear about your mother Jim."

"Why, what about my mother?" I asked.

She looked as if she was going to faint and I quickly said to her, "What has happened, what's wrong?"

Biting back the tears she said, "She died at four o'clock yesterday afternoon."

No one had told me.

Sharon knew all of this and told Napier about it.

"If Dad had been involved in the abuse of Katrina, he would hardly have admitted it was going on, to two Social Workers, who had not known anything about it. Nor would he have said he believed Katrina when she told him about my grandfather."

Napier made no comment about whether this made the abuse by me, more or less likely but he did promise to check the departmental files to see if there was any record of the meeting. The next week he contacted Sharon to confirm that the meeting had in fact taken place and, that I had said I believed Katrina. At the same time he asked her to attend another meeting with Yellowlees and Katrina the following week.

Sharon hoped that the fact of the existence of the file about my previous meeting with the Social Work Department, would cause Napier to have second thoughts but she was to be disappointed. It very quickly became obvious that as far as Napier was concerned, nothing had changed. Katrina was still opposed to the boys being told, despite Yellowlees arguing strongly for them to be brought into the arrangements for protecting the grandchildren. Napier agreed with Katrina, holding to his view they might have been brought up in a culture of abuse, in which case, the rest of the paedophile ring might find out and Katrina's life would be put in danger.

No one was now expressing any doubt about the existence of this paedophile ring. Napier's whole approach was predicated on its existence and the need to keep Katrina safe, all of which made her more afraid and uncertain she could be kept safe, particularly if the boys were told. Napier suggested that an "unofficial" approach could be made to the police to look at providing protection for Katrina and also to find out if there was any evidence against some of the names Katrina had provided. At this time Sharon had been given no names of any of the abusers outside of the family.

Sharon and Neil were now left under enormous pressure; not allowed to tell her brothers about the allegations and yet, given the responsibility to make sure the grandchildren were kept safe, from me and, from brothers who "could likely be abusers". There was no logic to the position being adopted by the Social Work Department. On top of that, Sharon continued to have meetings with Yellowlees because Katrina was still having flashbacks in which I figured. During one of those meetings Sharon had questioned Yellowlees about the alleged rapes in Katrina's flat, where I was supposed to have raped her at lunchtimes, frequently beating her at the same time.

When Sharon questioned Yellowlees how this could be possible that Katrina could stand being beaten and raped, yet be able to go to her work and have no memory of any of it. Yellowlees explained this away by claiming that Katrina would simply "dissociate" meaning, she would "close off her mind to what was happening and be in another place."

Sharon continued to protest that I was not the violent type and said,

"I just cannot imagine my father doing this kind of thing, it is so foreign to his nature."

Yellowlees's response was,

"Perhaps he dissociated too." In any case he saw no reason to doubt Katrina's flashbacks and continued to say she displayed all the signs of someone who had suffered years of severe physical and sexual abuse.

Stripped down to its essentials, Yellowlees was arguing that during these sessions when I was beating and raping Katrina, neither she nor I was fully aware of what was going on. The argument becomes even more ludicrous if it is properly examined. Some lunchtime, any lunchtime, every lunchtime, we are not certain; I would walk along to Katrina's flat, knock on the door and be allowed in. I would then beat and rape Katrina, during which time we were both "dissociated" so that we were totally unaware of what was happening. After the rape, I would go back to work as would Katrina and neither of us would have a clue it had happened. In the language of psychiatry, or at least of those who subscribe to this kind of theory, it is called "robust repression".

What is uncertain, is when exactly do I "dissociate"? Is it when I leave the office, knock on Katrina's door, after I enter the flat or when the rape begins? By the same token, when does Katrina dissociate? Is it before the rape, during the rape or when she hears the knock on the door? Needless to say, none of those perfectly logical questions were ever answered, beyond stating, "there can be an element of confusion in the claims being made," BUT "I have no doubt that the abuse took place" OR "In my professional opinion, I have no reason to doubt Katrina". The presence of other men during these lunchtime sessions was never explained.

It would be much later before Sharon had the time to really think about what she had been told. The pressure that had been put on her forced her to concentrate on the immediate situation and on persuading Katrina to speak to the boys. This was finally agreed and Sharon took Andrew and Jim to speak to Katrina, to hear from her, what had happened. Once the boys became involved, there were more questions asked and they expressed more scepticism about the validity of the claims. While Jim took Katrina back to the ward, on the day he and Andrew had been told, Andrew spoke at some length with Jenny Hogg.

He asked her how long the hospital had known, to which she had answered for some months.

"Is that why my parents have not been allowed to see Katrina?" he asked.

"Yes. I am so sorry this has happened, I realise it must come as a tremendous shock to you all."

"Do you think there could be any confusion, that Katrina has mistaken my Dad for someone else?" Andrew said.

"There is no confusion." Hogg was quite emphatic. "If you could witness her flashbacks you would have no doubt." she finished.

"What are Katrina's chances of recovery?" Andrew finally asked.

"Katrina will probably never fully recover as she is so badly damaged. What the hospital is trying to do is get her to put her experiences into little boxes and place them at the back of her mind. At the same time we want to teach her to cope with her flashbacks."

This is an assessment of Katrina that was to be repeated several times by others associated with her care. It was a mindset which Kay and I found quite disturbing and frightening.

Now that all the boys knew about the abuse, there were a number of decisions taken to try to get to the bottom of what had happened and more importantly, to help Katrina. The first thing that had to be done was to speak to Katrina, when they were all together and to question her more closely about the flashbacks and what they meant. A meeting was arranged at Sharon's house, which was to last for two hours and during which they all learned something new about the extent of the abuse that had been alleged.

Rather than make things clearer in their minds however, it left more questions than ever unanswered. The boys questioned Katrina about all aspects of her allegations and had it confirmed again, that she had no memories about my abuse, that everything she could tell them came from flashbacks.

To learn they had appeared as abusers, participating in turn when I was present, shocked and sickened them. Katrina had always been protected by her brothers who had spoiled her as a child and would not have let the wind blow on her if they could have stopped it. To be told now that they had helped to violate her was absolutely devastating. Sharon was also to learn for the first time that in one flashback, she had appeared being anally abused by me. The accounts of sodomy, and sexual abuse were gut wrenching to the point that Jim had to leave the room because he felt physically sick. As the names began to come out, one after the other, names of people known to all of them, they all began to feel there must be some other explanation, particularly when Jim Sillars was named as one of the abusers.

Andrew immediately picked Katrina up when she mentioned Jim. He had been the MP for Glasgow Govan and we both had been office bearers in the SNP for some years, sitting together on the National Executive of the party. Andrew knew that Jim and I were often on different sides of the debate, on some of the major policy issues in the party at that time, therefore he knew we were not that close personally, although we were on good enough terms. Of all the names that were mentioned, Jim was the only one Andrew knew for certain he had never met. A quick discussion established that none of them had met Jim and when this was pointed out to Katrina and she was pushed to say where the abuse involving Jim had taken place, she withdrew his name. She was absolutely adamant however that all the other names were genuine and they had all been involved. The other MP was well known to all of them and all of them had met him, more than once. Still, if one mistake could be made, there could very well be others. It was a start.

By the end of the meeting Katrina was exhausted and very upset. She was convinced the boys did not believe her and Sharon went to some length to impress on them that they had to support her. She took Katrina back to the hospital while the boys continued to debate what the next steps should be. For a start, they had been told by the Social Work Department, that the grandchildren would have to be questioned and, after objections were raised by the family, it was agreed they would conduct the questioning themselves, under the guidance of Social Work Department staff, who provided them with work books and a series of questions that were standard and used in all similar situations.

They also now knew that their cousin Susan, was supposed to have witnessed some of the abuse, as well as Katrina's ex-boyfriend, Steven. Andrew, Philip, Sharon and Jim were now in a position where they were being pushed by the Social Work Department to keep their children safe, there was pressure coming from Katrina to support her, backed by the psychiatric staff and finally, there was the possibility of police involvement before much more time had elapsed. They therefore decided they should divide the tasks, with Sharon having the sole responsibility of keeping contact with Katrina and making sure she was assured of all of their support. Jim was in a terrible state and was so distraught, they all felt he should be allowed to divorce himself from any involvement whatsoever. For him to start probing it was felt, could very well damage him and he and Anne were just married, and had two very young children, Susan being only four months old. Jim had more than enough on his plate.

That left Andrew and Philip to try to get as much information as possible from those they could approach. Susan was contacted and told what had been said by Katrina, who she knew was in hospital but had no idea of the seriousness of her illness. She said she had no idea what Katrina was talking about, there had been no abuse by me that she had ever witnessed, nor could she believe that I was an abuser. I had seen quite a bit of Susan when she was a youngster and she and Katrina had been friendly enough to keep in reasonably frequent contact, therefore she was someone who knew something about our family dynamics. Nevertheless she was questioned quite closely by Andrew until he was satisfied she knew exactly the position they were all in, particularly Katrina. Susan immediately volunteered to call the police in Perth and make a statement, which she did the next day.

Philip contacted Steven, Katrina's ex-boyfriend, who was now married. Steven knew the family because when he and Katrina had been going out together, he came to the house on occasion and was still on friendly terms with the boys, as well as with Katrina. Both he and his wife knew Katrina and when he was told what had happened and how ill she was, he was quite upset. He was even more upset when Philip told him why he was there. Steven had known about my father's abuse of Katrina but he was quite incredulous when he was told he was supposed to have witnessed my abusing her. He said to Philip that Katrina must be very ill if she was making this kind of accusation and both he and his wife, expressed their willingness to do anything they could if it could help. He was prepared to go to the police or to the hospital and make a statement to the effect that he had witnessed nothing and was not aware of any abuse by me at any time.

Each of the grandchildren was screened and questioned, with the older ones being asked about their feelings about me, without being asked directly. For example they were asked who they would like to take on holiday with them, or where they would like to go to stay. The family were given instructions about how to watch me with the children and which "signs" would be indicators of my "grooming" them. This caused a degree of conflict between the family members and they all found the exercise distasteful but they had been left in no doubt that if they did not question the children, the Social Work Department would do it and if I was not watched at all times, and reports presented, the children would be taken into care. Philip's wife Alison, who was training to be a social worker in the same department that was conducting the enquiry, found this to be particularly distasteful. After one session with her girls, which involved telling them about "good touching" and "bad touching", she turned on Philip and shouted, "All I ever see in your Dad's face is pure love".

Kay's and my regular visits every weekend, when we paid a short visit to each of the family's houses, caused real problems because the more that was revealed about the abuse, the greater the pressure coming from the psychiatrist to call in the police and the greater the pressure from the Social Work Department, the more difficult it was for them to pretend that everything was normal. To make things easier for themselves, they began to telephone each other to warn each of them we were on our way. As soon as we had left one house, to pop in to see another member of the family, they would receive a call so that, if it was possible, they could leave before we arrived. Anne began to leave the house just after five o'clock every night, so that she could avoid my frequent, if irregular short visits on my way home. Throughout August and September, Kay and I wondered often, without ever coming up with the real answer, why we met so many closed doors and empty houses.

The incident that was to be the final catalyst in forcing the confrontation involved Alison and the Social Work Department. As part of her training, Alison had to accompany a psychiatric social worker for a week in Murray Royal and Gilgal. By pure coincidence, she and her supervisor, visited the ward in which Katrina was housed, where a ward meeting was being held. Katrina's case was being discussed and Alison overheard some of the report, when it was said that a police investigation was being conducted on Katrina's abuse and that a Mr Fairlie – no first name given – was being investigated. The family had obviously known statements had been made to the police, but they had been given no information about an investigation, or who was being investigated, although that would have been fairly obvious. Nevertheless, things seemed to be happening that the family knew nothing about and when Alison told Philip and they all discussed the latest news, it was decided to telephone the police.

When Katrina made her statement to the police, Sharon had been persuaded to make a short statement in order to encourage Katrina, therefore she knew the woman police constable who had taken the statements. She called her the same evening and was surprised at the response. The police woman said,

"You are the second person who has called about this today."

"Why, who else called?" asked Sharon.

"I had Rhod Napier, from the Child Protection, on the telephone earlier today asking how far the investigation had gone," she replied.

Sharon reported this to the boys and it was decided to call Napier to find out what was going on. She had had more contact with Napier than any of the boys, who, after all, were under suspicion themselves as possible abusers, therefore she called him and was told that he had been acting under instructions from his boss, the Director of Social Work, Betty Bridgeford. She, Bridgeford, told him she had been approached by an SNP local councillor, to find out about the investigation. Napier's next statement almost floored Sharon. He said,

"Your father is obviously using his SNP contacts to find out how much the police know about the paedophile ring."

When Sharon put down the telephone she was visibly upset and when she told the boys what had been said, they felt quite stricken. The implications of Napier's statement were enormous. Throughout all the discussions that had taken place, no hard evidence had been provided by the psychiatrists, the Social Work Department or anyone else, that I had actually committed any of the abuse of which I was accused. Katrina herself, had no real memories, she had flashbacks and nightmares and the psychiatrist was basing his conclusions on the interpretation of what amounted to no more than dreams. But this was different. Some of the names Katrina had given were members of the SNP and now an SNP councillor was making enquiries on my behalf.

Andrew decided to telephone Napier the next day and when he did so, he was amazed at the reaction of Napier. He was furious that

Sharon had told the family because he had spoken to first of all the police, then Sharon, in confidence.

"I don't think I should be speaking to you at all." he said.

"That is not my concern," said Andrew, "but we have been told a SNP councillor is asking questions on behalf of my father and we want to know who the councillor is. Do you know his name?"

"Yes, I know who he is but I can't tell you that." said Napier.

"You must realise the position this puts us in," said Andrew, "How did the councillor find out about the investigation? You told Sharon my father must be using his contacts in the SNP to find out what is going on but how can you know that? That is why we want his name so that we can question him ourselves."

"That is the reason I can't give you his name. This investigation is being conducted with as little information as possible being passed on because of the people involved and the possible consequences. The only people in this department who know about it are the people who have been involved but suddenly Sharon is told by the police that they have been approached by a councillor and now you know. The whole investigation is being compromised and the more people who know, the greater the chance your father will find out and the more exposed Katrina will be. We are very concerned for her safety."

"But where did the councillor get the information?" persisted Andrew.

"There is only one place he could have got it," said Napier, "that is why I am convinced your father is using his contacts in the SNP to find out what is going on."

Andrew then asked if he should speak to Betty Brideford, the Director of Social Work and Napier's boss.

"That would not be a good idea for the reasons I have given you," said Napier, "the best thing you can do is to leave it to the police to get on with the investigation and to leave it to me to keep in touch with them."

The conversation with Napier left Andrew deeply unhappy and when he reported it to the rest of the family, they felt they had nowhere else to turn for explanations.

This changed everything. The need to confront me was now paramount but Andrew and Philip first of all wanted to speak to Yellowlees to ask him again about the nature of Katrina's flashbacks. Sharon called Yellowlees but he was not available and she could only leave a message for him to return the call as a matter of urgency. He called back within the hour but said he could not meet the family until the following week, which was not acceptable to any of them. When he was told of the unfolding situation he reiterated all he had said before about Katrina's flashbacks. They were genuine, he had no reason to doubt them, Katrina displayed all the symptoms of someone who had been severely physically and sexually abused over a very long time etc. After that telephone conversation there was no more the family could do. The decision to confront me was made for them.

CHAPTER TEN

October 17th 1995

As soon as I opened my eyes, I was wide awake. A quick look at my watch showed I had slept solidly for at least six hours and it was now 7 am. As the memories came flooding back, of the confrontation with the family the day before, the realisation of what was in front of me hit me hard. There was a knot in my stomach so tight, I could hardly breathe. I could not remember falling asleep and obviously had not moved a muscle all night because I was lying flat out in the self same position I could last remember. As I swung my legs over the side of the bed, my feet kicked something which slowly rolled into view. The empty Grouse bottle lay as silent testimony of how I had spent the evening and why I had no memory of falling asleep. Despite having consumed the entire bottle, my head was clear enough to be instantly aware of not only my surroundings and how I got there, but also of what I had to do first thing.

The brutality of the confrontation with the family had left me feeling raw and the wall of silence that confronted me when I tried to get information from the police and the hospital confused and irritated me yesterday, when I first encountered it. Now, that wall of silence was going to make it impossible to provide an explanation to my employers and the editor of the local paper. A quick shower freshened me up to an extent but putting on the same clothes I had had on all day yesterday, made me feel grubby and tainted, which somehow fitted my perception of how a pervert should feel. All that was missing was the shabby raincoat. That may sound melodramatic but dirty and unclean is exactly how I felt. Breakfast was out of the question but the tea making facilities in the room allowed me to have a cup of tea and therefore avoid meeting anybody else before I left.

My mind was still in turmoil, turning over the events of the previous day, when I arrived at my office and had the foolish notion that Alice, the receptionist, somehow knew what had happened. She didn't obviously, but I could not be my usual cheerful self when I spoke to her and therefore could not help wondering if she would notice something. I couldn't help thinking it might not be too long before everyone would know, if the police arrived to arrest me. As luck would have it, the partner I needed to speak to was engaged for the first half hour but when I finally made it into his office, he told me I could have no more than five minutes.

"I am afraid, it might take more than that," I said.

"Well excuse me while I sort out these papers but go ahead, I'm listening"

"Katrina has accused me of sexually abusing her." It was as well to be as direct as possible and it certainly caught his attention.

"What? Is this some kind of joke?" he asked.

"I wish it was," I replied, "The family, including Kay, confronted me yesterday."

I then went on to give him as much information as I had, including my attempts to speak to the police and the hospital. At a complete loss to give him any kind of explanation that made any sense, the whole sorry tale just sounded lame. The firm knew Katrina was in Gilgal and therefore they knew she had some kind of psychological problems, but this…

"What are you going to do?" he asked.

"I have to speak to the editor of the Perthshire Advertiser (PA) because I don't know if I am going to be arrested and if I am, it will hit the media pretty quickly. Then I have to go home and get some clothes and find some place to stay because I can't stay at home." I said.

"Surely Kay doesn't believe this, she must know there has to be some explanation," he replied.

"I have no bloody idea, but all she could say yesterday was "They say they have a lot of evidence." It looks as if she believes it all right," I said sharply. The thought of the way Kay had reacted had left a really bitter taste.

"I will tell the rest of the partners. You take whatever time you need but let us know what is happening, particularly if you get arrested," he smiled, but there was no humour in the looks we exchanged as I left his office.

As I passed Alice at the reception I stopped to tell her I was going along to the PA for a short time, that I would be leaving the office very soon after that and that I would not be in for the rest of the day. I also asked her to ask my secretary to come to my office as soon as I returned. There was going to be a great deal of juggling of appointments to be made and I had no idea how it was going to be done because I had no idea how long I would have before the police came to arrest me. How to explain my absence to Lara, my secretary, was going to cause problems of its own because normally she knew where to find me if I was out of the office for any length of time. There were also the telephone messages from the day before, that I had ignored.

I had been writing a social comment column for the PA for about eight years and a financial column for about five. The journalists were the usual mix in a local paper and Editorial was absolutely humming on the days just before going to press. My columns appeared on a Tuesday and a Friday, therefore I spent time in the office every week. The banter was infectious, sometimes cruel and always entertaining but it was the kind of place where you learned to retaliate first, if you wanted to hold your own. There was a mixture of political views represented and, given my long-established and high profile career with the SNP, I was a ready made target, whatever other excuses the staff could always find for a bit of mickey taking. That day was no different, but I managed to get to the editor's office without being sidetracked.

Robin Keay, the editor of the PA had become a friend in the years I had been writing for the paper, and was to prove to be someone I could talk to as my fight with the medical and legal establishment developed. He did not share my political views but gave me free reign when it came to the weekly column. Telling Robin was a great deal more comfortable than telling my employers, even although if I was arrested my position at the paper would be terminated with immediate effect. His immediate reaction was to get up and close the door, his face a complete mask and then to say,

"It is obviously not true but why did Katrina accuse you?"

"That is the problem Robin, I haven't a clue. I am not even sure what I am supposed to have done because no one will tell me anything. All I can tell you is that I have been accused of abusing Katrina. The family and Kay confronted me and told me I had been abusing Katrina for years, that a SNP councillor had been making enquiries on my behalf and that the police were involved and an investigation has been going on for some time, I don't know how long. Neither the hospital nor the police will speak to me but I have been told I'll be called in for questioning when they are ready."

Telling it like that simply underlined how little I did know. I did not even know how far the abuse had gone, what had happened to Katrina. After I finished, I just sat there and looked at him. He asked the same question as the partner had asked,

"Surely Kay doesn't believe it. What did she say when this was going on?"

"That's the problem, she said nothing other than", They say they have a lot of evidence," I replied with the same bitterness as before. "I didn't go home last night and I haven't spoken to her since but I am going home when I leave here, to get some things and I'll have a few things to say to her then."

We sat for a short time discussing the likely possibilities; Robin asking questions and getting the same answer to them all, "I don't know."

Suddenly he was all business,

"This is Tuesday and obviously there will be no column on Friday. I can say you are on holiday but we are going to have to work out what we are going to do for the next couple of weeks. It will be better if you have a break for the next two weeks and hopefully, something will be resolved by then. This is as far as this goes for now but you know what this place is like. If any of the staff pick up anything, I can field any questions for now but if it comes out we will have to cover it."

"I know the position this puts you in and I appreciate your giving me the benefit of the doubt but I honestly haven't a clue where the accusations have come from."

"I have absolutely no doubt you know nothing about it and I am sure, things will sort themselves out," he said, coming round his desk and shaking me warmly by the hand. It was only then I realised how much I needed to hear that.

When I walked in the door of my office a few minutes after leaving the PA, my secretary was in the reception and said,

"At last, you have at least half a dozen urgent calls you have to make. Where have you been?"

"I doesn't matter," I said, walking past her, heading for my office leaving her trailing behind. Once inside my own office with the door shut, I asked Lara to attend to all the outstanding calls, asked her to tell anyone else who was looking for me I wouldn't be in until the next day and then, without further explanation, told her I needed to make a private call and that I would see her the following day. It was right out of character for me to treat her in such an off-handed manner but it was obvious I was in no mood to discuss anything. I had started to ring home before the door to my office was properly closed.

Kay answered on the second ring, which meant she had the telephone beside her.

"Hello," she said, her voice little more than a whisper.

"I am leaving the office now..." I got no further before I was interrupted by Kay, whose voice had risen in volume as well as pitch.

"Jim, we have to talk. Are you alright?"

"I'm leaving the office now and will be home in about half an hour."

Whatever else Kay had intended to say or wanted to say, she was given no chance because I had hung up.

On the drive home to Crieff, about seventeen miles from my office in Perth, I was on auto-pilot, with little or no awareness of anything that might have happened or that I saw. I always took the back road, which was a good deal quieter than the main road, but which required more care because it was a bit narrower with some quite nasty bends. For the thirty minutes it took, my mind raced over the events of the previous day and the confrontation with the family. By the time I walked in the front door, the anger in me was just ready to explode. When I walked into the sitting room, Kay was standing obviously waiting for me. Her hands were clasped in front of her chest as she blurted out, her voice cracking with the effort,

"Jim, we have to talk."

"You had your chance yesterday and sat there and said nothing. No, you told me, they say they have a lot of evidence. What evidence? Evidence of what?" I said angrily.

"I know, I'm sorry. I wanted to come with you but I couldn't," she said, obviously finding it difficult to speak at all.

I was in no mood to listen to that kind of excuse,

"What do you mean you couldn't? What was to stop you? Why did you say nothing, not a thing? Do you believe any of that crap?"

"No, I don't believe any of it and I've told the family as well as Katrina I don't believe it. It didn't happen," Kay said, now desperate to get me to calm down.

I stood looking at her, trying hard to control the anger I felt.

"When did you tell them?"

"I called all of them this morning," Kay said.

"Why didn't you tell them yesterday? Why did you let me walk out of that house believing you all thought I had abused Katrina?" I shouted.

"I know, I'm sorry, I can't tell you how sorry I am but I don't know why I couldn't tell them yesterday. I don't know why I couldn't get up but I just couldn't." Kay was pleading now, upset at the way the conversation was heading and the anger in me.

"I found out just before you came to the house. I didn't have time to think about things, everything happened so fast and you left so quickly,"

The knot in my stomach was getting so tight I was having to force myself to take deeper breaths. It stopped my anger becoming uncontrollable and gave Kay a chance to speak.

"They didn't tell me much more than they told you yesterday. They just said they had a lot of evidence but even after you left, they told me very little else. They said the police are involved but they said patient confidentiality had stopped the police and the hospital telling them too much," she said.

"What did they tell you? What am I supposed to have done? I asked.

"They said you raped Katrina and beat her up." she said, watching my face, waiting for the reaction.

"For Christ's sake, I did what? And they believed it? How the hell could they believe that?" I shouted, absolutely furious.

"When is this supposed to have happened?" I shouted again.

"It has been happening since Katrina was just a wee girl and there are others involved." Kay then gave me some of the names of the other men that were supposed to be in a paedophile ring I controlled.

For the next ten minutes or so I fired questions at Kay, to most of which she did not know the answer but the picture she painted of me was so far removed from the truth I could not believe our own kids actually thought me capable of any of it. I was supposed to be violent, beating Katrina regularly and forcing her to have sex not just with me but with a list of other men who had given me drink and cigarettes. By this time I was quite visibly upset and when Kay finally said,

"They want nothing more to do with you."

I looked at her and suddenly the tears were running down my face. The more I tried to control them, the more distraught I became. As Kay reached out to put her arms around me I pushed her away; I could not bear to have her touch me for the first time since we were seventeen years of age.

For the next hour or so I was inconsolable. I walked back and forward from the sitting room to the kitchen, to the dining room and back again, sobbing and asking the same question over and over,

"How could they believe it? How could they?"

Finally, I had cried myself out but the tension in my body had me almost paralysed. The knot in my stomach was sore to the touch, so great was the tension and eventually Kay said she was going to call David Mitchell, our GP. She told me he had been in to see her the night before and had offered a part explanation for the accusations being made. He had suggested that Katrina had perhaps transferred the original abuse she had suffered at the hands of my father, to me. Kay said he had also wanted to know when I came home

When David Mitchell came in he said he was relieved to see me home and how horrified he had been to hear of the allegations. He could not expand on what he had said to Kay about how the allegations might have come about but he assured us there must be some explanation because he did not think for a minute it was true. He had given us a great deal of support throughout the time he had to deal with Katrina's illness and was to provide the same kind of support throughout the following years as both Kay and I suffered the consequences of the stress of fighting the medical and government establishments.

When he saw how tense I was he suggested he give me something to make me relax and perhaps help me to sleep. He got no objections to that and within a short time of having been given the injection, I had fallen sound asleep. While I was asleep both Philip and Andrew telephoned Kay to ask how she was and to find out if she had heard from me. Neither told the other they had been in touch with their mother because neither knew how the other would react. However, both had taken the opportunity to tell Kay a bit more of what had happened and how they had been affected.

It transpired they had been drip fed information by Yellowlees, usually via Sharon because of her constant contact with Katrina, and by the Social Work Department via Rhod Napier. The evidence they assured Kay was present, when they had confronted her the previous day, somehow now seemed to be unavailable. What the conversations divulged was just how little actual evidence they had. The had had assurances from Yellowlees and Napier the evidence was there but because of patient confidentiality, they had no real idea what it was. There were a number of instances that they had been told about that Kay was able to put into perspective and to show how they could not possibly be true, particularly in terms of timescale.

When Andrew had been told by Katrina about the drink and cigarettes being given to me by members of the paedophile ring, he remembered when he was young, an occasion when I came home from university in Dundee with a large number of cigarettes in my briefcase. At the time, listening to Katrina's account, that small incident which he had long forgotten about, suddenly became highly significant. The reality was a great deal simpler and much less sinister. A female student with whom I was friendly, did promotion work to earn extra cash to supplement her grant. On one occasion she had worked for a cigarette company and part of the perk was several hundred cigarettes which she sold to another student and me for a cut price.

At the time this took place, Katrina was not even born and as Andrew is only seven years older than her, he must have been very young at the time but his state of mind at the time of being told of my alleged abuse, had utterly confused him. They had also had the experience of being told by Yellowlees and others in the psychiatric team, mainly Jenny Hogg, that their own memories of events that conflicted with Katrina's, were childhood memories and simply dismissed. To the psychiatric team and the Social Work Department, the only member of the family whose memories were deemed to be valid, was Katrina.

Those first conversations with Kay, and others which she was to have over the next two or three weeks, highlighted to Andrew and Philip, how much fear had played a part in the way they were misled by both Yellowlees and the Social Work Department. After they were first told about the abuse, it was stressed very carefully to them how much Katrina's life was in danger, either from my hand or her own. She had made several suicide attempts and was terrified the paedophile ring I controlled would "get her" if they found out she had told anyone else. It was also impressed on them that their support was of vital importance to Katrina's health.

Their other fear of course, was for their own children. It had been made clear to Sharon first of all by Powrie, and then to Sharon and Neil by Napier, that the Social Work Department would have to be satisfied the grandchildren would be safe in the care of their parents, otherwise, "other steps might have to be taken". Sharon's experience of working in behavioural support, left her in no doubt what those "other steps" would be. Both the psychiatric team and the Social Work Department were so convinced I was not only an abuser, but that I controlled a ring of powerful people who were also abusers, that there was no room for argument or alternative views. That is, until the confrontation and the need to justify their behaviour to the person they had accused. Suddenly they couldn't wait to deny they had ever believed it, while at the same time, their every action said the exact opposite. But that would come much later.

After the conversations with Kay, Andrew called Philip and suggested they meet that day to discuss what to do next. Neither felt it was necessary to speak to either Jim or Sharon at that stage, knowing Sharon would have gone to the hospital to see Katrina and that Jim was in such a state that he was better left alone for the time being. Andrew and his wife Ashley drove up from Glasgow where they lived, to Philip and Alison's house in Perth. I had always felt very close to both Ashley and Alison and was very fond of both of them. Ashley's father had died only a short time before she and Andrew were married and in some respects I had become almost a surrogate father to her. Alison had come to the judo club, where I coached, as a youngster and had seemed to have been in and out of our house for years before she and Philip started going out together.

Neither Ashley nor Alison had wanted me to be confronted and had expressed doubts about the allegations from the outset. What had stopped their being more vocal was the feeling it was a family issue and that they were the in-laws, albeit, their children were the ones being screened and allegedly under threat from me. I had known both girls were fond of me and they were very shortly to prove it. As soon as Andrew and Ashley arrived and the discussion started, it was obvious to each of them they all shared the same view – they had made a monumental mistake. The problem now was how they were going to rectify it.

The girls had only the reports from Andrew and Philip of what had happened at the confrontation but on the basis of what they had been told, they both felt that Andrew and Philip had had all their preconceptions about the abuse, shattered. It was therefore a tremendous relief for them to have their own feelings about the allegations, confirmed. The abuse by me had never taken place. What had struck both Andrew and Philip at the confrontation was my reaction. Between first being told of the allegations and the confrontation the day before, the pressure on them had been so great they just wanted it ended.

Both were to explain to me later that they expected one of two things to happen. They had all had doubts from the outset, but little things like the cigarettes needed to be explained. The absolute certainty of the psychiatric team and the Social Workers, who had far more information than the family did, was difficult to counter. But the final straw, the one which had cut the feet from all of them, was the involvement of the SNP councillor, making enquiries on my behalf. For them, the confrontation would see me either admit it, in which case they would then have to deal with it, or, I would somehow explain what had happened. Either way, I was expected to make it go away and relieve them of the pressure.

Instead, they were faced with a man who obviously had no idea what was going on. Philip had been in the prison service for about five years and led one of the intervention teams which were called in to deal with prison riots. He had had his share of dealing with people who lied and cheated as a way of life and he felt confident he could tell whether or not someone was being genuine. They had all been told how I would likely react, that I would deny it at first but under pressure, would finally admit it. Instead, I had gone straight to the police. Now they were sick with guilt for what they had done but knew they could not leave it like this. They knew they had to do something to get to the bottom of what had really happened. They determined at that meeting they would now have to start pushing for answers and the place to get them was where it had all started – Gilgal and Yellowlees.

When I woke up in the early evening, whatever David Mitchell had given me had worn off and I felt more relaxed and refreshed. Kay and I were able to talk more calmly and she was able to give me more detail of what had happened. It was only then I was able to appreciate the pressure Kay had been under. At one point I stood and put my arms around her and asked,

"Are you sure you don't believe it? Are you absolutely certain?"

Kay looked me straight in the eyes and said,

"Yes, of course I'm certain it didn't happen. Do you honestly think I could live with a paedophile? Do you honestly believe I would expose the kids to that kind of abuse? I couldn't live with myself, never mind you."

We both cried for a short time but it was the last time Kay would ever see me shed a tear, although there were times I shed a few in private.

Kay made no mention of the telephone calls from Andrew and Philip. They had both asked that it should be left like that for a while until they could get some answers. The simple truth was they did not know how to face me, they were so eaten up with guilt and shame and they desperately wanted to put things right. We talked well into the night, going over and over the allegations, at least as far as we knew what they were. I decided to ask the firm for a couple of days off so that I could make a start to finding out what was happening.

I needed to speak to Yellowlees or someone at the hospital. I needed to speak to Napier or someone at the Social Work Department and I needed to speak to the police again. I had no desire to speak to the family, that would come later. Although I knew nothing about it at the time, the part played by Kay in keeping in touch with the boys, made the reconciliation with the family, that bit easier when it finally happened. In the event, it did not take too long before the barriers came down but the day after the confrontation, that was the furthest thing from my mind.

The one thing which did occur to both Kay and I, was that neither of us ever thought for one instant that Katrina was making the allegations out of some kind of malice. We had no idea why the allegations were made. I hadn't spoken to her but Kay had, and she was convinced Katrina believed absolutely that what she was saying was true. The fear and despair she was expressing was genuine, as her frequent attempts at suicide could confirm. Our concern for Katrina was as it had been from the outset, she was obviously desperately ill and there was no sign her condition was improving. It would be several years and several hospitals before we could even hope for improvement on that front.

CHAPTER ELEVEN

October 18th – November 5th

It was only the second day after the confrontation with the family and yet it seemed like a lifetime had passed. So much had happened, so many tears had been shed and so many hours had been spent talking and fretting over what had been said. Our lives had fallen apart and despite all of the talking and fretting, we still had no idea how it had happened. I had been accused of the most odious crime any father can be accused of and I had no idea how I could counter the allegations because I had no idea why they had been made. Kay and I spent the morning trying to make a list of priorities. Not knowing how long it may be before I was arrested, I was desperate to make some preparation but I had no idea what to prepare.

Eventually, we decided I would have to speak to the people most closely involved. I called the police and asked to speak to the WPC I had spoken to on the day of the confrontation. She gave me no further information and was not in the least helpful. I was told exactly the same as I had been told on the previous occasion viz. I would be brought in for questioning whenever they thought it appropriate but I would be given no further information until then. I still had no idea when or even if, I was going to be arrested.

The next call was to the hospital to speak to Yellowlees or, as on the previous occasion, Jenny Hogg. I now knew she had had a bit more to do with Katrina than I had first thought, therefore she might be able to tell be more. Despite being kept hanging on the line for several minutes, the message came back that neither Yellowlees nor Hogg was available to take calls but if I wanted to leave a message and a contact number, they would call me back. The number was left but no return call was made. Over the course of the rest of that day, I called another twice, only to be given the same answer each time, despite telling the receptionist I had already left a contact number but no return call had been made. I was assured the message would be passed on.

I had no better luck with the Social Work Department, when I called to speak to Rhod Napier. Never having met the man, I had no idea what to expect but on the basis of the little information I did have, I was not expecting any discussion to be pleasant. Kay and I had been told he was sure I was involved in Katrina's abuse, therefore he was unlikely to be sympathetic. It mattered little in the event because he was "not available", on any of the three attempts I made that day.

Over the next two days, until the weekend, I tried to speak to someone at the hospital and the Social Work Department at least three or four times each day, with the same response each time. It became very obvious no one was prepared to speak to me therefore I was going to have to try another tack. As the weekend arrived, I faced another problem to which I was definitely not looking forward. I was a member of the sports and leisure club at the Hydro Hotel, situated a matter of a few hundred yards from our house. It was where Kay and I had spent hours with the grandchildren at the swimming pool, the children's playground and the stables, where I rode every weekend and sometimes also through the week. The grandchildren were taken there regularly for pony rides.

I had been a regular at the stables for some years and was an experienced rider, so much so, that on occasion, I would help to ride out with guests at the hotel if the stables was particularly busy. I was on very friendly terms with not only the manageress and her staff, but with the other regular riders at the stables. The problem, as I saw it, was that I was the only man who attended the stables and who rode regularly. There were, on occasion, male guests who would ride out but I was the only male regular. The manageress had one or two young female apprentices with whom I was in regular contact but more importantly, there was a group of about a dozen young girls aged between twelve to sixteen years of age who helped out regularly at the stables in return for riding lessons.

I was popular at the stables with both the staff and the young girls who came because I was always willing to help with the heavy work and kept a watchful eye on them when we were riding out or jumping or doing cross country. There was also a group of regulars who were all experienced riders, who rode out every weekend on fast hacks across country. Every member of that group except me, was female. Kay was as well known as I was at the stable as we spent so much time there with the grandchildren, and both Sharon and Katrina had ridden out with me on occasion, therefore the family circumstances and dynamics were well known.

When I went to the stable on the Saturday morning and spoke to Liz Simpson, the manageress, her reaction was the same as that of Robin Keay the editor of the PA and David Mitchell, our GP. Liz was as horrified as they had been and knowing Katrina as she did, she could not believe she would willingly make such accusations out of malice. I had wanted to tell Liz because of the number of young women and girls with whom I came into regular contact at the stables and because I did not want to put her into a difficult situation if the whole sordid affair became known. She also had a responsibility for the welfare of the young girls who helped out, a responsibility she took very seriously. Liz set very high and exacting standards of behaviour at the yard and any girl who failed to observe them did not last long. For a start, she would not tolerate foul language and enforced that rule without favour, therefore to talk about the nature of the allegations was a great deal more embarrassing than it had been with Robin Keay.

It was Liz's decision not to tell the other women in the group until we knew how things would develop and assured me that she had absolutely no qualms about my continuing to go to the stable. She was quite prepared to take responsibility for any fall out, if and when the situation became known, but until then, she and I would be the only ones who knew. Liz's attitude and faith in me, touched me deeply and over the next couple of years, she would on occasion when I turned up for the regular weekend hack, tell me to just take my pick of the horses and go and come back when I was ready. She seemed to be able to tell when I just needed to be on my own and wanted to get as far away from people as I could get.

The four or five women who made up that regular group, I considered to be friends, therefore they were among the first group of people in whom I confided some weeks later and long before it became generally known. Each and every one of them was as appalled as Liz had been, which meant a great deal to me as I was still labelled a paedophile and rapist by the psychiatrist and the Social Work Department. I don't think that Liz and that group of women will ever fully appreciate how much their support did for Kay and I at that time and, as things developed later, the stable was to play an even greater part in my life.

Although no one would speak to me about the alleged assaults, both Andrew and Philip had better luck with Yellowlees who agreed to speak to both of them over the next few days. But first of all, there were a number of issues they wanted to speak to Kay about. There were dates that did not add up and try as they might, they could remember nothing from their own childhoods which gave any indication that any of the claims Katrina had made were true. The more they examined their own childhoods with Kay, the more they were all able to realise the claims could not possibly be true, either because of the timescale involved, such as the incident with the cigarettes, or because they were certain they had just never taken place.

When Andrew met Yellowlees, he went prepared to a far greater extent than he had been when he had last spoken to Jenny Hogg on the day Katrina had told him about my abuse.

First of all he told Yellowlees how surprised he had been by my reaction when confronted,

"My Dad's reaction when we confronted him, came as quite a shock. He was completely stunned and it was obvious he hadn't a clue what we were talking about." Andrew said. "The fact he then went straight to the police is hardly the action of someone who would be guilty of what we were accusing him of, is it? He asked.

"I don't think that is strange at all," said Yellowlees, "your father will want to get as much information as possible and the idea of him going to court is just nonsense. He will maybe take things as far as he dares, but he has too much to lose by pushing this himself."

Andrew persisted by pointing out that Katrina had withdrawn the allegations against Jim Sillars as soon as it had been pointed out to her that she had never met him, but Yellowlees countered by saying,"

"As Katrina's psychiatrist, I don't take everything she tells me at face value. For example when she told me about the abuse in the ward, I had it investigated and I am convinced it actually happened." He made no attempt to explain the allegations, later withdrawn, made against Jim Sillars.

Andrew continued to push him, "Why are you so certain the allegations are true when they came to light through flashbacks and nightmares?"

"Katrina is not mentally ill," said Yellowlees, "I have known examples of patients who have been mentally ill and who have made accusations which they later dropped, after they had received treatment but Katrina displays all the signs of someone who has been both physically and sexually abused. The consistency of her flashbacks and stories could not be acted out," said Yellowlees, repeating what had become the hospital's mantra for what was wrong with Katrina. What made him even more certain was his assessment that Katrina had improved greatly since she had started to disclose.

Andrew then told Yellowlees that despite examining his own childhood and, having no doubt about his grandfather's abuse of Katrina, he had been unable to see how I could possibly have been involved, to which Yellowlees replied,

"I can't say your father was the main abuser in Katrina's case because unfortunately there are no witnesses or evidence, but in my professional and clinical opinion, your father was involved in her abuse. I have interviewed Katrina and witnessed her flashbacks and as a result of them, I have no doubt your father was responsible for the damage done to Katrina's health. The damage which is so evident, is far beyond anything that would have been caused by the level of abuse carried out by your grandfather."

Andrew continued to press him and said that in order to believe I had been involved, he (Andrew) would have to remember something from his own childhood and asked about hypnotism. Yellowlees was very firm in advising him that that would not be a good idea. For a start, if things did go to court, whatever was divulged through hypnosis would not be acceptable. He also gave Andrew three possible reasons why he could remember nothing from his childhood that would incriminate me in Katrina's abuse.

The first was that Andrew was too young, that children remember very little under the age of four. The second was that the incidents were so traumatic that like Katrina, he had dissociated from the events and the safest way to bring back the memories would be to speak to a trained counsellor. Finally, the third reason for not remembering any incidents, was they did not happen. When Andrew told him he was supposed to be about nine to eleven years of age when he was supposed to be involved in the abuse of Katrina, Yellowlees told him it would be better if he did not remember and then went on to stress how important it was for the family to support Katrina.

Andrew said that that would happen in any case but as a parting shot asked Yellowlees his opinion of "guilt transference". When asked where he had heard the term, Andrew told him about David Michell's comments on hearing about the allegations, the day he had been called in to attend to me. Yellowlees then became very angry and said he found it unbelievable that any GP would pass comment on a case such as this without having access to the medical notes and, that GPs were not qualified to pass comment on cases of this nature. Yellowlees concluded the meeting by reminding Andrew how damaged Katrina was but that if the family continued to give her support, she would continue to make progress, as she had been doing. We were to learn later, through Sharon, that Yellowlees spoke to Katrina the following day, telling her of his conversation with Andrew and that Andrew did not believe the allegations.

Andrew then discussed the meeting with Philip and they both felt Yellowlees had told them no more than they already knew. They decided that Philip should try to speak to Yellowlees and put him under more pressure to explain not just the nature of flashbacks, but why Katrina's were considered so special. Yellowlees was not available until October 27th, which allowed Philip and Andrew to make more enquiries and further discuss things with Sharon, to whom they hadn't spoken for a couple of days. They were also keen to know how Katrina and Jim were coping. Sharon told them about Yellowlees's telling Katrina about the conversation he had had with Andrew which left her very distressed. They were all annoyed with Yellowlees because it made it difficult for them to discuss anything with him, if he intended to turn over the conversations to Katrina, while at the same time, impressing on the family how important it was to support Katrina.

Like Andrew, Philip was much better prepared now than he had been when the family felt forced to confront me. A number of things had been cleared up and they also had more information now, which he felt sure would make it more difficult for Yellowlees to simply brush his objections aside. Yellowlees had come to the meeting with what was obviously a prepared agenda and started out by beginning to explain the nature of flashbacks and memories and the difference between them. When he had finished his explanation and had gone as far as he obviously felt he needed to in order to justify the hospital's position, Philip said to him,

"We have two versions of how it came out, that my Dad was involved in Katrina's abuse. Were you aware that your staff had said to Katrina after she had come out of a flashback, "Are you aware your father was in that flashback?" That disturbed the family because to us, it looks as if Katrina is being guided to believe my Dad abused her?"

"You have to understand," said Yellowlees, "there are two different types of flashback. The first is when the patient is removed from what is happening and is "looking in" on events. They feel less traumatised and find it easier to relay what has happened to members of staff who are there to support and help them. The other type is when the person is reliving the event. This can be much more traumatic and more difficult to remember the details or the circumstances of what has happened. Katrina has often experienced the second type of flashback and staff would sometimes feel it was necessary to give her some information about what she had been experiencing in order to trigger her memory." Despite Philip's objections, Yellowlees saw nothing in that approach which might make it difficult for others to have faith in the validity of flashbacks of that type.

"There seems to be some confusion about this," said Yellowlees, "but I did not want to do disclosure work with Katrina when she first came into hospital, because I did not think she was emotionally strong enough to cope with it. But she insisted and disclosure work was started almost immediately."

"I also have to say," he continued, "that I have witnessed her flashbacks and one in particular, was so distressing that I asked Katrina to allow the staff to video her in a flashback but she refused. If you were to see those flashbacks, you would have no doubt about what happened to her."

He went on to repeat the same explanations to Philip, as he had given to Andrew and Sharon, about the symptoms of abuse displayed by Katrina, a factor which left him in no doubt about the nature and severity of the abuse. Philip therefore decided to try another approach.

"Have you noticed any similarity between Katrina's flashbacks and the experiences of two of the girls in the same ward, with whom Katrina has become very friendly?" Philip asked. "There is also her behaviour and the similarity between Katrina's behaviour and that of one of the other girls. Do you not feel there is a connection between the two, absconding from the ward and breaking up furniture and smashing windows?" Philip continued.

Yellowlees sighed and spoke to Philip as if he was speaking to someone who needed to have replies stated in words of one syllable,

"Katrina is a very badly damaged young girl and I have no doubt she is highly suggestible but that is merely consistent with the symptoms of someone who has been severely abused. I am aware of her behaviour and a member of staff has already commented on it, and its resemblance to the behaviour of another one of the girls. I am also aware she spends a great deal of time in the company of the other two girls and, if they are discussing their abuse, she may very well be affected by that."

"In that case," persisted Philip, "is it not possible she is suggestible enough to believe there are things that have happened to her, when in fact, they are the experiences of the other girls?"

Shaking his head, Yellowlees said,

"In certain circumstances, it might be possible but the fear and extreme concern displayed by Katrina at and around the time of your father's visits, suggests they are very real. She has also made remarkable improvement since he stopped visiting.

"I cannot say for certain what took place," he continued, "because I was not there, but given my experience of these cases and the consistency and detail of Katrina's recollections, I am of the opinion they are true and your father was her abuser."

He went further by telling Philip the incidents of abuse in the hospital were clear memories for Katrina, as was the incident that was witnessed by her boyfriend.

"I have asked Katrina to speak to that witness. If he could be persuaded to testify to the abuse, not only would we have proof that your father was an abuser but it will satisfy your doubts. This could be very important".

When Philip told him that he had already spoken to Katrina's boyfriend, who had denied witnessing any abuse but, because of his concern for Katrina's health, was willing to come to the hospital to speak to Yellowlees, the police or whoever, Yellowlees made no comment directly related to the witness. Instead, he launched into an explanation of confused memory and how incidents can become confused in the minds of patients, for different reasons. He then went on to explain, as he had done with Andrew, how he did not automatically believe everything Katrina told him and how he investigated her claims. When Philip pushed him to describe how he did this, his only example was to state that he would wait for a few days and then ask Katrina again, to relate what she had told him a few days before. He then added a slight qualification by saying he always allowed for "a degree of confusion".

By this time, Philip was beginning to feel that Yellowlees was shifting his position slightly, although there was no indication he was changing his opinions in any way whatsoever. He pushed Yellowlees further by saying,

"If Katrina believed her flashbacks and nightmares were true, even if they were not, would she not display those feelings of fear and apprehension in any case, would she not still feel afraid of my father and then lose that fear when he stopped visiting?"

"Yes, it is possible," said Yellowlees, "but I have known of cases when patients have made allegations and later retracted them after treatment because they suffered from a diagnosed mental illness. Katrina does not come into that category, she is suffering from Post Traumatic Stress Disorder (PTSD) and in those circumstances, the memories of patients will become clearer over time and less confused. The important point is that they remain relatively unchanged." Yellowlees went on to explain the nature and causes of PTSD and this was the first time the term had been used to describe Katrina's condition.

Philip continued to push and then told Yellowlees that their cousin Susan, had denied that she had ever witnessed any abuse by me or that any telephone conversation had taken place, when she and Katrina had discussed my abuse. Yellowlees again took the rather strange stance of saying he could not comment on whether or not the telephone conversation had taken place because he, "was not there". He then shook his head again and said,

"What a pity that those people who could corroborate Katrina's evidence are not willing to do so. Perhaps they have their own reasons for not coming forward."

"They are prepared to come forward," countered Philip, "Susan has already telephoned the police and Steven is willing to speak to you at any time. But they deny they ever witnessed any abuse, which is what Katrina is claiming."

Yellowlees then countered by saying that only time would tell and the family would have to make up its mind who it believed but then he gave an example of a family who had denied for ten years that abuse had taken place but eventually admitted it. In answer to Philip's scepticism about the alleged abuse in the hospital, he told him that there had been a case where a patient in the hospital, had been abused for over two years without the staff knowing anything about it.

"This went on right under our noses and we were totally unaware of it going on," said Yellowlees. Philip took these examples as an attempt by Yellowlees, to convince him that Katrina's claims were perfectly feasible. Yellowlees was to shift his stance on them quite considerably at a later meeting, which caused the family to doubt anything he told them and to seriously question his honesty.

Philip finally told him that what made it more difficult for the family to accept my guilt, was my reaction on being confronted and the fact I went to the police and told my employers the next day. Yellowlees dismissed all of that saying he could easily see my actions as those of a guilty man. According to him, I would go to the police to see what evidence they had against me and, it made sense to tell my employers because if the story came out, it would be in my interest to have told my side of the story first, to find out where my support, if any, lay. When he was again told I intended to take it to court and that the firm of solicitors for whom I worked, were to represent me, he actually laughed saying,

"If that is what I am up against, I have nothing to worry about. In any case, he can't sue me so who does that leave? Is he going to sue Katrina? As I told your brother, he will huff and puff for a while but he will soon drop it because he can't afford not to."

Yellowlees was to find he could not have been more wrong, or as ex-President Bush would have said, "He misunderestimated me" – and then some.

After the meeting Philip went to Sharon's house and told her that his meeting with Yellowlees had convinced him that things were not as cut and dried as the family had been led to believe. He told Sharon about what had been said about the possibilities of Katrina having confused the details of events and Yellowlees's admission that confusion was a possibility. Sharon telephoned Yellowlees immediately and questioned him about his conversation with Philip. After some time, she told Philip that Yellowlees said Philip had totally misunderstood what they had discussed, that there was no confusion as far as Katrina was concerned and that he, Yellowlees, had not changed his position one inch about my having abused Katrina. This led to Sharon and Philip having words which upset them both, and which led to Philip leaving the house in a fit of anger, but which was merely an indication that the tensions were beginning to drive wedges between the only people who were in a position to help Katrina.

The meetings between Yellowlees, Andrew and Philip established a number of things which were to have great bearing on later events, as the family began to fight back and try to discover what had really happened to Katrina while in the care of Yellowlees and his psychiatric staff. The conversations that took place between them, were to be later denied by Yellowlees, as he attempted to distance himself from the treatment Katrina had received. Unfortunately for him, the stances he took and the positions he adopted were to be confirmed by the medical notes so that his denials of what had taken place between him, Andrew and Philip merely confirmed him as a liar.

For a start, the conversations confirmed Yellowlees believed that memories could be suppressed only to resurface at some later date, under therapy. His whole diagnosis of Katrina's illness and his absolute belief that she had been abused, were predicated on his acceptance of repression. His telling Andrew that his memories could best be unlocked by speaking to a "trained counsellor" further confirmed his belief in repression. As we were to find out later, his own belief in repression of memories and their subsequent retrieval, was central to the type of therapy Katrina received. Nothing, it would seem, was going to shake his belief in my guilt, however much he again tried to distance himself from that position when the flack really started to fly. What was also established was his total conviction that Katrina's health had actually improved during her stay in Gilgal despite all the evidence to the contrary. As Professor Brandon was to remark later, "Not only the patients in Gilgal suffered from self-delusion."

However, all of that was to come later; for the moment Kay and I and the rest of the family were left to cope with the fallout of the confrontation and the fact I was still under investigation and suspicion. Every day seemed like a week and every week seemed like a year. Kay continued to keep contact with the boys while I continued, without success, to get someone at the hospital and the Social Work Department to answer my incessant telephone calls. The contact between Kay, Andrew and Philip was helping all of them, although I had still to speak to either of them. There had been no contact whatsoever between Sharon, Jim, Kay and me, while Kay spoke to Katrina on only two occasions.

Finally the contact which had been established between the boys and Kay paid dividends. She asked me one day shortly after Philip's meeting with Yellowlees if I would mind if he and Andrew called me on the telephone. I readily agreed.

The call from Andrew came first and the first tentative, "Hello" sounded as if it was being spoken by a child, it was so soft. It was difficult for both of us because I obviously did not want to say anything that would raise obstacles while at the same time, the last time I had been in Andrew's company, he had accused me of being a paedophile. That was not easily forgotten. From his point of view he was eaten up with guilt for what had been done and with his part in it. At that point, I knew he and Philip had spoken to Yellowlees, because they had told Kay, but I had no idea of what had been said. In the event we managed to stumble through a very brief conversation where neither of us was relaxed or able to speak in any way naturally. Andrew apologised and I accepted it but it was obvious that I was going to find it difficult to re-establish relationships which had meant the world to me. Philip called the same day with the same result. The calls had upset me because I had been unable to be natural and because it was exactly the opposite of what I had hoped for. Nevertheless, it was a start.

By far the most important telephone call I received within the space of those few days, was the one I received from the police three days after the call from Andrew and Philip. I was in the office when a call was put through by the receptionist, who said it was the police. My heart skipped half a dozen beats as I answered. The voice at the other end was not unfriendly but very matter of fact and business like.

"Can you call into the police station today," the female voice said.

"Yes, but can I ask you what it is for?" I asked.

"You'll be told when you arrive. When can you get here?"

"I can be there in ten minutes."

That was the end of the conversation and I made arrangements immediately to leave the office. I also called Kay because I had no idea if I would be able to call her after I had been to the police.

When I was shown into the interview room, the WPC who had taken Katrina's statement, was there, together with another WPC. As I entered the room, she smiled to me and said,

"You will notice I'm not switching on the tape."

I looked at her, slightly confused and said,

"What does that mean?"

"This is not an official interview," she said.

"What does that mean? Why am I here then?" I asked.

Her next comment caught me completely off guard,

"Katrina has withdrawn her allegations and we have finished our inquiries. This case is now finished."

I sat there and looked at her, relieved, astonished, bewildered and silent.

"I thought you would be pleased," she smiled again.

"After what we've been through over the past few weeks, pleased is putting it mildly, but I'm just caught off guard and surprised. Why did Katrina withdraw her allegations?" I asked

"We don't know that. All I know is that she called the office the day before yesterday and told us she was withdrawing the allegations and did not want the prosecution to proceed."

"But that would not have been up to her, would it, if you had found anything from your inquiries?" I said.

"No, that's right. If we had found any evidence that any of the claims she made had any truth in them, you would have been charged, whatever she said, particularly about the death of the little girl. But we didn't."

"I knew there was nothing to find but I was in the force, I have some idea how these things work. My concern was that I would be arrested anyway, given the nature of the allegations."

We discussed the reasons the police were called in because I wanted to establish the part played by Yellowlees. I was very interested in what he had to say as well as the statement that had been made by Jenny Hogg. The WPC was not in a position to tell me what I wanted to know at that stage and I asked if I could have a copy of Katrina's statement, which I was told Jenny Hogg had confirmed. I was told that decision would have to be made by a senior officer and that I would be contacted if and when I could pick it up, at which time we could discuss the other matters that were of concern to me. As that was as much as I was going to get, I stood up to leave, when the WPC said,

"You know, your daughter was very persuasive when she made her statement, but there were too many things which did not stand up to investigation. Even if she had not withdrawn her allegations, it is doubtful if you would have been charged."

"I hope you tell the psychiatrist and Social Work Department that; they still have to be convinced," I said.

It would be several weeks later before I received a copy of Katrina's police statement and learned of the full extent of what I was supposed to have done.

The news of Katrina's decision came as a tremendous relief to Kay. When I telephoned her from my office, she could hardly contain her excitement and said she was going to telephone Katrina as soon as I had hung up. My employers were equally pleased, although there was only one partner in the firm to whom I spoke.

"That will be it finished now," he said.

"Not by a long shot," I answered, "Katrina is still in hospital and obviously still very ill and, I have to find out why it happened. As far as I know, the Social Work Department and the psychiatrist still think I am guilty. There has been no retraction from them."

"But it won't go any further," he persisted, "If you are not going to be charged. Does it matter what the psychiatrist and the Social work Department think?"

I looked at him thinking,

"You really don't have a clue what this has done to the family and our relationships, or you wouldn't even think like that."

What I said, was,"

"I have no intention of spending the rest of my life on some grey list of suspected paedophiles, who only got away with it because of an alleged lack of evidence, just because some half-arsed quack of a psychiatrist got it wrong. I know how the police mind works and I may not be facing charges, but I am far from being innocent, in their minds.

When I was a raw recruit in the police," I continued, "I was often sent on the beat with a senior man, who would show me the vulnerable places where a break-in was most likely to happen, introduced me to local shopkeepers and so on. But one of the most important lessons I learned, was how they kept tabs on men they suspected of being "kiddy fiddlers" as we called them, no one ever spoke about paedophiles. They pointed out several men they suspected but were never able to catch. It was called the "grey list". There is no bloody way I am going to be on that list."

Andrew and Philip were equally delighted when they heard of Katrina's decision and although I still hadn't spoken to Sharon and Jim, nor had they made any attempt to speak to Kay, we were told they were pleased but surprised. Apparently Katrina had told no one of her decision but as more and more information began to seep out, the more the family spoke to each other, we learned that Katrina had never wanted to make a police statement in the first place. The pressure had come from Napier in the Social Work Department and Yellowlees, because of their own often stated fears for Katrina's life and the welfare of the grandchildren. Sharon had made a brief police statement, despite having nothing to tell them about my abuse, in order to help Katrina and that suggestion had first of all been made by Powrie. Later, they would all deny having played any part in putting pressure on either Sharon or Katrina but then, they would wouldn't they?

Despite Katrina's decision to withdraw the allegations, she continued to have flashbacks and I still was an ever-present figure in them. We learned Yellowlees was totally opposed to her withdrawing the allegations because of the continuing flashbacks and, it left Kay and I in a kind of Limbo, where nothing had really been resolved. Sharon was still spending as much time as she could with Katrina, who continued to be suicidal much of the time, and I still had no contact with Katrina at all. Jim caused Kay and I great concern because Andrew and Philip told us he was in a dreadful state. Jim worked as a shepherd on a thousand acre hill farm, where some of the ground was rocky and dangerous. He used a quad bike to get around the hill and Kay and I worried ourselves sick that his state of mind would lead to an accident on the hill, where he could lie for hours before anyone found him.

I resolved to go and speak to him and telephoned to tell him I was coming out to the farm. Jim had a beautiful nature and was one of the gentlest of men who doted on his own girls. When he and Anne had returned from honeymoon to learn of the allegations, their first concern was obviously for the two girls because Kay and I had baby sat while they were away. Jean, the eldest was still only two years old and when changing her on one of the first nights they were home, Anne discovered a slight rash in her genital area. Both she and Jim panicked and sick with worry, rushed Jean to the doctor, who diagnosed a urinary infection. I had always made a great fuss of Jean and she used to watch at the window of their cottage, for my car and would run to the door to meet me, giggling and holding up her arms to be lifted and given a swing. When the allegations came out, my behaviour with Jean was put down to my "grooming" her. Even something as innocent and pure as the love between a grandfather and his grandchild, was sullied and made to be obscene.

When Jim and I met at his cottage, we sat in the kitchen and I just let him talk at first, something he found extremely difficult to do because he couldn't stop crying. He admitted he had believed it because of the way they had been drip fed information, without actually ever being given any real evidence, although much was promised. He had panicked and felt so guilty because some of the abuse had allegedly happened in Dundee when I was campaigning as the SNP parliamentary candidate in that city, and he had been with Katrina on almost every occasion. When I started to question him about what had convinced him, he found it impossible to say, other than the accumulation of pressures, the fear Katrina had for her own safety, the alleged involvement of so many people he knew, and the clincher, the involvement of the SNP councillor, the explanation for which we still did not have.

As he became calmer, he said, "If they had told me you were dead, it would have been better. I had so much respect for you and looked up to you so much. Now...." he found it impossible to finish what he had been going to say.

I knew exactly how he felt because I had had to face my own father when I found out he had abused Katrina.

"Something died inside of me Jim, when I found out my own father had abused Katrina and that is a wound that has never healed," I told him. "I still have the same feelings of guilt for not having been aware it happened, of having done nothing to protect her. Your Mum and I still feel guilty."

"But how could you have known…?" he started to say when it dawned on him what he was about to offer was a defence for his mother's and my lack of action in Katrina's defence.

"Then," I interrupted him, "I made things a hell of a lot worse by choosing the wrong option to try and protect Nana. I still have a tremendous feeling of betrayal, by someone that I had been close to all my life. I spent far more time with my father, than with my mother, because of the horses. I still vividly remember my seventh birthday when he turned up at the school at four o'clock, with my first pony with a big red ribbon in its tail. There were all sorts of memories like that that were destroyed and soiled; and they always will be, no matter how much time has passed. I have never spoken to him again, and never will, because to me, that would be the final betrayal of Katrina. But I can't just forget all the good times, they can't just be wiped out."

I had never spoken about my own feelings, not even to Kay, when I found out about my father and when I told Jim this, it helped him to think I was taking him into my confidence about something that obviously still hurt deeply.

"There are no books to guide you through this kind of thing Jim," I said, "and no one can tell you how you should feel, which is what Yellowlees and his crew have been doing. I know exactly how you feel but only because I have been there and had to do what you and the rest of the family did, confront your worst nightmare. I cannot think of anything worse than having to confront your father with allegations of abusing your child, or your sister. In my case unfortunately, it was true but you can now put it behind you because it is not true. It is not going to be easy and I realise you will feel guilty for some time yet, that you believed that I had done the things I was accused of but time will make it easier."

That afternoon, we sat for several hours going over what had happened. I could offer no explanation for the involvement of the SNP councillor but I told Jim just how determined I was to get to the bottom of what had happened because as long as there were loose ends, there would be suspicion and that was something I could not live with, nor did I have any intention of doing so. By the time I took my leave, we both felt immeasurably better. We had spoken about things we hadn't spoken about for years but we both finished the meeting in absolutely no doubt about the depth of feeling there was between us and how close we had come to seeing it destroyed.

Thoughts of Katrina were never far from our minds and although Kay and I knew we were a long way from seeing her well, we did have hopes that she was making progress, particularly since she had decided to withdraw her allegations. That had come completely out of the blue and we kept hoping that her recovery might come as unexpectedly and quickly. Those hopes were completely dashed exactly five days after I was told by the police the allegations had been withdrawn. Sitting in my office, poring over some files, my mind was miles away from Katrina, Gilgal and allegations of abuse when the door was flung open and Katrina stepped into the room. I looked past her to see if there was anyone with her, but she was on her own and it was obvious she was highly agitated.

Before I could say a word, she asked,

"Why did you do it Dad, why did you abuse me?"

I just sat there and stared at her, not knowing what to do or say.

"How could you hurt me so much? What made you do it? Why did you let those other men abuse me as well?" By this time she had sat down on the chair on the opposite side of the desk, but she was perched on the edge of the seat, obviously very upset and with the tears welling in her eyes.

"Katrina, I know you believe I hurt and abused you and I don't know why. But it didn't happen dear. There was no abuse." I answered.

As I watched her, I lifted the telephone and dialled Sharon's number. She was still off work and I was hoping against hope she was at home. When she answered, I said very calmly and slowly,

"Katrina has just walked into my office. Can you come and collect her?"

Sharon did not ask for any explanation, she just said she would be right down and hung up.

I was very conscious of Katrina's agitation and I did not want to have to get up from the chair and go around to her side of the desk. Even in the unexpected situation I found myself, I was also aware of what might be said if for any reason at all, I had to restrain Katrina to keep her from leaving the office. I wanted there to be no possibility of being accused of any kind of assault. Again, I tried to assure her that no abuse had taken place but my main concern was to find out how she had arrived at the office.

"How did you get here and does the hospital know you have gone?" I asked. Katrina completely ignored the question and looking around her, her eyes darting all over the room, she again asked,

"Why did you abuse me Dad?" She was now in tears, and quite distraught, but before I could answer, Sharon appeared in the doorway and without saying anything to me other than,

"I'll look after her," she took Katrina by the arm and left the office.

After they had gone, I locked the door and sat with my head in my hands and quietly sobbed. I had never seen Katrina look so haunted and it broke my heart to think of the turmoil her mind must be in. She had withdrawn the allegations five days before and now, she had obviously run away from the hospital again, to confront me on her own. God knows what must have been going through her mind. I called Kay at home, told her what had happened and asked her to call the hospital to find out how Katrina was. We were told she had been sectioned and would be locked up for at least the next forty eight hours. Sharon told Kay she had had no problems with Katrina on the road to the hospital but we were furious that yet again, she had managed to leave the grounds and not a single member of staff had known about it.

Kay and I were sitting the Sunday following Katrina's visit to the office, quietly discussing what seemed to have been our sole topic of conversation for ever. I had been for the usual early morning hack, had showered and we were talking about the family and how things had developed. Kay had now spoken to all of the kids, including Sharon, who was the only one, except Katrina of course, I had had no contact with. She was still heavily involved with Katrina and any information we received generally came through Sharon. The telephone interrupted our discussion and Kay answered. I could hear her say,

"Slow down Andrew, I can hardly make out what you're saying. What does it say?"

There was a very brief conversation and when Kay put down the receiver, she said,

"Andrew wants us to get the Mail on Sunday, he says there is an article in it that will explain everything that has happened."

"What does he mean, explain everything?" I asked.

"He wouldn't say, he just insists we get the paper."

The newsagent was only minutes from the house and although I had already bought our usual Sunday papers, we did not normally take the Mail on Sunday.

We could hardly wait to see what was written and within a few minutes of finding and starting to read the article that had fired up Andrew so much, we hugged one another and could hardly contain ourselves in our hurry to read the whole thing.

We were staring at a photograph of a lovely young woman, obviously taken on her graduation day, under the headline,

"THERAPY OF DANGER"

How this sick girl came to believe that her loving parents abused her.

It was November 5th 1995 and that article was to open up a completely new chapter for us, starting us on the road that finally would lead to an explanation of what had happened to Katrina. It introduced us to the world of Recovered Memory Therapy and the "memory wars" so-called, that had been raging in the psychiatric profession for more than a decade.

CHAPTER TWELVE

THE FIGHTBACK BEGINS
November 1995 – December 1995

Kay and I could hardly believe what we were reading, the parallels to our own situation were so close, although the family caught up in the nightmare had had years of suffering as opposed to the few months of our own trauma. The article, written by Fiona Barton, related how a young university graduate, a brilliant scholar whose family were part of the Swan Hunter shipbuilding dynasty, had accused her family of the most sickening abuse, after undergoing therapy for an eating disorder. The girl, Anna Hunter had been told by the psychiatrist, Dr Robin Farqharson, that she had been raped by her father. He also told her he had no doubt she had been subjected to satanic abuse, because her recollections involved dismembered babies, a cross and slaughtered kittens.

"Evidence for these appalling allegations included a drawing she had made of a screwdriver, dreams interpreted by the psychiatrist and later – most frighteningly – the patient's denial that she had been abused. The family found proving their innocence was impossible in the face of the dogma of Recovered Memory Therapy. If they protested, they soon discovered, it meant they were "in denial", providing further evidence of abuse." the article went on, "The parents fought with the weapons of the middle classes – closely argued letters, appeals to common sense, and phone calls to MPs, councillors and pressure groups."

The father, Adrian Hunter says, "When an allegation of abuse is made there is absolutely no way to disprove it when all the proof is coming from therapy," and a psychiatrist points out, "Once it has been said, no one is going to believe you when you deny it because all perpetrators deny it. It is expected, so you are damned if you deny it and damned if you don't. All Anna did was relate her dreams, and draw pictures and write her feelings when she had been prescribed certain drugs to help her depression, which I understand may have enhanced her perceptions. And out of those musings of Anna's while in therapy came the interpretation from Dr Farquharson that she had been abused by her father and her step-grandfather."

The article went on to recount a whole series of accusations which were made against Anna's father, step-grandfather and mother, including one in which Anna told of a dream she had had where her father forced her to abuse her younger brother with a toy drill, when she was eight years old. Her brother had not been born when she was eight years old, but that alleged incident led to the involvement of Northumberland Social Services, who were called in to investigate whether the younger brother Ben, who by this time was fourteen years old, was under threat of being further abused.

Kay and I could not wait to tell the rest of the family about the article. As we pored over each line the similarities between what had happened to the Hunters and what had happened to us, seemed to leap from the pages at us. It gave us encouragement that we could at last get an explanation for what had happened, but it also dismayed us that we might have to go through the years of torment the Hunters had had to endure, with no real end in sight. They had been battling with the authorities for five years, had written to MPs and had other specialists in psychiatry and social work procedure examine their case and find in their favour. That had made no difference as far as Northumberland Social Services were concerned, the Hunters were still abusers and as far as the psychiatrist Dr Farquharson was concerned, "they would just have to agree to differ". It confirmed my feelings about the "grey list" but it provided us with another line of inquiry.

The following morning, I telephoned the Daily Mail first thing only to be told that Fiona Barton did not come into the office on a Monday and although I left my telephone number in the hope the office would get a message to her and that she would call me back, I had to call again on the Tuesday morning to speak to her. The rest of the Monday, was spent again poring over the article and discussing it with the family, all of whom had seen it by then. We were all excited over what it might mean but Sharon seemed to be less enthusiastic than the rest of us and cautioned us to wait until we had investigated it further. Although we did not know it at the time, she decided to make her own enquiries into the British False Memory Society, which had been mentioned in the article as having come to the aid of the Hunters.

When I finally spoke to Fiona Barton, I found myself being far more cautious than I had anticipated, in fact I had not given any thought to what I would do if asked to divulge my identity. In the event, I refused but questioned Fiona closely about the piece she had written.

"What has been the outcome of the case. Has the family been successful in proving their innocence?" I asked.

"It is not as simple as that. You have told me that no one in authority will speak to you, therefore you have already experienced the problems people in your situation face. The Hunters spent countless hours trying to get information, which the authorities simply refused to give them, until they made a final breakthrough and the article only scratches the surface of what they have gone through." Fiona answered. "They are still fighting and from what I know of Tania, Anna's mother, the fight will go on until they do prove their innocence, but it has been an uphill struggle. The authorities will do everything they can to stifle and stop any and every effort you make to find out what happened." At the time, I had no idea just how prophetic her comments would be.

"Can you tell me anything about the British False Memory Society, what are they and what do they do?" I asked.

"They are your best bet to get started because it is a pressure and support group for people who have been falsely accused by family members who have been in therapy. From what you have told me of your own situation, it sounds very much like you are a perfect example of the kind of people they were set up to help." she replied and then gave me the contact details.

Kay and I discussed my conversation with Fiona Barton and we agreed I should contact the British False Memory Society (BFMS). It was the best move we could have made because they provided us with a life-line. Without their help and the information they were able to provide, we would never have been able to fight back as effectively as we did, nor would we have ever been able to counter some of the more ludicrous arguments offered by the psychiatric and social work staff, as they found themselves increasingly under pressure to justify their actions. The more pressure they were put under, the more desperate their arguments became.

We will always be grateful to the BFMS for the help and support they have given over the years and we will always be just as grateful to the Hunters for having the courage to go public with their fight against authority. Without their story appearing in the Mail on Sunday, it might have taken years for us to find out about Recovered Memory Therapy (RMT) and the damage it has caused. When asked later, why I was prepared to go public with our own story, I always gave the example of the Hunters, arguing that if by reading about us, someone, somewhere can be helped to fight back against the same kind of false allegations, the publicity would be justified. As we were later to find out, the ramifications have been as I had hoped and the number of couples who have made contact runs well into double figures.

The telephone at the BFMS was answered by Roger Scotford, the Society's secretary and the man who started the group. He had been falsely accused of sexual abuse by his own daughters after he and his wife had divorced and having no idea why the allegations had been made, he was desperate to prove his innocence. An article about the setting up of the False Memory Syndrome Foundation in the USA, caught his eye and, on making inquiries, he found to his enormous relief, he had stumbled on a society which could help him. As a consequence he formed the British counterpart, the BFMS in 1993 and at the time I made contact, over four hundred families had already made contact and joined as members. At the time of writing this, that number has now swollen to over two thousand.

I related the details of our situation very briefly while Roger listened, asking questions from time to time. After a short period he asked my name and again, I found myself strangely reluctant to give it.

"OK," he said, "we can leave that for the time being"

Finally he said, "We can send you information and a number of articles which will explain the origins of RMT in the USA and how it was imported to this country. Having been started in the USA, the Americans have much greater experience than we have and, they are further advanced in fighting it. When you have had time to look at the material, if you want to contact us again, you have the contact number."

I said, "I would greatly appreciate that because we are at a loss right now to know where to turn."

"That is fine," said Roger, "give me your name and address."

There was silence for a moment or two before I replied,

"I'm not sure I want to do that."

There was another short silence, then he said,

"I'm going to find it difficult to send you anything if you don't tell me who you are and where you live."

Suddenly realising the stupidity of what I had said, I burst out laughing.

"I'm sorry," I stuttered through the laughter, "it just shows how uptight I've been over this." I then gave him my name and address.

"That is perfectly understandable and I know how it feels." said Roger, "I will have the stuff in the post today."

When the material arrived, we were amazed at the contents and even more amazed at the number of victims RMT had claimed in the USA, before the therapy had been imported to the UK, where it continued to create havoc. The story of the Hunter family was only one of over four hundred that had already contacted the BFMS and according to Roger Scotford, they were receiving more contacts every other week, from people, mainly men, totally confused, frightened and at a loss, like we were, to know where to get help. The thing that struck us most and certainly made the biggest impact on us, was the stupidity of some of the claims made by some of the alleged "victims" of abuse in the USA. But of even greater import was the fact that professional specialists in the medical and psychiatric professions either believed the claims being made or, were involved in the therapy that preceded the claims.

There were a number of bizarre claims that, in the USA, were cited by therapists, as genuine. One woman had memories going right back to her time in her mother's womb, when she could recount conversations she had heard. Another incident involved a woman who had been visited by an alien who impregnated her. The alien returned when she was several months pregnant and removed the foetus so that the half-human, half alien could be brought up by its alien family. The woman was visited when her "child" was about four years of age so that she could see it was prospering in its "alien" environment. Her therapist vouched for the strong likelihood that this account was true.

While it is easy to dismiss this kind of nonsense, there were countless other cases, where the bizarre nature of the claims did not reach the heights of alien abduction, but included satanic ritual abuse, where babies were sacrificed and "baby farms", where women were deliberately made pregnant to provide babies for sacrifice to Satan, were believed to exist but never found. The scale of abuse ranged from the truly "unbelievable" to the abnormal, where instruments and violence were commonplace. In fact, many of the cases cited were mirror images of the type of abuse of which I had been accused.

Stripped down to its basics, Recovered Memory therapy is based on a belief that memory can be "blocked" or repressed. Those who believe in repression, believe that "traumatic" events can be blocked because the mind, particularly the mind of the child, cannot cope with the knowledge. This process relies on the "video recorder" model of memory, in which the memory is lodged intact in the unconscious mind and can eventually be replayed essentially unchanged. Meanwhile it gives rise to symptoms, the origin of which is obscure to the patient. "Dissociation" is sometimes cited as an alternative explanation. The individual goes into a trance (sometimes this is claimed to be an automatic response, others claim that the individual, usually a child, learns how to go into a trance, and leave their body) at the time of the abuse. The traumatic memory is therefore stored in a separate mental compartment, gives rise to "symptoms" and remains essentially intact. Dissociated memories are said to be accessed through symptoms such as dreams and flashbacks.

While this "explained" to some extent what had happened to Katrina, particularly the notion of "dissociation" which it was alleged had also happened to me, it did nothing to explain why Katrina had displayed the symptoms in the first place. Nor did it explain why Katrina should have flashbacks about the alleged rapes in her flat, while I did not, although it was suggested we had both dissociated because we both found the experience so traumatic. Moreover, the more we read, the more ludicrous and nonsensical the whole farcical situation became. Despite years of clinical and laboratory research, no evidence had been found for the existence of repression, except in episodes of sexual abuse, which alone of traumatic events, seemed likely to create dissociation and repression. Why this should be so is never explained. Years of empirical research with Holocaust survivors and soldiers who went through the horrors of war, have found that far from forgetting their experiences, which many had done their best to do, they could not forget them and they impacted on their conscious mind to the point of causing serious mental problems. Why sexual abuse should be so special, is unknown and never explained.

The theory of repression is also subject to problems of logic and appears to run counter to common sense. It is apparently a basic concept of memory that repetition increases the likelihood of recall. However, adherents of the theory of "traumatic memory" argue that constant repetition increases the probability of "blocking" and that while a single act or instance of abuse may be remembered, a series of instances of abuse overwhelms the child's mind, leading to wholesale forgetting. At the time of our making contact with the BFMS, the Royal College of Psychiatrists had set up a working party to study the problems associated with RMT, and it had still to report. It did so in 1998 and debunked the whole idea of recovered memory, the problems of which were well known in the psychiatric profession, including the team that had treated Katrina, witness Yellowlees advice to Andrew not to allow himself to be hypnotised under any circumstances.

We learned that therapists who believed in repression and practised RMT, also believed there are a range of symptoms which are indicative of sexual abuse and which justify the search for buried memories, thus the insistence on "disclosure". The "symptoms" are non-specific and are common in the population at large. They are also features of common psychiatric conditions. Having embarked on a search for "memories" the patient may well start to have troubling dreams and nightmares, which are then taken as "evidence" that the trauma is about to surface or the patient is "reliving" the trauma. As we read further, we began to recognise the language that is common among RMT practitioners. For example, we read that it is common for therapists to inform their patients that, "they displayed all the signs of someone who has been sexually abused", while others will argue that any patient who cannot remember any abuse, is "in denial", which in itself, is "evidence" that abuse actually took place. The same concept of denial is applied to accused abusers who deny having committed abuse. Their denial is alleged to be "proof" that abuse was committed. With that kind of twisted logic, no accused person can possibly prove their innocence.

It all became frighteningly familiar and as we read, we discussed the conversations the family had had with Yellowlees, Hogg and Katrina herself, who had used many of the terms of RMT, the longer she was in hospital. But the problem we faced was the lack of contact with the psychiatric team and their absolute refusal to even acknowledge my telephone calls. Every conversation the family had had with Yellowlees led to his accusations, that previous "explanations" he had given were "misunderstood" or "misinterpreted" so that we were unable to come to any conclusions about any of the treatment to which Katrina had been subjected. No matter how often he had made the same points to either Andrew, Sharon or Philip, no matter how many times he had said Katrina "showed all the symptoms etc." it had been impossible to pin him down because he always claimed that he had been misunderstood.

As the weeks passed, I received more information from the BFMS and had several telephone conversations with Roger Scotford. Just to be able to speak to someone who had been through the same experiences made a tremendous difference. When I was first confronted and Kay and I seemed to be totally isolated from the family, it felt that what had happened to us had never happened before to anyone else. We actually took perverse comfort from knowing that after all, we were not alone, that it had happened to a great many other families and that there was a reason, there were factors that were responsible, albeit we did not understand fully just how they interacted to almost destroy Katrina's mind.

As November moved into December, we still had not met again as a family. There had been a series of disjointed telephone conversations between Kay and Andrew, Kay and Philip, Kay and Sharon; Philip and me, Andrew and me and Jim and I had spent one afternoon together, where we had talked for hours. Katrina was still in hospital and Sharon spent hours with her every week; but since the confrontation there had been no occasion when all of us, except Katrina, had sat down in the same room to talk things through. Since making contact with the BFMS, I felt there was a great deal more we could discuss. I had given everyone copies of the material I had received from Roger Scotford and relayed the details of the conversations I had had with him. Neither Kay nor I had actually met the family since the confrontation, therefore I suggested they all come to Crieff so that we could at least make a start to getting things back to normal.

It was agreed Sharon, Andrew, Philip and Jim would all come to the house one evening and unfortunately, the night on which the meeting had been arranged came immediately after a couple of days when I had had a miserable time with a heavy cold. I felt hellish, on top of which we had had reports from Sharon that Katrina was not at all well. Before they arrived I said to Kay, "We are going to have to be very careful and not lose our tempers tonight."

My concern was directed at Kay, although I didn't say as much, because I knew how angry she was about the fact I had been accused and the manner in which the confrontation had taken place. She readily agreed and before the family arrived, I made a list of questions I wanted to ask, just to clear up a number of points about what Yellowlees had said about certain allegations.

As soon as they arrived, the tension in the atmosphere was so great it was almost tangible. There were a few very nervous ,"Hellos" but no conversation, as they all waited for me to say something. I thought we would be able to get general agreement about the BFMS and the material it had sent but although the boys said very little, Sharon voiced her scepticism almost immediately. She said she had spoken to her psychologist friend, who had discussed it with other colleagues and they had told her the American Foundation had been started by a brother and sister who had been found guilty of incest. It had also been said the organisation was just a front for paedophiles. Sharon turned to me and asked,

"Do you know anything about these people?" meaning the BFMS.

"No", I said, "But I've read the material, as I hope you have, and the similarities in the Hunter case, to what happened to us, are far too many just to be ignored."

"Well, that's not what I've heard," said Sharon.

"Heard from whom?" I snarled "The man in the pub?"

Within seconds the atmosphere was like ice. I completely lost my temper and ripped into Sharon and, to a lesser extent the boys. Suddenly Sharon burst into tears and ran from the room, upstairs to the bathroom. We could hear her breaking her heart and at one point she was crying so hard we though she was ready to be sick. Philip went upstairs to her and gradually we could hear her calming down until all we could hear were their muffled voices, speaking very quietly. Jim had just sat saying nothing. He and Sharon were very close and I knew he was very upset for her. Andrew said,

"That is the first time Sharon has cried since this whole thing started. That has been coming for weeks and it will do her good to let it out."

Just then Philip popped his head round the sitting room door and said they should just go and get Sharon home. I asked where she was and he told me she had gone out to the car as she didn't trust herself to come back in, she was so upset.

After they had gone, I could barely speak to Kay I was so bitterly ashamed of myself. Sharon was thirty three years of age and I had never in all her life spoken to her, in the way I had that night. We had always enjoyed a very close relationship, although we debated, argued and discussed endlessly. If I said black, Sharon would say white, just for the sake of argument, but we had never fallen out over anything. I asked Kay to telephone Alison, Philip's wife, although I knew they would not be home yet, and ask if they would ask Sharon to meet me there the next day. If we did not get a telephone call that night and it didn't matter how late it was, I would assume it was agreed that we meet at lunchtime.

There was no call that night and I spoke to Kay until the early hours of the morning, as I poured my heart out about what a mess I had made of it. She tried to make me feel better by reminding me that Sharon wasn't the only one who had weeks of pent up emotion to get rid of, that I had probably needed to let rip at somebody. Unfortunately, I had picked Sharon and the boys when the people I really wanted to pummel, were Yellowlees and the social workers. As the weeks rolled into months and the months became years, there were countless times when I needed to let rip and I had to find other ways to do it. Fortunately I found release in physical effort but Kay was less fortunate and had to get rid of her frustrations and anger in other ways.

At lunchtime the following day, when I arrived at Alison and Philip's house, Sharon was already there and although Alison tried to excuse herself, we both asked her to stay because neither of us really wanted to deal with this on our own. I started by apologising for my outburst and found then I could not stop talking. Obviously I needed to get a great many things off my chest and with Alison's help Sharon and I were able to talk things through to the point where, before I finally left, I felt we had cleared the air completely. From then on, there was never a time when Sharon was on the outside of the rest of the family, although she continued to be Katrina's main support. She was to play an important role, as the boys also did, in future meetings with the Health Trust and the Social Work Department and having had such a close working contact with Katrina and Yellowlees, she had a great deal of information we were able to use to good effect later.

I continued to pursue Yellowlees and the Social Work Department throughout December and finally made a breakthrough with Napier at the Social Work Department, who agreed to meet me on December 21st at Rosslyn House, the head office of the department. Prior to agreeing to the meeting, which was on a Thursday, I had spent the previous week calling three or four times every day, with the same request and he had telephoned Sharon on the previous Friday, rather nervously asking why I wanted to speak to him. Sharon had told him it was surely rather obvious; I intended to sue the Local Authority as a consequence of his conduct therefore it might be in his own interest to meet me.

The meeting was arranged for 10am and when I arrived, was shown into a small interview room, shortly to be joined by Napier and a scribe. As I had never met the man, he introduced himself and asked my why I had asked for the meeting.

"I would have thought that was pretty obvious," I answered, "You are familiar with my case?"

"Yes," the response was short and gave nothing else away.

"I believe you think I abused my daughter Katrina, " I said.

Napier immediately looked away but said nothing.

"Well, do you?" I asked again. "Do you think I abused my daughter and if so, why?"

"I cannot answer that," replied Napier.

"Why can't you answer that?" I asked, "You have been involved in a case in which I have been accused of abusing my daughter and I have been told you believe that I abused her. Why?"

"No comment," he said again.

"You also think my sons have been brought up in a culture of abuse. Can you tell me why you think that?"

"No comment."

"You threatened to have my grandchildren taken into care, unless I was deprived of unsupervised access. Why?"

"No comment." By this time Napier was beginning to look decidedly uncomfortable. I have no idea what kind of meeting he expected but it was obvious things were not going as he thought they might. But I had no intention of letting up on him.

"You are aware, I take it, that my daughter accused seventeen other men?" I pushed.

"I can't comment on that."

"You are beginning to sound like an echo," I said and although there was a tightening of his face muscles and he was not pleased, there was still no reply.

"Why have you not investigated any of those other men?" By this time I was beginning to warm to the task of openly baiting him.

After the briefest of hesitations, the same reply

"No comment."

"Why did you agree to this meeting, if all you are going to say is "No comment?" I asked, then turning to the scribe, I said,

"I hope you are taking all of this down, particularly the responses from Mr Napier." She was as communicative as her boss and simply looked away.

"You told my daughter that I was using my contacts in the SNP to get information about how the police investigation was going. Why did you say that?"

A rather longer hesitation this time followed by another,

"No comment."

"Have you any idea how much trouble that remark caused? Have you any idea what that remark did to my family?"

This time, he looked at his feet and said,

"I am sorry but I cannot comment on that."

Suddenly, I threw at him,

"What is the name of the SNP councillor who spoke to your boss?"

"I can't tell you that."

I had lost patience by that time and in a voice that left him in no doubt how much contempt I felt, I said,

"You had plenty to say when you were faced with just my daughter. You threatened her and the rest of my family that their children would be taken into care unless they did what you told them to do. You created turmoil in my family by claiming I was using my contacts in the SNP to find out what was going on. But now, when you are faced with the person you accused, you have the gall to sit there and the best you can say is, "No comment".

I then told him that since he was such a complete waste of time, I wanted to see his boss, whose name I did not even know at that stage. Napier left the room accompanied by the scribe, without saying another word and after about ten minutes, he returned to tell me his boss, Mrs Betty Bridgeford, would see me.

A few moments later Mrs Bridgeford appeared, introduced herself and shook my hand. I asked her if she knew who I was and if she knew anything about me. Without even thinking about it she said,

"No, I have never heard of you. All I was told was that you wanted to see me."

Within fifteen seconds of meeting me, Bridgeford had told me her first lie and every word that came out of her mouth from then on in was a further series of lies. In fact, I don't think that woman said a single word to me that was anywhere near being the truth. The strange thing was, the lies were so obvious and so ridiculous, it must have been perfectly clear to her that she was going to be found out. But it didn't stop her.

As she claimed to know nothing about me, I began to tell her briefly what had happened with Katrina's allegations and how the Social Work Department had become involved. I had barely started to explain the circumstances when she interrupted me and said,

"A friend of your daughter Katrina was very concerned about her welfare while she was in the hospital and approached a local councillor to see if there was anything he could do."

"What friend of my daughter?" I asked

"I can't tell you that but she stayed in Auchterarder (a small town about fourteen miles from Perth)".

"Why would someone from Auchterarder approach a councillor from Perth about my daughter's health? What did she expect him to be able to do about it?"

"I can't tell you that, I am only telling you what happened." she replied, hurrying on to tell me the councillor then approached her, to ask her to investigate if I was under police investigation.

"Why would a councillor approach you, the Director of Social Work, to ask if I was under investigation, when he had been approached by some girl who was supposed to be concerned about my daughter's welfare?" I asked, completely puzzled by an explanation that made no sense.

"I can't tell you that, but as this was an official request from a councillor, I was obliged to find out for him, and therefore asked Mr Napier to speak to the police." she finished.

"Does it not strike you as strange, that some girl, whose name you cannot tell me, would approach a councillor who did not represent her ward and did not even live in the same town, to look into the welfare of my daughter and that he approached you about the police? The two things are not even connected", I said.

There was no reply to that despite waiting for several moments, therefore I made the same request I had made of Napier.

"What was the councillor's name?" I asked.

"I'm sorry I can't tell you that."

At that, I looked straight at Bridgeford, although getting any kind of eye contact was almost impossible.

"I have to tell you right now, I don't believe you and I fully intend to take this further but before I leave, I want to be certain I have this straight. You are telling me that some girl friend of my daughter, who you say comes from Aucheterarder, was so concerned about Katrina's health, that she approached a councillor from Perth, to ask him to intervene. He, in turn, asked you, the Director of Social Work, to find out if I was under police investigation and, because he was a councillor and it was an official request, you were obliged to find out for him. Is that right?" I asked.

"Yes, that is right," she answered.

As I made ready to leave, I suddenly turned to Bridgeford and said, "I want to see the file you have on me."

She was obviously taken aback, but quickly answered,

"There is no file."

"Then how could Mr Napier tell Sharon that I believed Katrina when I spoke to social workers in 1987?" I asked.

Bridgeford became very flustered, turning towards the door and turning the handle, obviously very keen to be rid of me,

"There is no file because there was no investigation."

"Are you seriously asking me to believe that there is no record of all the meetings where Napier and Powrie were involved with my family, to say nothing about the screening of the grandchildren?" I asked making no attempt to disguise my disbelief.

"There is no file." said Bridgeford obviously now in control of her voice.

I could hardly believe what I had been told. The story was such an obvious load of nonsense I felt insulted Bridgeford had had the audacity to give it to me as an explanation. What she had hoped to achieve was beyond me. When I arrived home, the first person I called, after I had spoken to Kay, was Sharon. I don't think she believed me at first.

"C'mon Dad, she said, "She has no obligation to tell a councillor anything, in fact she has an obligation ***not*** to tell anybody anything about an ongoing investigation."

"I know that perfectly well, but I was not going to contradict her because I wanted to hear what she had to say. I wanted to see how far she would go." I said. "Call her yourself and see what she tells you."

For the next hour, Kay and I discussed Bridgeford's explanation, even trying to think of any of Katrina's friends we knew, who stayed in Auchterarder. We were still at it when the telephone rang. It was Sharon.

"Well," I asked, "Was I right?"

"Yes, except that she told me that the girl who contacted the councillor, wasn't a friend of Katrina's. She knew a friend of Katrina's and had been told about Katrina being in Gilgal and she decided to contact the councillor."

"Why?" I asked, "Did you get any kind of rational explanation about what she thought he could do? And why a councillor from Perth, there are councillors in Auchterarder she could have contacted? Did you get his name?"

"No," said Sharon, "the rest of the story is the same as she gave to you but I told her she had no right to tell a councillor or anybody else anything, but she argued that she did. I know that is rubbish, she is lying."

"Good," I said, "I'm glad that has finally been established. The entire story from Napier and Bridgeford is a pack of lies. Why, we're going to find out because it just does not make sense. I am just glad you telephoned her yourself. It's a pity you weren't there when I saw Napier."

It was still early afternoon so I decided to have another go at telephoning Yellowlees and to my astonishment, he took my call. At first I was so surprised, I could barely get the words out when he answered and asked what he could do for me.

"I think it is time we discussed Katrina's situation, the last time we spoke was in April and a great deal has happened since then. For a start, Katrina has accused me of sexually abusing her, as well as some unspeakable crimes. You have told the family you believe that to be true. On what basis?" I asked

"There was a long silence and I had to ask him again before he responded,

"On the basis of my professional judgement and experience," he replied.

"But where is the evidence for any of it?" I asked.

"I don't need evidence, it is my judgement," he said.

That rattled me a bit.

"What do you mean, you don't need evidence? You can't encourage someone to accuse their father of rape and murder and then say, you don't need evidence. That is nonsense," I said.

"It is not my job to get evidence, it is my professional judgement based on Katrina's flashbacks and my experience of such things. Besides, she disclosed the abuse," he countered.

"But she has no memories of abuse, other than through the flashbacks and nightmares. That is the only basis of her disclosures."

There was no response to that so I tried something else,

"You told my daughter Sharon that you found me intimidating and imposing, despite the fact we had met only once and at that meeting, I hardly opened my mouth. Why did you say that?" I asked.

There was a slight pause before he said,

"That was Katrina's opinion of you, that was her assessment not mine."

Suddenly I knew Yellowlees was lying but I couldn't understand why.

"I don't believe you," I said. "That was your assessment, at least that is what you told Sharon."

"No, no," he stuttered, "That was Katrina's assessment, not mine."

Now that I knew he was lying, I pushed him harder.

"You are lying to me. Why? Why are you blaming Katrina for something you said? What is the purpose of lying about it?

"I am not lying and how dare you suggest I am. I am going to finish this conversation now," he said.

"I want a meeting," I said quickly, "It is important that we discuss this situation because it can't go on like this."

"Call my secretary," he said and hung up.

I again discussed the conversation with Kay and we were more confused than anything else, at Yellowlees's reaction.

"Why would he lie?" I asked.

"What is the point of lying?" she said, "There is nothing to be gained from it."

"That is the part I don't understand. But he definitely claimed that his assessment of me as "intimidating and imposing" was Katrina's opinion and not his. Can you imagine Katrina using that form of language?" I asked.

"Call Sharon and ask her if we perhaps picked her up wrongly. Maybe it was Katrina who said it, but I doubt it." Kay said.

When I called Sharon and gave her the details of the conversation with Yellowlees, her reaction was immediate.

"He's lying," she said. "That was definitely his opinion of you, Katrina's opinion did not come into it. He was explaining to me the impression you made on him, when I tried to tell him that violence was not part of your nature."

"Well, that is what he said but he agreed to a meeting and I have to call his secretary. Will you come as well?" I asked.

"You bet I will because he is making me out to be a liar," said Sharon, "Just fix any date you can get and I will fit in."

First thing the following morning, I called the secretary and a date of January 11th was fixed for the meeting, but our excitement over the prospect of getting a meeting at last, was soon flattened, when the morning mail arrived about lunchtime. There was a letter from Yellowlees which left us spitting with rage.

The letter read,

"Further to our recent telephone conversation, I have been advised to make you aware in writing of the effect that recent events in relation to her family are having on Miss Fairlie's mental health. The pressure she perceives herself to be under from the family clearly serves

to intensify her feelings of self injury, and at times, of suicide. In particular, she has made it clear to me that the family's recent request that she see a specialist in London was the main precipitant for her recent suicide attempt in which she intended to hang herself.

My primary concern is with Miss Fairlie's mental health and I therefore feel that I have a responsibility to make you fully aware of the situation."

Yours sincerely

Alex J Yellowlees.

"That bastard," I raged, "that letter must have been in the post just after we spoke on the telephone yesterday, for us to receive it today, and he never mentioned Katrina has tried to commit suicide again."

I wanted to telephone again straight away but Kay persuaded me to wait until I had calmed down. In the event, she called the hospital later that afternoon and was given only the briefest of details, that Katrina had made a half-hearted attempt on her life and was now sectioned. The staff did not feel it was serious enough to have called anyone to let them know.

"Not serious enough to let us know, but serious enough to tell us now because he wants to put the blame on us," I said, when Kay told me. She was very upset also and said,

"That is the first and only piece of correspondence we have had from that man since Katrina went into hospital over a year ago, and it is to tell us that it is our fault she tried to commit suicide. What about all the other attempts she has made in the last year? Who was responsible for them?"

We had to wait another two years until Katrina's medical records arrived, to get the answer to that question.

Kay called Sharon to tell her what we had learned about Katrina's suicide attempt and she was equally angry that she had not been informed, given how closely she felt she had worked with the hospital. I then called Philip to ask if he would come to the meeting with Yellowlees, when I had the date, and to tell him about Katrina. He agreed to call Andrew and Jim and was as furious as I had been. As a family, we were beginning to learn a bit more about the kind of people we were dealing with, but they were very soon going to learn a bit more about us. They were no longer dealing with frightened people and we determined that in any future dealings with them, we would be prepared because it was obvious we could not believe a word they said.

CHAPTER THIRTEEN

December 1995 – March 6th 1996

On December 23rd, we received yet another letter from Yellowlees postmarked December 22nd. It read

"Further to your telephone conversation with my secretary, I am writing to inform you that I would be pleased to meet you as you request. I understand that you wish to attend along with your solicitor. As a result, Dr Peter Connelly, Clinical Director, a legal representative and a scribe will also be in attendance.

We would request advance notice in writing of the points you wish to raise at the meeting. I will be writing to you in due course with a number of possible dates for the meeting."

This came as a great surprise because I had not expected any meeting to take place, particularly as Yellowlees had hung up on me. Kay and I discussed the import of what might come out of the meeting and after confirming that Sharon and Philip would attend along with me, Kay said she would like to see Katrina. She called Sharon and suggested that all three of them go out for lunch, Sharon arranged with the hospital to pick up Katrina at the hospital but the following day, which was the day before Christmas, she was delayed and asked Kay to collect Katrina in a taxi and bring her to the house. While Sharon was in the house waiting for Kay and Katrina to arrive, she received a telephone call. The voice on the other end belonged to a very agitated Dr. Yellowlees who, without any introduction, almost shouted,

"Do you know Katrina has just left here with your mother?

"Yes, of course I know," Sharon answered.

"Do you realise how much danger she could be in?" asked Yellowlees.

"Danger? What kind of danger?" Sharon asked.

"She will be taking her to your father, don't you realise that?" shouted Yellowlees.

"Mum is bringing Katrina here to my house and what kind of danger would she be in from my father?" Sharon asked.

She received no reply to that question, just a few muttered remarks about making sure that Katrina was brought back to the hospital before tea time, after which Yellowlees hung up.

Sharon was astounded at the telephone call and when she told Kay, who was furious, they did not know what to make of Yellowlees. On the one hand he was agreeing to a meeting and on the other, he was expressing concern that Katrina might be taken by her mother to meet me. Obviously he was convinced she would be abused. I was equally furious when I was told but decided to do nothing about it until we had the meeting in January, at which time there was an ever lengthening list of issues Yellowlees would be asked to address.

Christmas had always meant the family coming to our house on Christmas day. Andrew had spent several years in France and had only been back in Glasgow for the past two years. Christmas day was just another working day for him but the rest of the family, with the grandchildren, usually spent the day with us. In recent years, the numbers had swollen so that we needed the adults at one table and the children at a table of their own and it was a wonderful day full of laughter, music and fun. Christmas day 1995 had none of those things because although we had spoken to the family, they had been at our house only once since the confrontation and that had turned into a disaster. We hadn't seen the grandchildren for months and Katrina was still in Gilgal. I had neither seen nor spoken to her and she spent Christmas day in hospital. Jim and Anne went through to Glasgow to be with Anne's family.

We decided we were not ready to invite Sharon, Philip and their families to spend Christmas with us and we neither received nor sent cards. On Christmas morning, it would normally have been hectic, with our exchange of presents to each other, then making sure everything was in place for the family, who would start to arrive just after mid-day. On Christmas 1995, we did not even exchange presents with each other. We had no heart for celebration because there was nothing to celebrate. The house was dead, there were no family cards, no telephone calls, no presents.

We had decided to have dinner at a local hotel, where the atmosphere was artificially cheerful, with the rest of the guests looking as if they were enjoying themselves as much as we were. It was the first Christmas in our entire lives that Kay and I had spent on our own. Before we started going out together, we both came from large families, therefore family Christmases were the norm. For the four years we went together before we married, we had always had marvellous family Christmases with both our families and, every year since we were married we had had our own children. It was the most miserable Christmas we had ever spent and when we returned from the hotel, although it was still early evening, we locked the doors and drew the curtains. It was symbolic of our desire to just lock out the world and it became a nightly ritual for several years, as we seemed to fight the world on our own.

On December 28th, I responded to Yellowlees's letter of 22nd, giving him a list of the topics I wished covered at the meeting which had been planned for January 11th. I informed him that I would be accompanied by my solicitor as well as Sharon and Philip and that we would want the meeting recorded. The list of issues I wanted to discuss were as follows

- A diagnosis of Katrina's illness
- An explanation of the sequence of events from the time that Katrina had entered hospital, until the present time (including when she started flashbacks, dissociation and psychotic episodes)
- An explanation of and reasons for, Katrina's treatment

- Ÿ An assessment of the damage done to Katrina, as well as an assessment of the degree to which she has been abused
- Ÿ An explanation of the contents of Dr Yellowlees's letter of 21st inst.

A reply to that letter was received on the 5th January, in which confirmation of the meeting was agreed.

New Year came and went, with no change in our lives. Kay kept in touch with Katrina by telephone and I spoke to the family about the forthcoming meeting with Yellowlees. We had prepared a list of items, over and above those we had given in the letter of 28th December, therefore we expected a very lengthy discussion. About mid-morning of January 10th, the telephone rang in my office and the receptionist told me there was a Mr Sharp from the Central Legal Office wished to speak to me. When he was put through, he asked to whom he was speaking and seemed surprised when told it was me.

"Who did you think you were going to speak to?" I asked.

"The solicitor who is representing you," he answered.

"He is in court, which is probably why you were put through to me," I said, "can I help?"

"I wanted to discuss the meeting tomorrow, particularly the fact you want the proceedings recorded. That is most unusual and I cannot agree to it being done. I also have concerns about the length of the agenda as the time and effort it would take to get that information." he said.

"Why would you object to the meeting being recorded?" I asked.

"Well, for a start, Dr Yellowlees will not want his words thrown back at him at some later date." he answered.

"I can see why that might be," I said, "It is so much easier to deny everything, if there is no record of the actual words, but I would have thought in the interests of all concerned, a recording would be beneficial."

"That is not how I see it," he said, "and now that I have spoken to you, I don't think a meeting of any kind would be beneficial."

"Why, what have you got to hide?" I asked, "It took me weeks to get Yellowlees to even speak to me on the telephone. My daughter has been in his care for over a year and has made all kinds of allegations of abuse that could never have happened. My family has been thrown into turmoil as a consequence and I need some answers. The only person who can provide them is Dr Yellowlees."

"You have told me things I knew nothing about and before any meeting can take place, I will have to discuss things with Dr Yellowlees. I cannot agree to the meeting going ahead tomorrow therefore we will leave it there and I will be in touch."

With that, he hung up.

I had asked the court partner in the legal firm which employed me, to act for me and when I told him of the telephone conversation with the lawyer from the Central Legal Office, he said he was not in the least surprised as this was the kind of tactic they invariably used when dealing with this type of case. He further warned me to expect the meeting never to take place. When I had heard nothing by 17th January I wrote the following letter to Sharp. I have quoted from it extensively, as well as the reply I received in order to give a flavour of the kind of machinations with which we had to deal for the next two years and more, in attempting to have the Health Trust deal with our concerns, without having to revert to court action.

"Further to our telephone conversation of 10th inst. anent my daughter Katrina Fairlie, and in light of having had no further correspondence from either yourself or Dr Yellowlees, I hereby wish to make a formal complaint.

I find it astonishing that until our conversation of 10th inst. you were unaware of the gravity of Katrina's situation, despite having given earlier agreement to a meeting to take place on January 11th to address the agenda laid out in my correspondence of 28th December 1995.

I find it equally astonishing that your objection to that meeting being recorded is on the grounds that, "Dr Yellowlees did not want his words thrown back at him." That suggests that there is a distinct official nervousness at the prospect of a verbatim record being kept of such a meeting and obviously written notes are more easily challenged if they are produced at some later date.

It is difficult to understand your objections to the agenda on the grounds of the amount of time and research it would take to provide the information, as Dr Yellowlees assured me he had records of all telephone conversations he had held. Similarly there will be records of Katrina's care already in existence. Katrina has now been in the care of Dr Yellowlees for more than a year and her mental state is now worse than it was when she entered hospital.

Dr Yellowlees disputes this but he refuses to explain how Katrina can now believe she has suffered from abuse that never took place, at the hands of men she had never met. I must insist therefore that I receive notice of your intent...."

There was no reply from Yellowlees, Sharp or anyone else at the Central Legal Office until 2nd February, when the following letter arrived.

"I regret I am not clear as to the basis on which you want to make a complaint.

As far as I was concerned, I agreed to the meeting originally fixed for 11th January on the basis that Dr Yellowlees and I would be listening to what you had to say and I advised Dr Yellowlees to proceed with the meeting on that basis. I was obviously surprised therefore to receive your letter of 28th December, setting out a detailed agenda... Taping at a meeting is hardly likely to create an atmosphere of mutual trust, as I am sure your legal adviser will tell you. I have yet to discuss this at a meeting with Dr Yellowlees, therefore I will contact you at a later date."

In light of this letter, I wrote back immediately, pointing out that if there had never been any intention to do anything other than *listen* to what I had to say, there was hardly any need to have present the Clinical Director, a scribe and a legal representative as well as Dr Yellowlees, and to ask for prior notice of what I wanted to discuss. All of that could have been done by letter. I also pointed out that Katrina had been sectioned for two days prior to the meeting of 11th January, with no explanation other than that the doctors thought it was in her interests to be sectioned until after the meeting took place. Despite the meeting having been cancelled, she was kept sectioned until January 13th, again with no explanation.

As far as I was concerned that was an abuse and manipulation of Katrina for no apparent reason. Perhaps the most important issue was the fact that no matter what Dr Yellowlees said to individual members of the family, whenever they were raised at some later date, either he claimed he had not said them or, he claimed the family had misunderstood him. For that reason, the family felt their experience of Dr Yellowlees made it impossible to create "an atmosphere of mutual trust." There was no response until February 25th, when a letter arrived to tell me they had decided that "no useful purpose could be gained" from having a meeting and that Sharp and the Central Legal Office "could be of no further assistance".

Although the correspondence that passed between Yellowlees's legal advisers and the family, throughout February brought to an end our initial attempt to make progress with Yellowlees and the Health Trust, there was another letter at the very beginning of the month which lifted our spirits enormously. It was from Katrina, addressed to me and it arrived on February 1st. Katrina told us later that she had actually written the letter, which was not dated, towards the end of January but that she had had to pluck up the courage to send it. There were several items of mail that day and I did not notice the letter at first. Recognising the writing immediately, I was apprehensive at what it might say, therefore took it into another room to read, so that, depending on the contents, I would have time to decide how to tell Kay. It read,

"Dear Dad,

I've written you so many letters in the past year but none as hard as this one.

I've realised I was mistaken about you. All I can say is I'm so sorry. I don't know how I could ever have believed you could have hurt me so much. The things I accused you of are unforgivable. I'm sorry for putting you and Mum through hell this past year. I wasn't deliberately lying Dad, I genuinely did believe my memories and I don't have an explanation for my memories. Maybe I did put you in to protect me from Grandad. He did abuse me, he was violent to me and all I can say is you turned into an abuser too.

I know none of this makes real sense Dad. I can't explain it myself. All I know is I've come to my senses and again I'm so sorry for hurting you the way I have. I hope to see you soon but I'll understand if you don't want to.

Lots of love

Katrina.

I read it several times and went through the entire gamut of emotions from extreme sadness to exhilaration. As I read, the tears welled up and then started to run down my face. Not wanting Kay to see me crying, I went into the bathroom, just as she called to ask what had been in the mail. It took a few minutes to compose myself enough to take the letter to her but she could see in my face, what she took to be distress, when in fact, by that time I was feeling excited, delighted and bursting to share the news with her. She quickly took the letter and there was a look of sheer joy on her face when she read it. We hugged each other speaking over the top of each other in our eagerness to discuss what it meant. This was a major breakthrough and the best news we had received since Katrina went into hospital, more encouraging even, than her decision to drop her allegations to the police. It was not to last unfortunately and we had many episodes of heartache to go through, but we were not to know that then and for the moment, we simply revelled in our own expectations of the end of the nightmare.

We called the hospital but were told Katrina was asleep and it would be best not to waken her but left a message, asking that she be told we had called and that we would call back later. We found we were unable to speak to any of the family until later that night and share the good news, but were still unable to speak to Katrina because she was "unavailable" when we called back. Sharon did manage to speak to her however, and we learned that Katrina wanted to see me, but not at the hospital. She wanted to come to the house but there was going to be opposition from Yellowlees and his team. There was another problem, however, that was to postpone the meeting for some three weeks. I took pneumonia and pleurisy, which also prevented me from having a further meeting with Bridgeford from the Social Work Department and Bruce Crawford, the SNP leader of the local Perth & Kinross Council, Bridgeford's employer.

After the meeting with Napier and Bridgeford the previous December, I had asked for a further meeting. I was determined to find out why the Social Work Department had become involved in the first place. It was important to determine the chain of events because my intention to sue Yellowlees and the Health Trust necessitated the gathering of evidence that he had been instrumental in bringing in both the police and the Social Work Department. Sharon had told us what had happened, that Yellowlees had arranged the meeting between Sharon and Powrie and that Powrie had brought in Napier from the Child Protection Unit. From that time, the involvement of the police was inevitable. Our limited experience of Yellowlees however, had convinced us that he would lie until hell froze over, therefore we needed to get us much information as we could possibly get.

Two weeks into January 1996 and three weeks after the initial meeting with Bridgeford and Napier, despite several telephone calls, there had been no response; the telephone calls were not even returned. Napier had said absolutely nothing and Bridgeford had spun a story so ridiculous, it simply made us all the more determined to pursue the truth. The leader of Perth & Kinross Council was a councillor called Bruce Crawford. He was the leader of the Scottish National Party (SNP) which was the largest party in the council, which in turn, made him the Council leader. When I had contested the parliamentary seat of Perth & Kinross in 1987 for the SNP, Bruce Crawford was the chairman of one of the local SNP branches in the constituency, a councillor for his local ward, although without any position in the Council, and one of the most important people in the election team that fought the general election on my behalf. I had known him well for over fifteen years.

Crawford agreed to meet me in the third week of January and accompanied by Kay and Sharon, I gave him the details of Katrina's illness, the police investigation and the involvement of the SWD. Both Sharon and I gave him details of our discussions with Bridgeford, while Sharon was able to give him a great deal more information about Napier's involvement.

"I can't give you any of the names of the men Katrina accused Bruce because it would be unfair, but there were seventeen in total and two of the most important names were SNP MPs, well known to all of us." I said.

"I can hardly believe it," said Crawford, "But I have heard nothing about it."

"Is there any reason you would have heard about it?" I asked.

"No, no, I'm just saying I haven't heard, that's all," he muttered.

"You will appreciate the importance of finding out who it is Bruce because if there has been a councillor involved, who gave Bridgeford instructions to find out how the police investigation was going, there must have been a breach of confidentiality. If there was a breach, we need to know where it came from," I finished.

"The other thing you will appreciate Bruce," said Sharon, "Bridgeford had no right to find out anything on behalf of any councillor because no councillor has any right to know what is going on if there is a social work inquiry. Do they?" she said, looking directly at him.

"NO, no they don't," he said hurriedly.

As the story unfolded, Crawford had begun to look more and more uncomfortable, moving about in his chair, clenching and unclenching his hands and looking everywhere in the room except at whoever was speaking. He simply refused to make eye contact. Sharon had picked up on it, which is why she had been so direct in her last comment. We were midway through our explanation of what had happened and of why we thought it was important to find out who the SNP councillor was, if one existed, and how he/she had found out. Suddenly Crawford said,

"Maybe I can throw some light on this," he said.

"What do you mean?" we all said at once.

"I seem to remember meeting Betty Bridgeford at a social function, just before the control of the Social Work Department was transferred from the Region to the District Council. I had never met her before and I was going to have to work with her for the first time," he said.

"What does that have to do with Katrina's situation?" I asked.

"I have no idea but I told her I hoped the District would not inherit cases from the Region." he replied.

"Do you appreciate how important it is that Katrina and the family were told by Napier that this SNP councillor was making inquiries on my behalf. And that was held to be proof there was a paedophile ring with the majority of its members in the SNP. Have you any idea how important that claim became to Katrina and the family?" I pushed

"Oh yes," he said.

"So, how does your conversation with Bridgeford at a social function have any bearing on her claim to have been ***instructed*** by a SNP councillor to find out from the police, what was going on?" I pushed again.

"I have no idea," he said.

"In that case, we need to have another meeting with Bridgeford. Will you arrange it?" I asked him, although I made it sound very much like a demand.

"OK," he said, "I will be in touch after I speak to her tomorrow."

As soon as we left the meeting, Kay beat both Sharon and I by a whisker when she said,

"He is lying through his teeth. He knows a hell of a lot more about this than he admitted in there."

"There is no doubt about that," said Sharon, "Did you see him fidgeting? He could hardly sit still for a minute. All that nonsense about the meeting at the social function. He is as big a liar as Bridgeford."

It was to be several weeks before we could verify whether or not Crawford was being honest with us but he did manage to arrange a meeting with Bridgeford for February 7th. Unfortunately the week that Katrina's letter arrived, I attempted to work through a bad dose of influenza, not the "man flu"' beloved of female writers of fiction, but the real McCoy. The day before the meeting with Bridgeford, I barely made it home to Crieff before collapsing straight into bed. Kay could see I was ill and called the doctor, who diagnosed double pneumonia and pleurisy. For the past three months since the confrontation, the level of stress and hours I had been working had finally taken their toll. I was kept at home where Kay nursed me round the clock for the first few days, during which time a combination of drugs and high temperature, ensured I was in a world of my own. I raved like a lunatic half the time and suffered hallucinations and nightmares for the rest. It took a full fortnight before I was able to leave my bed.

Sharon and Philip went to the meeting with Bridgeford and Crawford, where they were subjected to another version of Bridgeford's fairy tale. She started by telling them that the girl who had contacted the councillor to express her concern about Katrina's health was Alison's step-sister.

"There is a relative of your father, who is currently training in the Social Work Department and her step-sister approached the SNP councillor to ask him to inquire about Katrina's health," said Bridgeford.

"What is the relative of my father called?" asked Sharon.

"Alison Fairlie," answered Bridgeford.

Sharon and Philip looked at each other but said nothing. Instead, Philip asked,

"What is the step-sister's name?"

"I don't have her name but I know she is related to Alison, who is related to your father," said Bridgeford.

"Why would Napier tell Sharon that the councillor was making inquiries on my father's behalf, if the original request for information came from a female relative?" asked Philip.

"Well I think that would be fairly obvious," said Bridgeford, "a relative of your father's making inquiries is pretty suspicious don't you think?"

"The problem is," said Sharon, "Napier made no mention of the inquiry coming from a relative of my father's. He said the inquiry came through a SNP councillor and then made the connection to my father, which was very damning as far as we were concerned at the time. Did Napier know the original inquiry came from a relative of my father? Did you tell him, because his instruction to ask the police came from you?" asked Sharon looking straight at Bridgeford.

Both Philip and Sharon had been watching Crawford who had said nothing, except muttering several times throughout the meeting and shaking his head,

"There has been a terrible mistake, there has been a terrible mistake."

But before they could say anything to him, Bridgeford sat back in her chair and said,

"I don't think we can take this any further…" but before she could say any more Philip interrupted her and said,

"Alison Fairlie does not have a step-sister, so where did this latest story come from?"

Although taken aback at being contradicted, Bridgeford said quickly, "I can assure you she does have a step-sister. Alison is currently training in my department and.."

Before she could get any further, Philip again interrupted her,

"Alison Fairlie is not a relative of my father.."

This time Bridgeford interrupted,

"Yes she is, her name is Alison Fairlie.."

"That is because she is my wife, not because she is a relative of my father," said Philip, "and I can assure you she does not have a step-sister. So, who is this mysterious girl who keeps cropping up in your version of events? You told my father she was a friend of Katrina's. You told Sharon, she was a friend of a friend of Katrina's. Now you are telling us she is my wife's step-sister. So, if she exists at all who is she and where does she fit in?"

Both Bridgeford and Crawford sat stunned by Philip's outburst. Bridgeford was the first to recover and said,

"Obviously there has been a mistake and certain assumptions have been made."

"What is the name of the councillor who made the original inquiry of you," Sharon asked Bridgeford. "It is perfectly obvious that this mysterious girl does not exist, other than in your imagination for the purpose of this nonsense of a story you have been giving us."

"I can't tell you that," said Bridgeford.

"Do you know who it is Bruce?" asked Philip.

"I can't tell you either," answered Crawford.

At that point, Sharon and Philip realised that anything else they were told would in all likelihood be more lies and that they were not going to get any more information. As they made preparation to leave and stood up, Crawford uttered the last words he would say. Attempting to introduce some levity to the meeting, although it was obvious he actually wanted to know, he said,

"The SNP members Katrina named Sharon, I don't suppose my name was among them," he said with a slight laugh.

Sharon looked at Philip before she looked back at Crawford and said, stony faced,

"You will be told in time Bruce."

With that they both walked out without another word.

As soon as I was able to get back on my feet for a few hours at a time, Kay made arrangements for Katrina to come to the house to see me. Jim's wife Anne, agreed to bring Katrina to Crieff and the day she came out, I made sure I was showered and shaved as for much of the time I had been ill, my face hadn't seen a razor and after a few days I looked like a man looking through a hedge. When we saw the car draw up at the front of the house, Kay let me go to the door myself so that I was waiting for Anne and Katrina, with the door open by the time they got out of the car. Anne passed me in the porch and left Katrina and me on our own. Neither of us said a word at first, we just stood and hugged. Eventually I told Katrina I loved her and took her into the house to see her mother.

We sat for about two hours and chatted about all sorts of things but did not touch on the allegations or the abuse or anything that was likely to be upsetting. There were two things I did want to find out however. Katrina had mentioned in her letter that she had written several letters to me over the past year but none had been received. She explained she had not posted any of them, that it was part of her therapy to write letters to the family telling them how she felt.

"But how can it help if you don't post them?" I asked.

"I have them all in my diary, the one I have to keep when I write down what is in the flashbacks," she said.

This was the first time Katrina had said what was in the diaries, other than fleeting mentions right at the beginning before she had become so ill that conversation had been reduced to monosyllabic responses to our questions. Neither Kay nor I had seen her in almost a year, therefore we were keen to know what had been happening but were afraid to push too much in case it upset her.

"What do you say in the letters?" Kay asked.

"All sorts of things," Katrina answered, "I write about what was in the flashbacks and sometimes just things I feel."

"A lot of it can't be very pleasant," Kay said.

I looked at her, wondering what she was going to say.

"No it isn't," Katrina said.

"I sometimes write to you in them before…" she hesitated, "before I try to commit suicide" she finished.

Anne, Kay and I all looked shocked and Kay said,

"You don't really want to talk about that Katrina."

"No, I'm all right," said Katrina. "It helps sometimes to talk about it."

Very quietly, I asked her,

"What happened just before Christmas? We got a letter from Yellowlees, telling us it was our fault you had tried to commit suicide but we were given no details about what had happened, other than to say it wasn't serious."

"Is that what they said, it wasn't serious?" asked Katrina. "I was very low and had a session with Charlotte Proctor, the psychologist that I see. I told her I had been thinking about suicide and she told me it was my right to commit suicide if I wanted to but that I should prepare myself first by writing letters to the family. They are in my diary."

"She actually told you that?" asked Kay, the look on her face expressing the horror she obviously felt.

"Yes, she has said it to me a few times," said Katrina.

"How soon after your meeting with Proctor, did you attempt suicide?" Kay asked.

"The next day," answered Katrina.

I was so angry I couldn't speak. I just looked at Kay and Anne. Katrina sat with her eyes down and Kay signed she did not want this conversation to go any further. We suggested that it was probably time Katrina went back to the hospital before she became too tired. After they left, I asked Kay,

"Do you think the psychologist actually said that to her?"

"I don't know what to think," said Kay, "If she did, she has a lot to answer for but I don't know if we can believe Katrina. It may be another of her stories."

"In a way, I hope it is," I said, "But if it is, she is obviously still far from well but if it isn't, the bloody psychologist is more in need of treatment than Katrina is. She must be nuts to tell someone as vulnerable as Katrina it is OK to commit suicide. What if she does it again and Katrina succeeds the next time?"

It suddenly dawned on Kay, the importance of what we had just been told.

"Do you realise," she asked, "that Proctor had her meeting with Katrina just twenty four hours before Katrina tried to hang herself, but Yellowlees wrote to us the next day and blamed us for putting Katrina under pressure to get a second opinion, and that was the reason she had tried to kill herself? If what Katrina said was true, that Proctor has said this to her on more than one occasion, I wonder how many times it was said just before Katrina made the attempt."

"We have to get her away from there Kay, or one of those days she is going to succeed," I said. That would happen much more quickly than we expected but there was another shock yet to come.

A few days later the police finally contacted me to tell me that the copy of Katrina's statement I had asked for was ready for me to pick up. When I arrived at the station, I was shown into the same interview room with the same two WPCs. I was given a copy of handwritten notes, obviously taken by the WPC, when she actually took the statement from Katrina, something she verified when I asked her. As I flicked through them, there were obvious gaps,

"Any reference to other men Katrina named has been removed," I was told. "What you have there, are mainly the accusations made against you."

"That is fine, I have no need of proof of the names of the other men because I know who they are." I said, "but that is not all that seems to be missing."

"There are one or two other items that have been removed but they are unimportant from your point of view", said one of the WPCs. "they were just side notes I made at the time."

I looked at them but it was obvious there were going to be no more details given.

"Is this it finally finished?" I asked. When they nodded I said,

"What about the grey list?"

"What grey list?" at which I looked at them, smiled and said,

"I was in the force, for a short time granted, but you know what I mean."

They both just shrugged but then one of them said,

"I told you the last time that it would have been unlikely you would have been charged because there were too many things that did not add up."

"All that means," I said, "is that there was not enough evidence to charge me. It doesn't keep me off the grey list."

"What do you intend to do now?" she asked.

"I intend to sue both the Health Trust and the local council," I said, proceeding to tell them some of the problems we had faced up to that point, in dealing with both of them, outlining the number of times we had been told a pack of lies.

"It is the fact we can't get anyone to tell us the truth and that some of the lies we have been told are so stupid they are an insult to our intelligence, that makes us so determined to get to the bottom of what really happened. We now know a great deal more about the kind of therapy we think Katrina was given and it is not even pseudo-science. The stuff we are dealing with is no more than junk science, including reports of alien abduction in the USA." They both laughed at that and stood to indicate the meeting was over.

"Before I go," I said, "I was told the last time that Jenny Hogg confirmed Katrina's statement, is that correct? She actually confirmed Katrina was telling the truth, rather than simply witnessed the statement?"

"Obviously she could not confirm what she did not witness," said the WPC, "but those parts she could confirm, yes, she confirmed rather than simply witnessed the statement."

"Thank you," I said, "I just need to have that *confirmed,* you might say."

Both WPCs shook my hand and wished me luck before I left the station, but not for the last time.

On the road home to Crieff, I drew in to the side of the road to read the statement before going home. Before I had read more than three pages I had to leave the car and be sick at the side of the road. I still hadn't shaken off the effects of the pneumonia, was still off work and still on medication. That might have had an effect but what I read, about the things I was supposed to have done, the use of instruments, the violence and the beatings just horrified me. If even a fraction of it had been true – and I knew it did happen in some families – I would have deserved to have been locked up and the key thrown away. But Katrina had given accounts of rape as early as when she was three years old, when children are not supposed to have any memory properly developed. Kay was also accused of having on occasion, brought me the instruments to use.

It was a tale of sickness and depravity that should have been confined to the pages of some horror story but it was the accusations of my own daughter of what her mother and I were supposed to have done to her, from the time she was a small child. Kay has never read the police statement; I wouldn't let her, destroying it shortly after so that the contents would never be seen, even by accident. When I returned home, Kay was obviously curious to know what the statement said and she was given a sanitised version because that is all she needed to know. It was bad enough that I had seen it, that I finally knew what I had been accused of and it made me all the more determined that no quack of a psychiatrist and his half-witted team, no social work director who seemed to be pathologically incapable of telling the truth, were going to be allowed to destroy my life and the lives of my entire family.

CHAPTER FOURTEEN

October 17th 1995 – March 6th 1996

My confinement in the secure unit after the confrontation with Dad and my telephone conversation with Mum the day after, was short lived. I calmed down quite quickly and was allowed back to the general ward, where I discussed what had happened with the other girls Everyone was very supportive but I had vomited some blood and there was some blood in a discharge that had developed. I asked for an interview with Dr O'Shea, to whom I had always found it easy to talk.

"Why did you try to abscond from the unit?" Dr O'Shea asked.

"Because I just want to get away from everything. I can see no future now. My Mum doesn't believe me, my brothers don't believe me and the only person left in my family who still supports me is Sharon. How can I have any future?" I replied.

"You know the staff support you and you really should try to think of the positive things that you can do." replied the Dr. "We are also going to have to concentrate on your eating problems because the blood in your vomit is being caused by the retching. Unless you allow me to examine you, I can't say what is causing the discharge but I can give you some medication that should sort that out."

The following day, I was allowed time out with a member of staff and we decided to spend it in Perth. As we approached the centre of the town, where the main City Hall is situated, I became aware of the streets suddenly becoming very crowded. There were large groups of people walking together in the pedestrian precinct, all wearing identity badges on their jackets and coats, when I suddenly froze, then panicked, stopping dead and grasping the nurse by the arm,

"What is it?" she exclaimed.

"Those people," I said," they are members of the SNP and I am sure I saw a couple of the people who abused me."

"Where are they?" she said quickly, looking around as if she would recognise them.

"They just disappeared among that crowd that walked down the High Street," I said.

"We have to get away from here, back to the hospital."

The hospital lay in the opposite direction from the City Hall, where the SNP were obviously having one of their conferences. As we quickly walked away, the crowds were being left further and further behind and I began to relax, but I was desperate to get back to the hospital, where I knew I would be safe.

"Are you sure you recognised them?" Are you sure they were some of the people who abused you?" the nurse asked.

"I am positive, although I don't know any of their names," I answered.

When we reached the hospital, the nurse immediately reported the incident to Dr Yellowlees, who spoke to me briefly, asking if I was going to be all right.

"I am fine now," I said, "but I was frightened in case any of them saw me," I replied.

"They couldn't have done anything in the street," he said, "but you are safe now."

"But am I ever really going to be safe?" I asked, "What happens when I leave here, who will keep me safe then?"

For the next few days, I stayed in the hospital although Sharon visited me and we discussed Mum and her decision to support Dad.

"Does Mum know how much that upsets me Sharon?"

"Yes, but she is determined that the abuse could never have happened and she told you that she will give you as much support as she can but she is not going to encourage you to believe you were abused by Dad, when she claims it didn't happen." said Sharon.

"But how can she be sure it didn't happen? She wasn't with me twenty four hours a day," I said.

"But you yourself have said you have no memories of Dad abusing you, that you only have the flashbacks to rely on," said Sharon.

"Yes, but Yellowlees is convinced the flashbacks are memories and so are the rest of the staff. They keep telling me they believe me. Why won't my own family believe me?"

Every day was the same as the day before in the ward. The people were the same, the conversations were the same, the staff were the same and my moods were the same. My mind was in a constant turmoil, particularly since the confrontation with my Dad and the statement I made to the police. Dad hadn't been arrested and Sharon told me he was more determined than ever to sue the hospital, although Dr Yellowlees was convinced nothing would come of it and the staff kept telling me not to worry. No matter how much they tried to reassure me, the fear never left me, even when I was in the hospital where I knew Dad could not get near me. The fear was totally irrational but at the time it completely dominated every waking hour.

On October 25th the police asked me to go over the statement again because there were a number of things they felt were unclear. They were particularly unclear about the part played by Mum, the fact I had accused my Mum of giving Dad the instruments to use on me. As the police probed, I became very uncomfortable because as I kept trying to explain to them, all of the "memories" I had of all the abuse my Dad was supposed to have committed, were the product of nightmares and flashbacks. The more they probed the more uncomfortable I became because I felt they did not believe me. They didn't tell me that, they didn't say anything that allowed me to say what they believed, I just became more concerned about the allegations I had made, despite the number of times Dad still appeared in my flashbacks.

After the police left, I went into the ward and lay on the bed, crying quietly until one of the staff came to ask me how I felt. I admitted I was very depressed and was beginning to feel I had made a mistake in speaking to the police. The more I thought of the discussion with them, the more I became convinced they did not believe me. Yellowlees had persuaded Sharon and I it was for the best, but all that it had achieved was the division of the family. Mum did not believe me, the boys did not believe because Andrew had said as much when he spoke to Yellowlees after the confrontation. It now looked as if the police did not believe me either. The loneliness of my position began to hit home as it became clear that only Sharon, out of my whole family, still believed and supported me.

The following day, Yellowlees asked me to go to his room, where he told me that Philip had asked to speak to him. Philip had told him there were a number of issues he wanted to discuss, which might mean Yellowlees would need to tell him about treatment and other information he needed my permission to divulge. I told him he could tell Philip whatever he asked and also told him how uncomfortable I was feeling.

"You are going to feel like this for a while and it is only natural that you should," said Yellowlees. "It took courage to speak to the police but it was necessary for your own protection and for the protection of the grandchildren."

"But it has meant I have lost my family. Sharon is the only one who supports me now." I said.

"Then you have to ask yourself why they would support your father," Yellowlees said. "He abused you. Do you think they are right to support him, even after what he did?"

"No, I don't but it doesn't help me and I can't help how I feel. I am now just so alone."

After Philip spoke to Yellowlees, I asked what Philip had said.

"He covered a lot of old ground and asked many of the same questions that Andrew asked," said Yellowlees.

"Then he doesn't believe me either does he?" I asked.

Yellowlees did not answer that, he told me to try to relax and forget what the boys were saying.

The short talk with Yellowlees decided me to speak to the police again and withdraw my statement. I had been given the telephone number when they came to the hospital to see me, and was told to call them at any time. When I was put through to WPC Anderson, who had taken my original statement and had come to see me a few days earlier, I told her I wanted to withdraw my statement.

"I want to withdraw the allegations against my father," I said. "I think I made a mistake in speaking to you."

"What do you mean you made a mistake? Are you saying your father didn't rape and abuse you?" WPC Anderson asked.

I wasn't sure how to answer that because I still believed he had, and that was not why I was withdrawing the statement.

"No, I just think it would be better if I withdrew the statement," I said.

"Have you discussed this with the doctor?" I was asked.

"No, I just want to do it. I can withdraw it, can't I?" I asked.

"Yes, it is up to you but I want to be sure you have not been put under any pressure to withdraw the statement. Have you?" WPC Anderson asked sharply.

"No, I haven't but I am not happy and I haven't been happy since I spoke to you," I replied.

"You are perfectly free to withdraw the statement, but I will speak to the doctor before I make it official," said WPC Anderson finally.

As soon as I put down the telephone, I asked to speak to Dr O'Shea, and told her how unhappy I was, that I had withdrawn the police statement but that now I wasn't sure whether I had done the right thing. I desperately wanted and needed reassurance but all Dr O'Shea said was, "I can't tell you whether or not you did the right thing. But it is important you always remember that whatever decision you take, the doctors and staff will support you and help you all we can."

That didn't help much. It was not what I wanted to hear.

"It won't matter I have dropped the statement, Dad is still going to sue the hospital." I said.

"That has nothing to do with you and it won't affect you," Dr O'Shea said.

"Yes it will," I replied, "It must affect me. It is because of me he is suing the hospital. It must affect me."

"I think you should speak to the duty staff just now Katrina. I will ask for stronger medication to calm you down."

"Do you have a pill that will make all of this go away?" I asked.

Two days later, I had been so upset after speaking to the police, I decided to go and face Dad at his office. I was not supposed to leave the hospital but no one saw me sneak out and walk down the hill to his office. I knew the receptionist and spent a short time speaking to her when she told me Dad wasn't in and wasn't expected back for some time. I was angry that he was out, so angry I walked round the corner to the chemist and bought a bottle of paracetamol. After swallowing the entire contents of the bottle, an estimated 50 tablets, I called the hospital and spoke to Jenny Hogg. I still have no idea why I did it, whether I was getting back at Dad, or the hospital or Jenny Hogg who had cancelled our appointment that morning. The staff found me sitting at the side of the road and took me to casualty at PRI, where they pumped my stomach. Released a short time later, I was sectioned after being returned to Gilgal.

I was absolutely determined to face Dad and despite being under observation the whole time, I managed to sneak away again, about two days later. This time I was successful and managed to confront Dad again. The receptionist had been on the telephone when I went in to the front office so I didn't bother to wait, I simply walked past her and into Dad's office. He was alone and looked astounded to see me, asking why I had come to see him.

"Why did you do it Dad? Why did you abuse me?"

Dad barely moved behind his desk and muttered something about his knowing I thought he had abused me, but he then assured me he hadn't. I desperately wanted him to admit it to me because I was still getting the flashbacks, I still saw the images. If he didn't do it, I thought I must be losing my mind. We were alone, without witnesses; he could have admitted it and then denied it later but I needed him to admit it to me, just to me.

He didn't, instead I remember him lifting the telephone and speaking into it briefly. I could feel myself beginning to go into a flashback and tried to remember the things I was supposed to do to cope. I remember I began to see fairies, the black ones that frightened me and I started to look for a way out. I just needed to get away now. Suddenly the door opened and Sharon came in, as I started to rise from my seat. I don't remember saying anything, just Sharon taking me by the arm and leading me from the office to her car. I cried all the way to the hospital where I was immediately taken to the secure unit and locked in.

The whole of November and much of the early part of December was almost a complete blur. I know I had begun to self harm quite seriously, cutting my arms and on occasion my face. A large part of this period, I spent locked up in the secure unit because I persisted in walking away from the hospital grounds. I didn't feel safe when by myself and repeatedly told the doctors how suicidal I felt. On one occasion I caused real panic among the staff when I ran away up to the top of Kinnoull Hill. I don't honestly know if I would have thrown myself over the cliff because I was caught before I got to the top. Fortunately another patient had seen me going in that direction and told the duty staff who raised the alarm. Dr O'Shea spent a great deal of time talking to me, encouraging me to rely on the staff and much of the time, I felt very comfortable with her.

Sharon continued to take me to her house for weekend passes and sometimes, I had flashbacks that were so serious that she and Neil had to take me back to Gilgal early. I have no idea how they coped with me or how they had the patience to put up with it. We were all very concerned that Euan and Craig did not witness the flashbacks, which posed serious difficulties on occasion because they could come on quickly and without warning. I realise I clung to Sharon, becoming far more dependent on her than I should have been but she was my only support at that time. Mum telephoned every week but there were times I didn't want to speak to her, because she supported Dad. The boys were the same so I didn't feel I wanted to speak to them either.

Mum asked to come to the hospital to see me about the middle of December and, as I had been feeling much better for a few days, I agreed. It was an awkward visit because I asked Mum if Dad still intended to sue the hospital.

"Is Dad still going to sue the hospital Mum? Even after I have dropped the statement to the police?"

"He is more determined than ever to sue Katrina, and what difference does it make whether or not you made a statement to the police? Your Dad thinks the hospital have to be made to justify what they did and the only way to do that is to sue."

"Is he still going to take me to court?" I asked. Mum just looked at me, the astonishment written all over her face.

"Where in Heavens name did you get that idea? Your Dad never had any intention of taking you to court." Mum said.

"I don't know," I muttered. "It was something Yellowlees said about Dad not being able to sue him and the only person he could sue would be me."

"That is complete nonsense," said Mum, "We don't blame you for what has happened. There is only one person to blame for what happened and that is Yellowlees. We are going after the Social Work Department as well because of what they did to the rest of the family, but Yellowlees is responsible for what happened to you."

In fact, she told me now that they had more information about the type of treatment they thought I had been given, Dad was more determined than ever. I became quite upset at this because I had hoped it would all go away once I had dropped the police statement.

"Mum, why can't Dad just let it drop? Nothing is going to happen to him now because the police statement has been withdrawn and it means everyone is going to know what has happened," I said.

Mum looked at me, taking my hand and said,

What happened to your Dad Katrina, is the worst thing that can happen to a man. It is the worst accusation you can possibly make of a man. Your Dad needs to clear his name because he is determined it does not go on to the grey list of suspected paedophiles. Do you understand that?"

"What is the grey list?" I asked.

"It is the list of men the police suspect of being paedophiles, but they don't have enough evidence to prove it. Your Dad could not live with that suspicion hanging over his head."

I became even more upset and said,

"I caused all of this. I accused Dad but Mum, I still see him abusing me in the flashbacks and I have to keep telling myself it is not true."

"You did not cause it Katrina," Mum said, "We still don't know what happened but we are determined to find out."

Mum also told me Andrew and Philip had spoken to Yellowlees and they weren't happy with the answers they had been given.

"Andrew and Philip have both spoken to Yellowlees and they are convinced he has not told them the truth, that there is more to what happened than they have been told." Mum said.

"Yellowlees told me he had spoken to Andrew and that Andrew did not believe me," I said. "The only person who now supports me is Sharon."

"That is not true Katrina." said Mum quickly and firmly. "We all support you, even your Dad supports you but we know the abuse did not happen. We would like you to see another doctor to try and explain what has happened. There is something far wrong but we need to find someone else to tell us what it is."

I told both Dr O'Shea and Yellowlees about the meeting, that it upset me and that I didn't want a second opinion. The last thing I wanted was to go over all the old ground about abuse with someone I had never met and who didn't know me. The flashbacks continued, as did the self-harming and the suicidal feelings so I felt pretty miserable for a great deal of the time during this period, just before Christmas, to which I was definitely not looking forward. For some time, I had been working with a psychologist called Charlotte Proctor. I didn't like her much because I was supposed to do disclosure work with her, which meant discussing the abuse endlessly, which was supposed to help me but simply kept reminding me of what had happened. The original abuse by my grandfather was never discussed, it was all about Dad and the contents of the flashbacks.

During one of the sessions with Proctor I was feeling particularly low and suicidal. I could not see any hope of things improving and told her.

"You know Katrina," she said, "It is your right to commit suicide if you feel that is the only solution. But you should prepare properly and write letters to your family."

"What good would that do?" I asked.

"It would make you think about what you were doing and it would explain to your family why you did it," she said.

We prepared the letters together in my diary. I wrote one each to Mum and Dad and Sharon, trying to put my thoughts together about why I could see no end to the torment I was going through, why I was sure it would be best for everyone if I ended my life. When I returned to the ward, the staff could see I was upset and when I asked for extra medication, it was given without question. The following morning I felt very low and when one of the duty staff left the ward, I went into my room and tried to hang myself from the wardrobe door, using the cord from my dressing gown.

When I regained consciousness, two of the staff were standing over me, trying to bring me round. I have no idea how they found me before I was successful but the attempt cost me my freedom again, as I was locked up in the secure unit for a few days. Between that attempt and Christmas, I had sessions with Drs Yellowlees, O'Shea and Proctor, but nothing was resolved because nothing could be resolved. I continued to vomit, sometimes several times a day and was eating very little so my weight began to plummet, which caused the staff further concern.

"Katrina if you continue to force yourself to be sick, you are going to damage your throat and stomach lining permanently," Dr O'Shea told me.

"I don't make myself vomit all the time," I said, "sometimes It just happens."

"But that is because you force yourself at other times," she said, "Why do you want to keep your weight down?"

"Because I think I am too fat," I said.

"How heavy do you think you are?" she asked.

"Nine stone," I answered.

"Do you realise that when we weighed you last week, you were only seven and a half stone?" she asked.

"Then that is fine," I answered," because that is the weight I want to be."

"Why?" Dr O'Shea asked, "What is so special about being seven and a half stone?"

"Nothing," I said, "but the more weight I lose, the sooner I'll die."

As I was under one to one observation for such long periods, there were no further attempts to commit suicide but I talked about it to all three doctors at different times. Dr O'Shea tried to make me realise how upsetting it would be not only to the family, but also to those who had nursed and looked after me. Reluctantly, they allowed me to spend Christmas with Sharon and Neil and the boys. I spoke to Mum on the telephone and to Dad for just a few minutes but the only family members I saw were Sharon, Neil and the boys. The few days I did spend with them were fine but as soon as I returned to the hospital, the depressive moods set in very quickly.

After New Year, Yellowlees told me that a meeting had been arranged between him and Dad. He said Dad wanted to have his solicitor present and that a date had been set for January 11th. I called Sharon to find out what was happening.

"Dad has been told that Yellowlees, the lawyer for the hospital and the clinical director, are all going to meet Dad and his solicitor but he wants me to go as well," said Sharon. "Dad wanted to have the meeting recorded but the hospital wouldn't agree," she continued.

"Why would Dad want to do that?" I asked, taken aback.

"Because he thinks Yellowlees lied to him and he doesn't trust him," said Sharon. "He says it is the only way to be sure of being able to prove what Yellowlees says at the meeting."

I could understand Dad's anger at the hospital and Yellowlees, but I found it embarrassing that he kept pushing to have his lawyers involved. I kept asking Sharon what was happening but she just kept telling me that nothing was happening until the meeting took place on January 11th. She had started to suggest it was possible I had imposed Dad into my flashbacks as a protector, and that in the confused state of mind I was in, he had suddenly become the abuser. I told Yellowlees about it but he simply dismissed it as nonsense. As the arranged meeting drew nearer, I became more up tight and unsettled. Two days before the date of the meeting, that is on January 9th, I was sent to the enclosed unit, without explanation, other than being told I was to remain there until after the meeting. On the afternoon of January 11th I asked what had happened at the meeting, only to be told it had been cancelled. When I protested to the staff about being kept in the secure unit, I was told it had nothing to do with them, that I would have to speak to Yellowlees. I was not released back to the ward until January 13th but received no explanation for having been held there.

"Sharon, why was the meeting cancelled?" I asked. Sharon had come up to see me after my release from the unit.

"I have no idea but Mum and Dad are livid because the meeting was cancelled at the last minute. Dad is convinced the hospital have too much to hide to allow him to have a meeting with Yellowlees." said Sharon. "Why were you put to the unit?" she asked.

"I don't know, I was just told it was in my interest and that I would be kept there until after the meeting," I replied.

"Were you having flashbacks and nightmares that were any worse? Did you try to run away again?" Sharon asked, looking at me accusingly.

"No," I said heatedly, "I hadn't done anything since I saw Dad at his office. But the flashbacks and nightmares are always there. I hate the idea of Dad taking the hospital to court."

"I think he is right to sue them Katrina," said Sharon for the first time. "They are obviously trying to hide something and you should not still be having flashbacks after all this time."

Sharon's change of attitude upset me because it looked as if I was losing her support as well.

"Don't you believe me?" I asked.

Sharon looked away and said,

"It is not about whether or not I believe you. We are all just desperate to see you get well."

Several days after Sharon's visit, I decided to write to Dad. I had written several letters to him and Mum but just in my diary. This time I intended to post it in the hope he would forgive me. The pressure from Sharon and the family to see another doctor, the flashbacks and the staff telling me they believed that I had been abused, left me utterly confused. I had no idea if I had actually been abused by Dad but the flashbacks and nightmares said I had been. Yellowlees and the staff believed I had been and the conflict between the two tore me apart. I was prepared to do anything to bring it to an end. I was genuinely deeply sorry for what I had done to Dad and just wanted things to go back to what they had been before I became ill. It took another week before I picked up the courage to post it.

Sharon told me Mum and Dad had been delighted to receive the letter and had tried to telephone me but that I had been asleep.

"What did Dad say?" I asked, "Does he blame me for this?"

"No," said Sharon, "he doesn't blame you. Neither Mum nor Dad has ever blamed you and you are going to have to accept that Katrina. Try to put it behind you now."

"That is a lot easier said than done," I replied. "I want to see Dad now. Do you think he will see me?"

"Yes he will see you but when he came home from work on Friday, he collapsed. He has pleurisy and pneumonia and I haven't seen him but Mum says he is very ill just now. You will have to wait."

When I told Yellowlees I had written to Dad and wanted to go and see him, he was not pleased.

"I don't think that would be a good idea Katrina. You are rushing things too quickly," he said.

"I need to see him but he is ill just now and I won't be able to see him for another week or so." I said.

"That will give you time to think about things a bit more. He is still appearing in all your flashbacks, which have been more serious than ever, since the beginning of January," said Yellowlees. What did you say in your letter?"

"I told him I was sorry for accusing him and asked him to forgive me," I replied.

Yellowlees looked at me closely and asked,

"Why would you apologise to him, after what he did to you?" he asked. "I am also very unhappy about the pressure your family appear to be putting you under, especially at this time when you have been having such severe flashbacks, all of them with your father in them."

"I have lost my family because I have accused Dad and I want them back. I am not going to see another doctor but I need my family back. I also want my Dad and as soon as he is better, I am going to see him." I replied and Yellowlees said nothing more.

When Ann collected me at the hospital to go and see Dad, I was feeling sick with nerves.

"Do you think he will speak to me Ann?" I asked.

"Of course he will speak to you," said Ann, laughing as she looked across at me. "Your Mum and Dad are desperate to see you, particularly since you wrote to your Dad."

"I just hope everything will be OK," I said, "but I am really nervous because I don't know what I am going to say to him."

After a few minutes of driving in silence, Ann asked,

"What are you hoping for when you see your Dad?"

I thought for a minute before answering,

"I just want him to give me a hug. I have really missed him but I'm so scared that something will go wrong or I say the wrong thing. I told him in the letter that I couldn't explain why I accused him and I still don't know why. I just hope he understands."

"I don't know that any of us understand Katrina but I do know your Dad doesn't blame you and wants to see you as much as you want to see him."

The first meeting with Dad for almost ten months and after everything that had happened, went as well as I could have hoped for. Ann left me at the porch with him and he gave me a long hug before we both went in to the house. That very obvious show of his love said a great deal more to me than anything he might have said. As children, we were always used to being hugged by Dad and it was that closeness that I had missed so much while in hospital. The two hours we spent talking seemed to pass in a flash, with the only sour note being struck when I told them about Charlotte Proctor and my attempted suicide. It was obvious that all three of them were astonished that Proctor should have told me it was my right to commit suicide, but I was not going to allow that to spoil what had been a wonderful meeting for me.

Unfortunately, the feelings of euphoria were not to last. Within a few days I was experiencing the same flashbacks and nightmares, with the result the feelings of despair returned as did my depression. The lower my mood became, the more flashbacks I experienced, some of them very severe. After another two weeks of swinging between the depths of despair and levels of normality I hadn't felt in months, I finally decided I had had enough. I made up my mind that if I was going to get better, I had to get away from the environment of the hospital, the constant contact with people who did nothing else but speak about sexual abuse. I had to fight to get away from Gilgal, to go back to live with my parents. Within a few weeks, they were having to fight to have me re-admitted. They were about to have to endure another twelve months of nightmare that must have felt as if it was never going to end.

CHAPTER FIFTEEN

PROFESSIONAL ARROGANCE AND BUREAUCRATIC INDIFFERENCE
March 6th 1996 – December 1996

The year 1996 will be forever burned into the memories of Katrina, Kay and I in particular but the family in general because during that period we were pushed to the very limit of our endurance in both physical and emotional terms. This is the year we spent going through the absolute farce of the internal inquiries conducted by Perth & Kinross Council and Perth & Kinross Healthcare NHS Trust, while we desperately looked for help in dealing with Katrina's deteriorating health. Such was the degree to which her mental health had been damaged, I could not be on my own with her in the same room, or in the car, in case she had another flashback which included me, which the Health Trust and Social Work Department could then use as "evidence" that abuse could have taken place. If the opportunity to commit abuse never arose, it could never be said it happened, therefore I was never in Katrina's company under any circumstances, without another member of the family being present. Naturally, she found this very hurtful. But we were to find that even the presence of independent witnesses, was not enough to persuade some of the more idiotic of the psychiatric staff, that abuse could not have taken place.

But there was another aspect of family life which was sullied and debauched as a consequence of the determination of both the Health Trust and Social Work Department to continue to maintain they were right in what they did. After Christmas 1995, Kay and I began to see the grandchildren more often. It is impossible to explain the sheer delight of hearing the sound of their feet scampering to meet us at the door, or their squeals of excitement at the prospect of being with us. However I refused to be in a room on my own with them and I particularly watched how they sat on my knee. Whereas before, they had been used to the rough and tumble of wrestling with me and climbing all over me, I now became ultra careful about how that could be interpreted. I never took them to the toilet, nor saw them in their bath or without their clothes on while undressing for bed. I would not even help them into their costumes when we went swimming and the innocence of a normal relationship between a grandfather and his grandchildren had been destroyed for ever.

It was brought home to our own children, the first time we were asked to babysit by Philip and Alison, who lived in Perth, about seventeen miles from where Kay and I lived in Crieff. They were still getting ready to go out when we arrived, so Kay and I put the three children to bed and read them their customary story, by which time Philip and Alison were ready to leave. When I put my jacket on, Philip asked,

"Are you going out for something?" He had no idea I was going home.

"No," I replied, "I am going home."

"Are you not staying with Mum?" he asked, surprised.

"No, it would be better if I go home and come back later," I replied.

He and Alison looked at each other as it dawned on them what was happening. Both were acutely embarrassed.

"You don't have to do that," said Alison, "you can't drive all the way back to Crieff and come back again. It's not right."

"I am not going to put myself in a position where it can ever be said I had an opportunity to commit abuse," I said, feeling the anger mounting.

"But we don't think you're an abuser," said Alison, looking desperately at Philip, who joined in the protest by saying,

"Come on Dad, this is daft. You can't go home."

"I'm sorry son," I replied shaking my head, "It doesn't matter what you think. You have to remember your Mum was accused of helping me to abuse Katrina and there is no way I am going to give them any opportunity of suggesting abuse was a possibility. Until we get this settled, I am afraid this is how it is going to have to be."

Alison and Philip accepted the logic of what I said, while objecting strongly to the practical application of it.

After the meeting with Katrina, she had had another two or three weeks back on the rollercoaster that had been her life since first going into Gilgal in December 1994. By the beginning of March she had had enough and on March 6th 1996, she discharged herself from Gilgal *Against Medical Advice.* The discharge letter from Dr Yellowlees said that Katrina was suffering from

1. Severe Complex Post Traumatic Stress Disorder relating to long standing physical and sexual abuse
2. Dissociation Disorder relating to the above
3. Episodes of Depression with accompanying suicidal ideation
4. Eating Disorder of Anorexia Nervosa type.

Katrina had gone into hospital fifteen months previously with none of those disorders and suffering from no more than withdrawal symptoms of coming off drugs which she had been prescribed by the medical team at the PRI, after undergoing two abdominal operations neither of which had been necessary, according to the medical staff. Yellowlees and his team were repeatedly asked to explain what had happened to Katrina, during her fifteen months under his care, that would account for such a severe deterioration in her mental health. The great problem we faced was that according to Yellowlees, Katrina's health had improved and she was actually better than she had been when she went in, despite the rather inconvenient fact she now believed she had been raped and abused by a total of seventeen different men, some of whom she had never met, over a period of some twenty years. She was also convinced she had witnessed the rape and murder of her six year old friend, whose identity was unknown. Katrina moved into our house in Crieff for the first few weeks, before moving into her own flat. Neither move was a success and we went through months of sheer hell. At the same time, we had to deal with the Health Trust and the Social Work Department.

After Sharon and Philip had met with Bridgeford and Crawford, I questioned them about what had been said. We had to laugh at the stupidity of Bridgeford to come up with yet another version of events, leading to her instructing Napier, the Head of Child Protection, to question the police.

"What was Crawford's attitude?" I asked.

They had both known Crawford for several years because of our involvement with the SNP and had always been on friendly terms with him. For that reason, there was no reason for personal hostility and none was shown by either side, therefore he should have felt perfectly relaxed.

"He was like a cat on hot bricks," said Philip and Sharon just laughed.

"It was quite funny watching him," she said, "there was obviously something bothering him right from the start. He was very uncomfortable being there," she said.

"He was a damn site worse when I pointed out Alison was my wife," said Philip, "both Bridgeford and him could have died. He just kept muttering, "There's been a terrible mistake.""

"He didn't give you any indication who the councillor was?" I asked curiously.

"No, he admitted he knew who it was but refused to tell us," Philip said.

"That is the bit that makes no sense to me," said Sharon, "What difference does it make to them if we know who it was. We only want to find out why he wanted to know if you were under investigation Dad, and more importantly, how he found out?"

"It makes no sense to me either," I said shaking my head.

The obvious answer did not strike any of us.

It annoyed me that I had been unable to attend the meeting because there were still a number of issues I needed to clear with Bridgeford. For a start, I wanted an assurance there was no file kept on me. In the absence of any further contact from Bridgeford, I pushed Crawford for another meeting and eventually on April 17th a letter arrived from Bridgeford, dated the day before, April 16th. It had taken three goes at Crawford and ten weeks to get Bridgeford to respond. It is important that the full text is given of both the letters from Bridgeford and my reply, for reasons that will become obvious. Bridgeford's letter read as follows;

Dear Mr Fairlie

I write in response to concerns raised by you regarding an enquiry carried out by members of Tayside Region's Social Work Department into allegations of sexual abuse in 1994. As you will be aware, at that time, information was conveyed to this Department by an adult member of your family indicating they had been sexually abused by you as a child. This information inevitably raised questions as to the possible safety and well-being of other children who are currently members of your extended family. Under Section 37 of the Social Work (Scotland) Act 1968, as amended by Section 85 of the Children Act 1975, Local Authorities have a duty to cause inquiries to be made "where information is received suggesting a child may be in need of compulsory measures of care." (Child Protection Policy, Practise and Procedure – Directors of Social Work in Scotland HMSO 1992) In light of this requirement, preliminary enquiries were conducted by experienced staff into the substance of these allegations. This said, a measured approach was adopted in light of the antiquity of the allegations, and of the absence of any contemporary corroborative information.

In accordance with Departmental procedure, and with the recommendations of Lord Clyde's Report into the Orkney Inquiry, information was shared with police colleagues, and a planned approach was adopted in order to test the information provided – without proceeding to interview any children directly. This decision led to interviews with certain adult members of your extended family regarding the care and protection of their children. These interviews elicited no corroborative concerns regarding these or other children.

In light of these developments, Tayside police decided to take no criminal proceedings, and this Department similarly decided to take no further action. No formal Child Protection Investigation involving interviews with children was conducted. No referral was made to the Reporter to the Children's Hearings. No Child Protection Case Conference was convened in the light of this inquiry. The matter was, and remains closed. On hearing directly that you had concerns about how this situation was handled, I commissioned an independent internal audit into the conduct of the enquiry. I am satisfied that the relevant staff acted in an appropriate manner in the conduct of their duties.

On a quite separate matter, I note your concern regarding the manner in which information concerning this inquiry came to be shared with the Convener of the Council. I regret that this stemmed from certain similarities between those suggestions that had been made regarding your self, and separate allegations of a similar character in a quite different case. Basic information regarding the nature of the allegations was provided, but no names were exchanged in an effort to preserve the principle of confidentiality. Unfortunately, pursuit of this same principle appears to have led to the aforementioned confusion.

Having mistakenly believed that this was a Council enquiry into allegations concerning yourself, information was then sought from relevant Social Work staff in order to respond to the councillor's enquiry. I would wish to give you my assurance that at no time did any member of this Department seek out a Councillor with whom to share this information. I would also wish to affirm that no detail of the above enquiry concerning yourself was shared between myself and the Convener. I do not know exactly who first informed a member of your family that a Councillor had enquired into the conduct of the case concerning yourself. I am able to affirm, however, that it was not a member of this Department.

In conclusion, I would wish to reiterate that there are no ongoing enquiries within this Department, in relation to yourself. I trust that this information will serve to clarify the situation for you, and to allay any outstanding concerns as to the manner in which limited aspects of this enquiry came to be known to a member of the council.

Yours sincerely

Mrs Betty Bridgeford
Director of Social Work.

As an example of bureaucrat-speak, this is a classic. It is also a classic of a bureaucrat attempting to cover her backside, with a mixture of misinformation, half-truths and out and out lies. When Kay and I read it, we could not help but laugh at Bridgeford's effort to impress and intimidate us with the references to Social Work legislation, none of which was in the least relevant. The letter was so transparent and such an obvious con, we were tempted to be insulted but since the woman did not even have the wit to know when she was contradicting herself in the same paragraph, it would have been a waste of time to have pointed it out to her. I replied the next day and the following is an abridged version;

Dear Mrs Bridgeford,

Your letter of 16th inst falls far short of "allaying my fears" and tells me nothing other than that there is no on-going enquiry. I seek clarification of the following;

1. *Mr Napier, a member of your Department, first told my daughter Sharon that he had been instructed by you to ask the police about the progress of the police inquiry on me. He also said you had been approached by a SNP Councillor, whose name he refused to divulge. You claim "no names were exchanged". If that is true, how did you know the Councillor was asking about me? I only ask because you also claim that you and councillor Crawford had a conversation about two different people, allegedly having committed two entirely*

> *different offences, the circumstances of which were entirely different, that you did not exchange names and that you came away from the meeting convinced you were both speaking about the same person, and you thought that person was me.*
> 2. *Can you explain to me what legislation requires that you furnish any Councillor with any information, about any investigation that is being conducted by your Department?*
> 3. *Can you explain what has happened to the mysterious girl, who has had three different identities, first when you spoke to me on December 21st last year, second when you spoke to my daughter Sharon on the same day, and third when you spoke to Sharon and Philip on February 7th this year? This young lady now seems to have disappeared altogether.*

It must now be obvious to you that my family has been given three different versions of the same story by you and another different version, of the same story by Mr Napier, that none of the stories either make sense or stand up to examination. I would now appreciate the truth at your earliest convenience.

Yours etc.

Three weeks later I had still had no reply and contacted the Scottish Office to ask what action I could take. I was informed that the proper procedure would be to contact the Chief Executive of the Perth & Kinross Council to make an official complaint. This I did on May 9th. writing to the Chief Executive, Mr Harry Robertson and enclosing the correspondence relating to the complaint up to that point but pointing out that there was a great deal more to the case than was contained in the correspondence and that I would provide any information requested. The reply to that complaint was dated May 10th. and arrived two days later. It read,

Dear Mr Fairlie,

I am in receipt of your letter of 18th April 1996 and acknowledge its contents. I regret that you appear to find the contents of my earlier communication unsatisfactory. Accordingly, I would offer the following by way of further clarification:-

1. *Towards the end of the summer last year I was advised of the allegations relating to you and your family by Mr Napier. This is standard practice in cases of particular sensitivity, such as those involving enquiries of a delicate and complex nature concerning adults who hold, or have held political office.*
2. *I was subsequently approached by Councillor Bruce Crawford who asked me if a Councillor was under investigation. He did not identify this person by name, and to date I do not know to whom he referred.*
3. *In light of Mr Napier's briefing, I mistakenly took Councillor Crawford to be referring to you and your family, as one of the reasons for my being briefed concerned the former involvement of a member of your family in local politics. I did not mention any names, assuming that we were both talking about the same case. It would not have been appropriate to embark upon more detailed discussion as this might have entailed a breach of confidentiality.*
4. *After this brief discussion, I naturally asked Mr Napier to establish what stage the enquiry had reached. This he did, by contacting colleagues in the Social Work Department and Tayside Police.*
5. *I advised Councillor Crawford at a later date that no Councillor was under investigation. Again, no names were exchanged and he did not indicate whether he had any information to identify the Councillor to whom he had made reference at our earlier meeting.*

I am satisfied that, to the best of my recollection this is a true account of the relevant events.

*If, inadvertently confusing the route of our own enquiry that that of Councillor Crawford I have caused you personal anxiety, I would sincerely apologise. As will now be evident, however, no Councillor made an enquiry specifically naming you or your family. I would regret any possible contribution to this confusion, but would consider it important to stress that, after careful and proper consideration by both police and Social Work Officers, **there was deemed to be insufficient evidence on which to proceed to formal investigation.** (my italics) I consider this a full and satisfactory explanation of my actions. Should you wish to correspond further on this matter, I should be grateful if you could direct any communication to the Director of Law and Administration at 2 High Street, Perth.*

Yours sincerely
Mrs Betty Bridgeford

Kay, Sharon, Philip, Andrew and I all discussed the letter from Bridgeford and not surprisingly, we all came to the same conclusion. The woman was obviously lying but we did not know why. In some ways it was hilarious the lengths to which she and Crawford had gone to hide the name of the Councillor who had approached her and now, she had confirmed it was Crawford. He had sat through two separate meetings with Kay, Sharon, Philip and myself, either refusing to say who the Councillor was or claiming he did not know who it was. Why, why was it necessary for him to do that if a genuine mistake had been made? Why perjure himself in such a stupid fashion? If he had any gumption – which was doubtful – he must have known it would come out eventually, but we had no doubt he would never have thought his fellow conspirator in a pack of stupid lies would be the one to drop him in it.

I had discussed the prospects of succeeding in my case against the Health Trust, with the Court Partner in my own firm but more importantly, I had been provided with material from the most important case to date, which had been settled in the United States. It involved a winery executive in the Napa Valley in California, by the name of Garry Ramona. Ramona's eldest daughter had undergone Recovered Memory Therapy because she had been under stress while at college and the therapist was convinced her concerns and depression were the result of long buried sexual abuse. The girl accused her father of raping her and forcing her to have sex with the family dog.

Garry Ramona had been warned that he would never succeed in bringing a case against the therapist, because it had never been done. If I continued with my intention to sue Yellowlees and the Health Trust, it would be the first case of its kind in the UK, and I had been told exactly the same. The Ramona case hinged on the fact

1. That the therapist had encouraged the daughter to believe her father had raped her.
2. That she should first of all tell her mother and then;
3. Tell the police.

As a consequence, Ramona's wife divorced him, he lost his job, his house and his family. He won his case in court in 1994 and started the movement that alerted America that therapists could be sued successfully.

We discussed Bridgeford's letters in light of the Ramona case.

"We have to be able to prove that Yellowlees involved the Social Workers," I said.

"But we have the proof he did, because he arranged the meeting with Powrie for me," said Sharon.

"Can we prove it?" I asked.

"Well I didn't ask to see her, it was arranged for me," repeated Sharon.

"Will Powrie admit as much though?" I insisted. "Look at Bridgeford's letter where she claims, *"information was conveyed to this Department by an adult member of your family indicating that they had been abused by you as a child."* Who is she talking about? Katrina didn't ask the social workers to become involved and she is the only one claiming I abused her."

"But Yellowlees told the social workers, Sharon knew nothing about the abuse and Powrie had attended ward meetings in Katrina's ward," said Philip.

"Can we prove it?" I asked again. "This is really important and despite the stupidity of Bridgeford's claims, we have to be able to prove the family did not ask the Social Work Department to become involved."

"There is the other point she makes in her second letter *"that there was insufficient evidence etc...."* I said. "There is NO EVIDENCE but that is classic social work modus operandi and it leaves me as a prime target for the grey list, which is what I was afraid of." I said. "There is no evidence other than the so-called professional opinion of Yellowlees and Bridgeford's lies."

"How do you propose we get the proof we need?" asked Philip.

"I don't know yet but the first thing we are going to do is reply to this letter from Bridgeford," I said.

I did that by writing another letter to the Chief Executive of Perth & Kinross Council, Harry Robertson, on May 14th.

Dear Mr Robertson,

You will note that Mrs Bridgeford's latest explanation differs quite radically from her previous attempts and gives a quite contrary explanation from that offered by Councillor Bruce Crawford. Not least among the many curiosities in Mrs Bridgeford's various explanations, is the complete disappearance of the mysterious young lady who was alleged to have made the original enquiry of the equally mysterious SNP Councillor.

You should be aware that there is currently another investigation into the conduct of the Consultant psychiatrist in charge of my daughter's case. He has already admitted lying and we have evidence that his staff made a false statement to the police. The degree of collusion between the hospital and the Social Work Department, therefore has very obvious implications. (this will be covered in the next chapter)

Mrs Bridgeford has not helped the situation by providing a series of explanations which are, to say the least, highly inconsistent. An early resolution to this debacle would be in the interest of all concerned and I look forward to a more satisfactory response than has been provided so far.

Yours etc.

The next letter I received, dated 3rd June, came from the Director of Law and Administration of Perth & Kinross Council, Mr R W Jackson. He repeated the story given to us by Bridgeford, without mention of the mysterious girl, claimed that Crawford and her had become "confused" and expressed his "sincere apologies" for any "personal anxiety" I may have been caused. However, there was a much more important paragraph, which I intended to have cleared up. It read as follows:

"I have noted from the terms of your letter dated 14th May, 1996 that you have stated that there is currently another investigation into the conduct of the consultant psychiatrist in charge of your daughter's case, that he has admitted lying and that you have evidence that his staff made a false statement to the police. You then suggest that there has been a degree of collusion between the hospital and the Social Work Department. As you will be aware these allegations are extremely serious and potentially defamatory and I am not aware of any evidence which would suggest such a conclusion. If you are suggesting that this is a separate issue which requires to be investigated by the council then I will arrange for this to be done on receipt of any relevant evidence."

As soon as I read the letter, I called Jackson's office and surprisingly, he immediately took my call.

"I have just read your letter and would like to meet you to discuss it," I said.

"The only time I can see you over the next fortnight is at 4pm this afternoon," he replied. "If you can't make it then, I have no idea when I can see you."

"Fine I'll be there," I replied.

Without any further conversation Jackson hung up, after which I called both Philip and Sharon. Sharon couldn't make it but Philip could and we agreed to meet at lunch time to discuss the letter's contents and to decide how to approach Jackson.

"I think we will just have to play it by ear," I said, "although his talk of defamation gives us a clue to how he intends to approach things."

"Do you know him?" asked Philip.

Only by reputation," I replied, "and from what I have heard he is a bully who puts the fear of death into the female staff."

"Oh well, it should be interesting," said Philip with a laugh. We had been dealing with his kind since this whole thing started.

Jackson was pleasant enough when we were shown into his office. He introduced himself, shook our hands and offered us a seat but that was where the pleasantries ended. He was a big man, slightly over six feet and heavily built, with black designer stubble and black hair, which he wore on the long side. He had no sooner taken his own seat on the other side of his desk than he started with,

"I want to make it clear from the start that you are not going to come into this office making demands. Am I clear?" His voice had a slight rasp and matched his physique.

Philip and I looked at each other then we both just nodded. I don't know whether Jackson took this as an indication he had already intimidated us but he then continued,

"You are not going to be allowed to make demands, nor am I going to allow you to make accusations about social work staff, for which there is no evidence. Am I clear?"

We nodded again, without saying anything.

"I have spoken to both Mrs Bridgeford and Councillor Crawford and they both say they made a mistake for which they have apologised and as far as I am concerned, the matter is closed."

said Jackson, moving in the chair as if to stand and bring the meeting to a close.

Both Philip and I had been waiting for an opportunity to speak and before Jackson could lever himself up from his seat, I threw a large brown envelope on to his desk and said,

"You may think the matter is closed but we have a number of questions that need to be answered. I came here this afternoon looking to have a civilised conversation, not to be spoken to like a member of your staff or some schoolboy. If you want to continue the way you started, I am quite happy to argue the case with you, but I am determined before I leave here, I am going to have some answers."

Jackson did not appreciate being spoken to like that but then, neither had Philip and I and he certainly did not intimidate us. He looked at us as if he intended making a fight of it, but he settled back down in his chair and said,

"What is it you have to say?"

I picked up the brown envelope and shook out the contents, which was the correspondence that had passed between Bridgeford and me, as well as the letter he had sent that had arrived that morning. Philip had copies of all the correspondence and we had agreed the order in which we intended to tackle this.

"In your letter you talk about defamation. Are you suggesting that my claim that the social workers and the hospital were colluding is defamatory?" I asked.

"That is exactly what I am saying," he said drawing himself up in the chair.

"Why would that be defamatory?" I asked.

"Given the circumstances of this case, that could be potentially defamatory." he replied

"Only potentially defamatory now?" I asked.

Jackson hesitated and looked from Philip to me and then said,

"The claim that the hospital and the Social Work Department were colluding, which means they were acting together in secret, makes it defamatory."

"But they were working in secret, before they eventually told my family," I said.

Jackson looked down at the letters he had on his desk and it was obvious he was struggling. Before he could say anything else, I said,

"Supposing it was defamatory, although that is a nonsense as far as I am concerned, but supposing it was, what would you do about it?"

Jackson immediately looked a bit more comfortable and said,

"I think you should be aware that defamation is actionable and we will pursue it in the court, if necessary,"

"Good," I replied, "whether you sue me, or I sue you, as I fully intend to, this is going to go to court. So we are agreed on that?"

I then asked,

"Can we now discuss the correspondence from Mrs Bridgeford? On the basis of the contents of her letters, that woman is either thick or lying. I happen to think she is both."

I wasn't deliberately trying to get under Jackson's skin but it was clear that I was. His face turned livid but he didn't rise to the jibe. Instead he turned over the letters from Bridgeford and before I said anything, he picked up her first letter and said,

"I don't know that we have to discuss this letter, it is meaningless."

"We are not going to get very far if you persist in trying to dictate what is discussed, because we did not come here to be dictated to," I said, while Philip interjected with,

"Bridgeford's letters are inconsistent and that needs to be explained, not dismissed as being meaningless."

Jackson shifted again in his chair, picked up the letter and looked at it but I doubt if he could see a single word, he was so obviously angry.

"Why do you say it is meaningless?" I asked

"There is too much emphasis on legislation, which I doubt you know anything about," said Jackson.

"Well, that is something you can explain to us, but the first thing we want to know is why the Social Work Department became involved," I said.

"Your daughter asked us to become involved," Jackson answered.

"Which daughter?"

"The one who is in hospital, Katrina."

"No, she didn't, Katrina did not even want her brothers and sister to know."

"Then it must have been your other daughter... I am sorry I don't know her name. I know it was one of your daughters." answered Jackson, who was beginning to look uncomfortable again.

"Her name is Sharon," I said, "but she did not ask to have you involved. The first appointment was made for her with Mrs Powrie, by Yellowlees...."

Jackson interrupted to point to Bridgeford's first letter, where it stated that the information had been "*conveyed to the Department by an adult member of my family*"

"Mrs Bridgeford's letter suggests it was Katrina," he said, "In any case, does it matter why we became involved, or the circumstances of the involvement? In situations where allegations of abuse have been made, we are always involved."

"It matters if the allegations are false, which it is now clear they were. Do you normally just accept the opinions of psychiatrists so readily and without question?" I asked. "So the question still remains, why did you become involved?"

Jackson was obviously struggling to come up with an answer and to keep him on the back foot, I asked,

"Why was I the only person to be investigated?"

"What do you mean?" he asked.

"Katrina accused seventeen men, your Head of Child Protection was convinced there was a major paedophile ring involved, so why were none of the other men investigated?" Philip asked. "Napier even suggested that my brothers and I were also abusers."

Jackson attempted to regain control by asserting strongly,

"You have no idea how many men were investigated, unless you are claiming to have seen social work files."

"We not only know the other men who were named, we know the names of the children they are in contact with on a daily basis. I can assure you not one of them was investigated. Should you not have screened their children, the way you screened my grandchildren?"

"You are not going to tell me how the Social Work Department should do its job," Jackson blustered, getting more annoyed by the minute.

"I have no intention of telling you how the Department should do its job. I am just asking a question," I said, beginning to enjoy myself.

As we had arranged before we went in Philip suddenly intervened, completely changing the line of questioning.

"Who was the girl who first approached Bruce Crawford?" he asked.

"I am sorry, I don't understand. What girl?" said Jackson

"Bridgeford claimed that a girl approached Bruce Crawford and told him she was concerned about Katrina's health. She first told my father that the girl was a friend of Katrina's. She told Sharon on the same day, it was a friend of a friend of Katrina's and then, when she and Crawford met with Sharon and me, she claimed it was Alison Fairlie. So we have had three different versions of who this girl is and you will see from the letters, there is no mention of the girl at all. Can you shed any light on it and tell us who she was?"

It was obvious Jackson did not have a clue what Philip was talking about but we did not make it any easier for him by elaborating further. We just sat in silence until finally he said,

"I am afraid I have no knowledge of that."

"Perhaps you can explain then, under what legislation was Bridgeford obliged to tell Crawford, or any other councillor for that matter, about any on-going investigation, particularly since there is so much emphasis on confidentiality in her second letter?" I pushed.

By this time Jackson's face was puce coloured as he struggled to control his temper. As he hesitated longer than we thought was necessary, both Philip and I said at the same time,

"Well?"

"There is no legislation," he finally answered although we could hardly make it out.

"Then does that mean Bridgeford was lying in her first letter?" I asked.

There was no response so Philip asked again,

"Was she lying?"

There was still no response and Jackson began to shuffle the papers on his desk.

I asked him for a third time and finally he said,

"She was misquoting Council policy."

"Misquoting or lying," I said, "you are confirming there is no obligation to tell any councillor anything...." but by this time Jackson had had enough. When Philip and I had arrived at his office his whole demeanour showed that he had no intention of giving us the time of day but as the meeting had progressed and he became more and more uncomfortable, it was obvious things were not moving quite how he had planned. He stood up and said,

"We will leave things there for the moment but I will have your complaint investigated. It will be done by a lawyer who will contact you when he wants to speak to you."

The meeting was over. Jackson showed us to the door with no attempt to observe the normal courtesies and with no handshake or acknowledgement, we found ourselves in the corridor outside his office, where we burst out laughing. Unfortunately Jackson would have the last laugh.

Having managed to get an agreement that there would be an investigation into the conduct of the Social work Department, we did not intend to let things slip. We all discussed the ramifications of some of the things we had learned from the meeting with Jackson. It had become obvious as the meeting progressed that he did not have all the information and equally obvious he did not expect us to be quite so aggressive. Bridgeford and Crawford apparently had been less than completely truthful in whatever they had told him, which suggested that we could make things even more uncomfortable for them. Having never had experience of dealing with this kind of situation, we had no idea of just how devious public authorities could be when challenged. I thought I knew a bit about the system, and I did know a great deal more than anyone who had never been involved in politics at the level at which I had operated; but I soon found I was a babe in arms compared to those charged with the defence mechanism available to the public sector.

The very next day, June 5th, I wrote to Jackson, listing the points we had discussed and the areas the family wanted examined. They could be summarised as follows:-

1. The reason for the Social Work involvement, given that we had agreed that neither Katrina nor Sharon had asked them to do anything.
2. Why the other seventeen men who were accused, had not been investigated
3. The duty of the Department to report details of any case under investigation, to any Councillor or any other person not connected to the department.
4. The identity of the mysterious girl who, it was claimed, approached Crawford
5. The part played by Powrie and Napier and the latter's claim that I had been using my contacts with the SNP to find out how far the police investigation had gone.
6. The part played by Bridgeford and the very obvious attempt by her to deliberately mislead us.

I emphasised the effect the Department involvement had had on the family and its dynamics, particularly Napier's comments and pointed out that Jackson had not been given all the information available to Bridgeford and Crawford. I also emphasised the impact that Bridgeford's lies had had on Katrina's health and the difficulty that created. Finally I made it very clear that we were aware of the Scottish Office guidelines for the speed with which Councils were required to attend to complaints, and that we expected those guidelines to be adhered to.

Before the end of June I was contacted by a George Harper, a lawyer from the legal department of Perth & Kinross council, who had been given the responsibility of conducting the investigation. We agreed to meet within the next few days, so that I could give him an overview of what had happened. I liked Harper immediately and he was sympathetic to my position.

"It must have put you in a hellish situation and I honestly don't know what I would have done in your position," he said.

"I don't think you would have taken long to make up your mind," I said, "that kind of accusation tends to concentrate your thoughts."

"Well, I have been given the task of looking at your complaint and to do that, I will have to speak to you and the other members of the family who were involved. Do you see any problem with that?" he asked.

"None at all," I answered, "the family will be only too happy to tell you what happened because to date, we have had nothing but a pack of lies and obstruction. Obviously we want to get to the bottom of what happened, particularly the part played by Bridgeford, whose explanation of her discussion with Crawford is risible, to say the least."

"I want to stop you there," he said, "so that I can explain my obligations and my position with regard to this inquiry. My job is to take statements from everyone involved and that includes social work staff. It is not my job to evaluate what is said, merely to report what is said. That report will then be sent to Mr Jackson, Head of Law and Administration and he will decide what is to be done."

The look on my face must have conveyed my feelings because Harper continued,

"I am sorry but that is how it has to be."

"Will we have an opportunity to contest the statements made by the social work staff because if they run true to form, very little of what they say will be the truth," I asked.

"Yes, but they will also have the opportunity to contest your version. That is only fair," Harper said.

"That is fair enough," I said. "There is one thing I want to find out, which I consider very important. I want to know if there is a file on me and I would also like to see any notes that have been taken during the time we have been involved with the social workers. Can you do that?" I asked.

"I can't see why not but I will have to check that," he said. "If it is OK, I will have them for the next meeting."

I looked at him and smiled,

"Given your remit, it is obvious where this is going to end but I want to make sure that if this goes to court, I can't be accused of being unwilling to cooperate. For that reason and that reason only, we will give you as much help as we can."

We spent the next hour going over the details of the social work involvement and the nature of my complaint, and arranged to meet the following week, by which time Harper would have arranged to speak to the social work staff. He also hoped to have spoken to Sharon and the boys. We agreed the areas on which Harper's enquiry would focus, which were those same areas I had asked Jackson to investigate, with particular emphasis on Bridgeford. Harper agreed to this and I took it for granted he had the authority to determine the nature and extent of his investigations. When we met the following week, unfortunately Harper had been unable to see nearly as many of the others as he had hoped, but he did have some news that astounded me.

"What was the problem with the social work staff?" I asked.

"Shift work and emergency call outs," he explained. "This might take a bit longer than I expected."

"What about the file and the notes?" I asked

Harper looked at me and I could tell straight away, there was something wrong.

"You are not going to like this," he said, shaking his head, "all the original notes have been shredded, although I have been assured that these were made contemporaneously."

With that, he took a thin bundle of A4 paper, printed on one side, from his briefcase and handed it to me. There were eight sheets of paper and I quickly looked for anything about my meeting with Bridgeford. There was nothing. I then looked for details of the meeting with Napier which, although he had told me nothing, had lasted for forty-five minutes, during which time the scribe wrote down every word spoken. There was a single line which read,

"At his request, met with Mr Fairlie. His queries were noted and general information given (see record).

Of course, there was no record and for some unexplained reason, at the top of the sheet it said,

Client name:- Sharon Johnston.

I did not bother to read the rest, that could wait until I saw Sharon and the boys. I looked at Harper, who could not meet my gaze,

"Is this it?" I asked.

"Yes, that is all there was. I was told that is the only file they have on you."

"They have shredded every original note?" I asked, the contempt in my voice quite obvious.

"I was told that is normal practice," he said.

"And you believe them?" I asked. "No, don't bother to answer that, it doesn't matter a damn whether or not you believe them. I don't believe them. Not a bloody word they say do I believe because they are incapable of telling the truth."

I was too disgusted and angry to continue with the meeting. I told Harper I would call him after the family had seen the notes he had given me.

"I haven't read them yet," I said, "but I bet you a pound to a penny they will not be accurate."

Sharon, the boys and I agreed to meet the following week, to go over the Social Work Department notes together, what little there was of them. I said nothing until they had all read them. Sharon was the first to comment.

"They are trying to make out that I instigated the whole thing, that I asked the social workers to become involved," she exploded. She was raging and started to go through the pages one at a time.

"The reference to the meetings we had with Napier that Yellowlees organized," she said, "that is a complete fabrication. Neil, you were there," she said, turning to her husband Neil, "Is that anything like what took place?"

"No, it's not even close," said Neil, "It says Napier was asked to check previous records to see if any reference was made to you (Sharon) as a victim. That is a lie. Napier was asked to check the records to see if your Dad had said he believed Katrina and he reported back to us that your Dad had. That was when you asked Napier if your Dad was abusing Katrina, why would he have reported his own father."

Sharon then looked at the reference to what would happen to the grandchildren if I was given unsupervised access.

"Look at that. That is a downright lie. They say they "offered advice". Is that what it sounded like to you Neil? Those shits threatened us. Napier left us in no doubt that the kids would be taken into care."

Neil was as angry as Sharon.

"Look at this bit," he said, "it says, and this refers to Napier, 'I suggested that SWD staff could meet with family members to advise of protective action they could take if they felt children to be at risk.' If WE felt children were at risk," he shouted. "They were the ones who thought the kids were at risk. It was Yellowlees and Powrie who started all of this. They are the ones who kept telling us that the kids were at risk and we had a DUTY to do something about it."

As we went through the notes it became perfectly obvious what was being done here. Every single sheet had at its heading – **Client; Sharon Johnston**. The name of Yellowlees did not appear once, despite the fact he was the consultant psychiatrist and had been instrumental in arranging the first meeting with Powrie and Sharon and was present and provided the venue when Napier met Sharon and Neil for the first time at the hospital. There was a difference of opinion between him and Napier, at that meeting, about whether or not the police should be involved and when it would be best to have me arrested. Yellowlees wanted me arrested as soon as possible but Napier urged caution because "it would alert the paedophile ring". Sharon and Neil had been mere bystanders for much of that meeting. It was obvious that the fact that Sharon and Neil could corroborate each other's statement, was of no concern to them. The arrogance of what was being done was astonishing but as we were to find later, it was arrogance founded on the knowledge that their defences mechanism would back them, whatever lies they told and however obvious and stupid the lies were.

What really infuriated Sharon was the claim by Napier that, *"Sharon seems to set some store by Katrina's statement to her…"* and Powrie's entry that, *"She believes Katrina and is prepared to confront her father once Katrina gives her consent."* Powrie made a further entry to the effect that, *"Sharon does not want further counselling from me but will get in touch if she changes her mind."*

"That bitch," she exploded, "what counselling did I have? Do they really think they are going to get away with this? I never at any time said I believed Katrina."

The entry that was of greatest interest to me was the one from Napier which referred to Bridgeford's instructions to him to approach the police to find out how far the investigation had gone. An entry of 3.10.95 states,

> *"1. Approached by AD (Assistant Director) who advises that she has been approached by a Councillor enquiring re action taken by Department*
> *2. At her request, I contact Rona Anderson Police and inform of development."*

Napier was making sure his back was covered and however much these notes had been the creation of several fertile imaginations, Napier was obviously determined he was not going to be hung out to dry. The reference to *being instructed* to contact the police, made sure he was not going to be held responsible.

Sharon immediately wrote to Harper on August 7th 1996, objecting in the strongest possible terms at the notes she had seen. She reminded him that Powrie had admitted to attending ward meetings where Katrina's case had been discussed, that she did not initiate any of the meetings that were arranged, that the first meeting had been at the insistence of Yellowlees and from then on, the Social Work Department. She pointed out to him the weakness of the family's position in that their father was the subject of serious allegations of sexually abusing and raping his youngest daughter, of having committed murder, of controlling a paedophile ring composed of some very powerful and influential men. And yet, the Social Work Department were claiming they intervened **ONLY** because Sharon had asked them to and for no other reason. They were trying to give the impression they had almost to be forced to take action.

Harper sent her letter to Napier and Powrie, both of whom denied all the charges Sharon made. Napier's contribution was short and sweet, writing on the 29th August,

"In the context of the interviews which were conducted with Mrs Johnston I can confirm that she gave no indication at the time or immediately after the interviews of being anything other than satisfied that she had had the opportunity to discuss the situation and to reflect on what course of action she should take.

In this regard the case recording, which I now understand you have copied to her, remains an accurate reflection of the discussions which took place."

Powrie covered each point in turn but still denied everything. According to her, Sharon had instigated everything and all meetings had been arranged at her request. She did concede that the first meeting with her had been arranged via Yellowlees but, it was at Sharon's request. Yellowlees may very well have told Powrie that Sharon had asked for the meeting but she, Powrie, had attended other meetings at which Napier had been present and where Sharon and Neil were given no choice about what was going to happen.

We were unable to meet Harper again until the 9th October, when it was agreed we would attempt to bring the enquiry to a conclusion, after which Harper would submit his report to Jackson at Law and Administration. Sharon came with me and she was determined to have her say. Harper started the meeting.

"I have to admit there are certain problems in trying to bring this enquiry to some sort of conclusion," he said.

"Why?" we both asked at the same time.

"There are quite big disparities in what you have told me and what I have been told by the social workers involved.." he started, but before he was able to finish, Sharon interrupted,

"But they are lying," she said.

"I can't say that," he said, "there are obvious differences of opinion about what happened and I have to take their word at face value."

"But we have shown where they can't possibly be telling the truth," Sharon argued heatedly.

"I still have to accept their version of what happened. I explained my job is not to evaluate what is said, it is simply to report."

"A fat lot of good that is," said Sharon who by this time, had become really angry.

Suddenly Harper snapped,

"I told you before, you have more information than I do but if you continue with that attitude, I will stop the meeting now."

I put a restraining hand on Sharon's arm and asked her to be patient.

"What is your next step now?" I asked Harper.

"I will report to Mr Jackson and he will contact you," he replied.

"You will be reporting on Mrs Bridgeford?" I asked.

Harper took a minute or two before answering, as if he was weighing his response.

"I have to admit, I could make nothing of Mrs Bridgeford's explanation of what happened," he said. "I have interviewed her twice and each time I questioned her closely but at the end of each session, I could not make head or tail of what she said. Nothing she said made any sense."

"Will you tell Jackson that?" I asked

"I will tell Mr Jackson exactly what I have told you," he replied.

We parted with the agreement that Harper would telephone me the day he submitted his report to Jackson.

Harper did not call me until the 12th December. He told me nothing I did not already know, except – the most important thing to me, the part I had been waiting for and the reason I had pushed for the enquiry to take place, was missing.

"What did you say about Bridgeford?" I asked.

There was silence at the other end.

"Hello," I said, thinking I had been cut off.

"Yes," came the reply.

"What did you say about Bridgeford," I asked again.

"I said nothing about her," he replied.

"What do you mean you said nothing about her?" I asked, my voice rising noticeably.

There was another short silence, before Harper finally said,

"I said nothing about Mrs Bridgeford because I was told she was no longer part of the remit."

"What?" I roared, "do you mean that bastard has just decided to wipe the slate clean on her? Are you telling me that she is going to get away with telling a pack of lies and nothing is going to be done about it?"

"I am really sorry," said Harper, " but I was only told the day before I sent in the report."

I was livid but there was no point in ranting at Harper.

"When will I get a copy of the report?" I said.

"You won't get a copy, at least not from me. My job was to furnish the report for Jackson. It is up to him whether or not you get a copy." said Harper.

I knew then we were being stitched up. I knew there was no way Jackson would give me any report, what I would get would be some anodyne letter running to two or three paragraphs, about how everyone had performed beautifully and how pleased they all were with themselves.

That is exactly what I got and the single page of A4 arrived on December 17th. The first paragraph read,

"I refer to my letter of 16th May and have now received the report by Mr G Harper of his investigation into your complaint and advise that I am satisfied that the Social Work Department acted appropriately in the circumstances."

It then continued,

"It has been noted by Mr Harper that Mrs Johnston described Social Work staff as being "very supportive", "good at keeping me informed" and "acting entirely properly throughout the investigation", which is indicative I would suggest of an acknowledgement and acceptance of the grounds for Social Work involvement.

Mr Harper does advise however that a number of conflicting statements were made by yourself, Mrs S Johnston and Social Work staff....

I responded as follows;

I acknowledge receipt of your letter of 16th inst.

Having had no sight of the report made by Mr Harper, I am at a disadvantage. However given that you say, '..a number of conflicting statements were made..' I would like an explanation of how you arrived at your judgement that the Social Work Department 'acted appropriately...'

We were not given a satisfactory reason for the Social Work Department involvement but we showed without a shadow of a doubt, that it was not by invitation by Mrs Johnston or any other member of my family. Mrs Johnston's description of Social Work staff as being 'supportive' was in response to a direct question that had absolutely nothing to do with their involvement. You know that perfectly well and are using the remark completely out of context."

I wrote at some length in reply to Jackson's letter, leaving him in no doubt as to my opinion of him and the Social Work Department, particularly its Director, Mrs Bridgeford. I pointed out that:-

"...you referred to Mrs Bridgeford's letters to me of 16th April and 10th May as being 'meaningless'. You also stated that she was 'misquoting' policy.

At several meetings with Mr Harper he said he could neither defend nor explain Mrs Bridgeford's behaviour or her correspondence. I would like to see sight of the procedures of the Social Work Department which allow the Director to lie with impunity. I use the word 'lie' quite deliberately because it is inconceivable that the Director of Social Work could inadvertently 'misquote' Social Work policy not once, not twice but no fewer than six times..

At my first meeting with Mrs Bridgeford on 21st December 1995, she 'misquoted' policy. She later did likewise to Mrs Johnston on December 22nd. At a meeting on 7th February, at which she met with Mr Crawford, Mrs Johnston and Philip Fairlie, she 'misquoted' policy for a third time. In her letters of 16th April 1996 and 10th May 1996, she 'misquoted' policy for a fourth and fifth time and she confirmed her version of events to Mr Harper, thereby 'misquoting' policy for the sixth time.

There is no doubt in my mind that Mrs Bridgeford set out from the very first meeting, to mislead us and did so quite deliberately. The question that I asked to be addressed was the reason for her behaviour. You decided to remove her behaviour from Mr Harper's remit, only after Mr Harper discovered the degree of Mrs Bridgeford's mendacity and reported same to you. You are therefore guilty of instructing a cover up of, what I suspect, was a gross breach of confidentiality of which not even Mr Napier was aware. His interpretation of my non-existant contact with an SNP Councillor – 'that I was using my contacts to gain information' – had a devastating effect on my family, including Katrina and the grandchildren, for whose welfare you claimed to be concerned.

Finally I want to draw your attention to the case notes which exist, case notes, which I was assured by Mrs Bridgeford, did not exist. They run to eight pages, six of which refer to me either by name or family relationship. All references dwell on the alleged sexual abuse of my daughter Katrina, by me. Nowhere in the notes is there any references to the successive challenges made to the SWD, for more than a year, to provide any evidence to support the allegations. Anyone, unfamiliar with this case and reading the notes for the first time, would be led to believe that I had been accused by my entire family of sexually abusing their youngest sister and that they had sought SWD advice on how to protect their own children from similar abuse. I now demand an assurance that those records will be set straight."

I received no reply to that letter, in fact there was no further contact with anyone associated with Perth & Kinross Council.

From then on, the battle was conducted with their legal advisers through the Court of Session in Edinburgh. My letter had done no more than allow me to let off steam. Jackson had had the last laugh – at least for the time being, as he would find out when I later went to the media.

CHAPTER SIXTEEN

March 6th 1996 – December 1996

The street lights threw off a rather dim, orange coloured glow, which left large parts of the street and pavements in shadow. I could see the three figures approaching about fifty yards away and there was something about their demeanour and body language that gave off warning signs. Part of self-defence training is learning to be aware of your surroundings, your company; to learn to anticipate trouble, without helping to create it. I knew this trio spelled trouble and, as they came closer, they confirmed it by taking up positions that left me no alternative but to face them.

As we drew closer, they walked three abreast, taking up the whole width of the pavement and I knew exactly what was coming and relaxed my upper body. Not a word was spoken but suddenly, they had split up so that I had one on each side, who took hold of my arms and slammed me up against the wall. The third pushed me in the chest to help position me. There had still been nothing said, not a sound had passed between them and, as I knew what was coming I completely relaxed my arms, so that there was no resistance for the pair that were holding on to them.

As the one facing me readied himself to start pummelling me, he took a short step forward, at the same time drawing back his right arm, making a fist of his right hand. As his arm drew back I suddenly grabbed a part of the clothing of the two who were holding my arms and using the leverage this created, I swung my right foot in a kick to the undefended left side of the third assailant's head. I was wearing leather-soled shoes with a pronounced and heavy welt and the toe connected with the angle of his jaw, just under the ear and just where I had aimed. I saw his face change shape as the jaw dislocated and he was unconscious before he hit the ground. I changed my grip on the one holding my right arm and grabbed his testicles, crushing them so that he curled up to try to avoid the pain. I then kneed him in the face, smashing his nose to a pulp. That left the third assailant, who by this time was struggling to get away from the grip I had on his shirt front.

I began to punch him, hard and deliberately. I knew exactly where I wanted to hit him, first of all in the short ribs to knock the wind out of him and cause as much pain as possible. As he doubled up I switched to his head and the same angle of his jaw that had floored the first one. I really wanted to hurt him and punched and punched. Suddenly the lights were on and I was sitting in the middle of the floor in the bedroom, surrounded by the duvet which had been over my head. Kay was sitting up in bed, her eyes like saucers and her hands up to her mouth. I was soaked with sweat, the rivulets running down my bare upper body. I had been roaring my head off and was quite breathless, but with the realisation of where I was, I burst out laughing. It was sheer relief of tension.

I had had another of the nightmares that had started not long after I recovered from the pneumonia that floored me at the beginning of February 1996. In the nightmares, I was always being attacked and physically assaulted. I always fought back and I wasn't interested in just defending myself, I wanted to hurt my attackers, really hurt them. The years of judo training taught me how to and I broke arms and legs without a thought. Unfortunately, Kay was on the receiving end of much of the retaliation and many a night she had to leave the bed as I thrashed around, frequently landing blows on her back or head, that fortunately never did do any serious damage but hurt nevertheless.

When my temperature was at its highest and I was at my lowest during the bout of pneumonia, I believed I was walking along a country road when I came upon a large wrought iron gate, which opened on to a wide, tree-lined avenue, leading to a large country house. I entered the house, which seemed to be deserted but on walking through the large entrance hall, I could hear the sound of someone sobbing. Looking into the large room on my right, I saw a figure in rags, hunched over a table, their head in their arms and sobbing their heart out. The room was dilapidated, as was the other parts of the house I had seen, with broken window shutters hanging at different angles from the broken window frames. Clothes, old newspapers and rubbish were strewn everywhere.

I approached the sobbing figure and gently lifted the head, which was covered with thick, matted and filthy hair, which at one time might have been blond. As I tilted the head so that I could see the face, I recognised the woman as a friend of mine who was a journalist with the local newspaper for which I wrote regular columns. She had been badly beaten and her face was swollen and bruised. When I asked her what had happened, she only sobbed harder and shook her head. Reaching into my pocket, I took out a Cadbury's cream egg which I put into her hand. Suddenly the whole scene was transformed. Maureen became the lovely, impeccably groomed woman she always was, the room became a beautifully furnished and decorated sitting room. It was a standing joke in the newspaper that Maureen always had cream eggs on her desk and it caused some hilarity when I later told her of the hallucination.

I had spoken to the doctor about the nightmares and he put it down to the stress we were experiencing at the time. I mention it because I can still remember every detail of those nightmares, just as I can remember the details of the hallucinations and dreams I had when my temperature was sky high during the bout of pneumonia. The fact that I can, and the fact that they were so vivid at the time I was experiencing them, made me appreciate how Katrina felt and how she must have suffered as a consequence of the nightmares she had experienced, of rape and abuse. The big difference however, is that I know none of it happened. I was never assaulted, nor did I break any arms and to my knowledge, not even Cadburys has claimed such magical powers for their cream eggs. Even after the therapy ended, Katrina was left with the images, the horror of what was supposed to have happened to her. That became the most difficult part for her as she was recovering, having the images and having to keep telling herself it didn't happen.

There are good and decent people in all walks of life – and then there is the dross. As a family we have been fortunate enough to have seen the very best of the NHS, where dedicated practitioners have gone the extra mile on our behalf, where the nursing staff have nurtured and cared for those of us for whom they were called on to offer care. We could not have asked for greater support and attention from our own GPs in Crieff, who have offered outstanding service since the very first day of confrontation. When our eldest son Andrew, was diagnosed with a brain tumour in 2005, he could not have asked for more from the surgeon and staff at Glasgow's Southern General Hospital, whose skill ensured he made a complete recovery. For many reasons and over many years, we have had a great deal to be thankful for in our dealings with people whose professionalism could not be faulted.

Unfortunately there are others whom I once described as scum and in the thirteen long years during which Katrina was first of all treated by them, and we then had to deal with their behaviour as they lied at every turn in order to cover up their mistakes, aided and abetted by their legal advisers, they have done nothing which has made me alter my opinion. If my daughter-in-law Alison is any kind of example, there are undoubtedly many social workers who do a very difficult job, with all the dedication and commitment to their profession that is required, in order to pick up the pieces of lives shattered by modern society. We were never lucky enough to encounter any of them.

On 21st December 2003, the Sunday Times printed an article by Kenny Farquharson, in which he wrote, *"Given all he has been through, all the gut-curdling grief of 10 awful years, Jim Fairlie comes across as a level-headed man of good humour. But ask the polite financial adviser from Crieff his opinion of the medical profession and his bitterness and anger seep rapidly to the surface."*

My opinion was anything but complimentary;

> *"My view of the profession is that the culture of mendacity is so engrained it is endemic. Its modus operandi is that it didn't happen. And if it did happen, I didn't do it. And if I did do it, it wasn't my fault. And if it was my fault, I couldn't help it. And even if I could help it I don't owe you a duty of care, so tough."*

That may sound hard and unjust but anyone who has suffered from medical negligence in the UK and has attempted to seek redress through the legal processes will immediately recognise the format. It is often said we live in a "blame culture", where someone has to be blamed for anything that might go wrong. The precise opposite applies in the public sector, where no one will ever accept responsibility for anything unless absolutely forced to do so, where the first line of defence is to lie – and to continue to lie, whatever evidence is presented to show their guilt is beyond question. Anyone who doubts that judgement need only look at the high profile cases involving the medical profession and social work departments from Orkney and Cleveland, to Shieldfield, to Ayrshire, to Alder Hey to Haringay. The names of Sally Clark, Trupti Patel, Angela Canning, Christopher Lillie and Dawn Reed, Victoria Climbie and Baby P, should long be remembered as the victims of medical and social work negligence, or as the victims of miscarriages of justice as a consequence of the same type of negligence. By the same token, the names of those who were responsible for that negligence, should always live in infamy.

I also said in another newspaper article, that I could not think of a word in either Scots or English, that would adequately express the utter contempt I have for the medical and social work practitioners who were responsible for Katrina's treatment and the subsequent trauma to which we were all subjected over many years. Arrogance and stupidity provide a heady cocktail and unfortunately those with whom we were forced to deal had both in abundance, and felt obliged to display them at every opportunity. My disdain for these people arises not from the fact they made a mistake, but from the fact they were prepared to destroy the lives of twenty people – our immediate family – rather than admit their mistake. What will always remain unforgivable is that the psychiatric team, aided and abetted by their legal advisers and their so-called "expert witnesses", deliberately tried to convince Katrina that she had been abused by me, when every iota of evidence that existed proved the abuse could not have taken place.

That they knew perfectly well that not only had they made a mistake, but the nature of the mistake, finally became evident. Had they come to Kay and I and said,

"Look, we have made a dreadful mistake here and we cannot say how sorry we are. But it can be rectified and it would be of great help to us if you would work with us to restore Katrina's health," there would have been no attempt by us to seek redress through the courts. Our concern was Katrina and why she was ill. We knew, as her parents, there had to be a reason for her to accuse me of the most despicable crimes against her. By continuing to lie, both the Health Trust and the Social Work Department, made that approach impossible and prolonged Katrina's illness.

As soon as I had recovered from the pneumonia at the beginning of February, we began to look for other ways to carry forward our complaint with Yellowlees and Murray Royal/Gilgal. When the meeting with Yellowlees had been cancelled by the legal advisers at the Central Legal Office, we had no idea where to turn to, either to further the complaint or even to seek advice. Fortunately, on one of her visits to see Katrina, Sharon had picked up a booklet at the hospital door, which gave the address of the Mental Welfare Commission, as a body that handled complaints and looked after the interests of patients. I wrote to The Secretary in Edinburgh, on 27th February, enclosing the correspondence we had exchanged with Sharp, at the Central Legal Office, together with a very brief summary of what had happened up to that time.

The reply from the Mental Welfare Commission, came speedily enough, arriving on 7th March but simply asked if we had gone through the local complaints procedure at the hospital, which apparently was the proper way to make a complaint. Unfortunately, there were no instructions as to how that could be done. My next letter to them could have been a lot more tactful, as I accused them of employing delaying tactics, but having no idea of procedure and at the end of my tether having to deal with bureaucrats who were not in the least interested in what I had to say, I was not overly interested in being tactful. Nevertheless, I received another reply from the Commission on 21st March, giving me the name of the Clinical Director for Mental Health, who was also the Complaints Manager at Murray Royal. At last, we had a focus for our complaint.

In my second letter to the Commission I wrote,

"I would prefer to be told quickly and from the outset, whether or not you intend to pursue this matter further."

In their letter to me of 5th March, the Commission had also said,

"I confirm it is the Commission's view that your complaint does not fall within our remit which relates 'specifically to the welfare of people with a mental disorder' rather than relatives. You might nevertheless, wish to keep the Commission informed of the progress of your complaint."

Taking them at their word, that their interest lay in the care of patients rather than their relatives, I again wrote to the Commission on 21st May, reminding them that they had asked to be kept informed. By that time, there had been a number of developments and further correspondence between the Health Trust and the family. We were desperate at this time, to find someone, anyone who could or would help, and wrote,

"My daughter Katrina was re-admitted to hospital on Monday 13th inst. She almost succeeded in hanging herself on Thursday 16th inst. And made another attempt yesterday, Monday 20th. My family and I are at a complete loss to understand how it can be said, as Drs

Yellowlees and Proctor insist on saying, that Katrina is improving or that her treatment is appropriate... I am sure that you will be able to gage from the enclosures the degree to which Katrina's family are concerned about her welfare. Our greatest fear is that she will succeed in killing herself before we are able to have someone else talk to her. For that reason, I would ask you to give this your immediate attention, even if it is to say you can do nothing."

A full month later, on the 25th June, I received the following reply,

"The commission remains of the opinion that your complaint lies outwith the remit of the Commission though, because of the nature of the issues you have raised we would be interested to be kept informed of any further steps you take. The Commission, as a separate matter, continues of course, to have an interest in the welfare of your daughter in relation to any psychiatric assessment or treatment which she has."

Not only were we desperate because of Katrina's continued deterioration, which we were now having to deal with outwith the hospital, we were utterly confused about the function and remit of the Mental Welfare Commission, in 1at July, I again wrote to them, this time laying out in as clear a fashion as possible, that we were seeking help and advice:-

"You state in your letter of 25th June, '...your complaint lies outwith the remit of the Commission.....although we would be interested to be kept informed' 'The Commission continues to have an interest in the welfare of your daughter...'

That raises a number of points which perhaps you can clarify:-
1. *What exactly is the remit of the Commission?*
2. *What exactly does the Commission think is the nature of my complaint?*
3. *Why do you wish to be kept informed if my complaint is outwith your remit?*

> 4. *If the welfare of my daughter is of interest to the Commission, why have you made no attempt to ascertain whether or not she has improved since becoming a patient of Dr Yellowlees? I have drawn attention to the fact my daughter believes she has been the victim of abuse that did not take place and, unfortunately the problem is on-going. My daughter left hospital on June 13th at the end of a twenty-eight day section. Two days later, while waiting for a bus, she saw a man she believes abused her and became so hysterical she had to be taken into a shop until help arrived. She has since had hallucinations which involved being abused by me, at times, when we were miles apart, with witnesses to prove it.*
> 5. *Dr Yellowlees still insists my daughter's health is improving. From the information with which you have been provided, are you in a position to make even an educated guess as to whether or not there has been any improvement? If not, what does it take for the Commission to intervene, to become involved, to do something other than write letters telling me it wants to be kept informed about events it claims are outwith its remit? At what point does your professed interest in my daughter's health provoke a reaction?*

On the 19th July, the Commission wrote back, stating for the first time, the actual nature and extent of their remit.

> *With regard to the questions you raise:-*
>
> 1. *The Commission has a duty to make enquiry into any case where it appears to them there may be 'ill-treatment, deficiency in care or treatment, or improper detention'.*
> 2. *We wish to be kept informed because there are references in your letters to the care and treatment of your daughter which therefore, lie within our remit. We therefore, have to keep the matter of further enquiries open.*

> 3. I hope this clarifies the Commission's position and continued interest. It is, of course, entirely up to yourself whether you keep the Commission informed of the progress of your complaint. The information you have given has been of assistance in helping us to decide what further enquiries might need to be made but we would, of course, be considering this in any case.

I replied to that letter on 24th July expressing my frustration and reiterating the nature of our complaint and the continuing problems of dealing with the Health Trust. In sheer exasperation I finally asked,

"If the overall handling of Katrina's care does not fall into the category of 'deficiency in care or treatment', can you explain how much worse it has to get before someone in the Commission is moved to act?"

By the 8th August, there had still been no reply, therefore I wrote asking if the Commission intended replying. Their final communication dated 14th August ran to one sentence.

"Thank you for your further letter and enclosures of 8th August 1996."

During the entire time I was in communication with the Commission, the family was going through the internal complaints procedure with the officials of the Health Trust, which also involved several letters and reports, all of which were sent to the Commission so that they were kept informed, at every stage of the proceedings, of everything that was said and done. Despite several attempts to get a response from them that would tell us if and when and under what circumstances the Commission would be moved to intervene, we got nowhere. I still have no idea if the Commission would ever have intervened, nor do I have the foggiest idea what function, if any it fulfils. From our own experience, it would seem it has no function other than to write letters.

On the 1st April I wrote to the Clinical Director of the Health Trust, as had been suggested by the Mental Welfare Commission and received a reply by return from the Chief Executive, Frank Brown, who suggested I should meet with Mrs Caroline Inwood, Director of Nursing and Quality on an informal basis. That meeting took place on 16th April and was attended by Caroline Inwood, Mr McGuinness, Deputy Mental Health Services Manager, Sharon, Kay and myself. The usual pleasantries were exchanged before we got down to discussing the reason for being there.

"I believe you have concerns about the care of your daughter Katrina, who is being looked after by Dr Yellowlees, consultant psychiatrist," said Inwood.

"That is correct and you will be aware we have correspondence from Mr Sharp at the Central Legal Office," I replied, "He cancelled a previously arranged meeting at 24 hours notice on the grounds that he saw no useful purpose in having the meeting."

"We think that it would be better if there is cooperation all round," said Inwood, "Now can you give me the details of your complaint."

"If you have seen the correspondence, you will know the nature of our concerns." I said, "the first is that Dr Yellowlees lied to me, that Katrina believes she was abused by men she never met, her health has deteriorated since she came into hospital and that we are repeatedly told that she is improving when she quite clearly is not."

"There are several questions we need to ask Dr Yellowlees and Dr Proctor," said Kay, "Therefore we want a meeting with them as soon as possible. Katrina had no memories of any abuse by her father until she came into hospital and then the allegations came about only after a series of flashbacks in which her father appeared."

"Katrina has been told that flashbacks are recalled memories but we have been told that other people can be imposed into flashbacks, which negates any notion they can be accurate memories," I said.

For the first time, McGuinness spoke and said,

"There is no evidence that someone can impose other people into a flashback."

Kay, Sharon and I looked at each other because the implication of what McGuinness was saying was immediately clear to each one of us.

"Are you saying then, that Jim abused Katrina?" asked Kay sharply, looking hard at McGuinness, who repeated his claim,

"There is no evidence that someone can impose other people into a flashback."

Both Kay and Sharon bridled at that but before either of them could say anything more, I said,

"How do you explain the claims of alien abduction in the USA? Professionals in mental health have testified that it is a possibility. Do you believe in aliens?"

McGuinness did not answer, so I asked him again,

"Patients in the USA have claimed to have flashbacks of being abducted by aliens and their psychiatrists and psychologists have said it is possible. Do you also believe in aliens?"

McGuinness looked as if he could have struck me but still did not answer, so I asked him for a third time and still received no answer. However, Inwood intervened hurriedly at this point and said,

"Some people would say they could and some would say they couldn't."

"And that is your answer? Which is it in this hospital?" Sharon asked.

No one answered that question either and as we were there to discuss meeting Yellowlees and having our concerns addressed, I did not want this meeting to get bogged down. It was agreed that Caroline Inwood would make arrangements for a meeting to take place and that she would contact us when that was done. As we made our way along the corridor to the front door, accompanied by Inwood, McGuinness had taken his leave, she said,

"You know, I have spoken to Dr Yellowlees and he did not believe you abused Katrina."

Both Sharon and Kay turned on her immediately,

"That is not the impression he gave us and was quite clear, that there was no other explanation for Katrina's condition," Sharon said angrily.

"Well I know he did not believe it," repeated Inwood.

"Why does he not tell Katrina that, if he does not believe it?" asked Kay.

That was the end of the conversation as Inwood chose not to answer and, as we had reached the front door, we took our leave.

The meeting was arranged for 2nd May and it was agreed that Sharon and Philip would accompany me. Caroline Inwood, Yellowlees and Proctor were there for the Hospital. We had agreed on the approach we intended to take and had prepared a number of questions, which we would take it in turns to ask, because we had all been involved with Yellowlees and his staff at different periods and we thought it best that we would each tackle Yellowlees on the parts where we were involved personally. The others would take notes while each of us took it in turn to speak, so that nothing from the meeting would be lost. I had wanted to have my solicitor present, which Inwood refused, because of Yellowlees's tendency to deny previous statements he had made, or to claim he had been misunderstood. Inwood wanted the meeting to be kept as informal as possible.

When we were all seated, Caroline Inwood asked me to start the meeting as I had expressed concerns about the treatment Katrina had received.

"I would like Dr Yellowlees to clarify his diagnosis of Katrina, both when she entered hospital in November 1994 and when she left in March 1996," I said.

"She came into hospital suffering from addiction to drugs which were prescribed and she left in March suffering from four different ailments, none of which were the problems she had when she came in."

Yellowlees confirmed both diagnosis. I then asked him,

"Can you explain the deterioration in her health? Why is she worse now than she was when she came in?"

"Katrina has improved since coming into hospital," Yellowlees said. "She came in suffering from psychogenic pain and that has cleared up."

"The pain has gone but she now believes she was raped by me and seventeen other men, some of whom she has never met, that her three brothers abused her and that her mother participated in the abuse." I said, "Are you seriously asking us to believe that is an improvement?"

Yellowlees just looked at me and did not answer.

I then asked him to explain flashbacks and both he and Proctor, confirmed that flashbacks were fragments of memory. When asked if it was possible to include others into the flashback, who were not present at the original event, whatever it was, both admitted it was possible. As soon as they heard this both Sharon and Philip interrupted.

"That is not what you told us. You insisted there was no other explanation for Katrina's condition and at no time did you ever suggest that the flashbacks could be no more than imaginary." said Philip.

"That is not what I said," replied Yellowlees, "you have misunderstood me."

"What did you say then?" asked Sharon.

Yellowlees looked at both Sharon and Philip and insisted again that they had misunderstood him and that was all he would say.

"Can you verify that Katrina reported to the hospital that she had been raped in the shower at Sharon's house?" I asked.

"I remember Katrina returned to the hospital particularly distressed and immediately went into flashback. That is when the rape in the shower came to light, but I have no idea where she had been," Yellowlees replied.

"The rape in the shower came in a flashback?" I asked, surprised. "Have you any idea when it is supposed to have happened?"

"No, I have no idea, it could have happened any time," Yellowlees answered.

"Or not happened at all?" said Philip, "now that you have admitted that the contents of the flashbacks might be nothing more than a bad dream."

"That confirms that Jenny Hogg made a false statement about me to the police," I said. "When asked if Katrina reported being raped in the shower, when she returned to the hospital, Jenny Hogg told the police she had. But that is not what we are hearing now."

"Can you confirm the rape even took place?" asked Sharon.

After much hesitation and a second request from Sharon, Yellowlees admitted he couldn't. Sharon, Philip and I just looked at each other. This was moving in a direction we really hadn't expected. Yellowlees was all over the place and his whole treatment of Katrina was beginning to look very suspect. Caroline Inwood sat with her head lowered throughout the exchange, while Proctor sat nodding, although it was difficult to know why. I decided to push Yellowlees on the rape.

"This alleged rape has caused serious concerns in the family and you are now telling us you have no idea if it even took place. Did you question Katrina about it at all?" I asked

"No, I didn't," responded Yellowlees, "I always have to be mindful of the therapeutic relationship and accept what is said at face value."

"Are you telling us you simply accept everything without question because to do other wise would harm the therapeutic relationship?" I asked astounded.

"I always question her," he answered defensively.

"But do you ever say that something couldn't have happened?" I asked.

"That is not how it works," he replied. "I offered Katrina a physical examination but she refused."

"What happened then?" I asked.

"She was given a pregnancy test." Yellowlees replied.

Sharon, Philip and I looked at each other again in disbelief.

"What message do you think that would have given to Katrina?" I asked. "Why in Heaven's name would you give her a pregnancy test for an alleged rape that you cannot even say actually happened?"

"It was negative," Yellowlees replied.

It was a classic non sequitor, a non answer from someone who was obviously struggling to keep his head above water. Sharon decided to keep on the rape theme and questioned Yellowlees on the alleged rape in the hospital grounds, which he had told her he believed had actually taken place. Yellowlees vehemently denied he had said anything of the kind and also denied he had told Andrew the same thing. Philip then took up the challenge.

"Do you remember the conversation you and I had about this alleged rape Dr Yellowlees?"

"Yes, I remember the conversation," he replied

"Do you remember telling me you thought it was perfectly possible for it to have happened in the hospital grounds and then, when I questioned you further, you told me of a patient who had been assaulted by a relative 'right under your noses' in the hospital for two years?" asked Philip

"Yes, but the patient was in the community when it happened," said Yellowlees hurriedly.

"But that was not what you said to me," said Philip, "you led me to believe it happened in the hospital…"

"No, no," interrupted Yellowlees, "the patient was in the community. I remember the conversation we had."

Philip hesitated for a moment before he said,

"Then why did you give it as an example of how it was possible for my father to have raped Katrina in the hospital grounds?"

Yellowlees just stared at Philip but said nothing, so Philip asked him again. He asked him three times in total and Yellowlees simply sat and stared at him, refusing to answer. I again took up the questioning.

"When we had our telephone conversation in December, I accused you of lying to me about Katrina's description of me as 'intimidating and imposing' and you insisted that was her description. Sharon has since confirmed that you said it. Would you still confirm it was Katrina that said it?" I asked.

"Yes, I would confirm it was Katrina's opinion of you," answered Yellowlees.

"That is not what you told me," said Sharon, "you said that was how you had found my father when I said he was not a violent man. You definitely did not say it was Katrina's opinion."

"It was Katrina's opinion and not mine. That is what I said," Yellowlees retorted.

I was about to have another go at him and call him a liar again but suddenly he said very quickly,

"All right, I was less than honest during that telephone call."

"Would you care to explain that?" I asked

"Yes, I found the conversation intimidating and I wanted it to finish. That is why I blamed Katrina." he answered.

"How could you be intimidated on the telephone?" I asked, "What could I possibly do to you while speaking on the telephone?"

"You underestimate your ability to intimidate people," he replied in a small voice.

Caroline Inwood's face was a picture, she looked as if she would prefer to be anywhere but in that room. The three of us looked at each other and knew we had Yellowlees now. His entire credibility had been shot during this meeting but there was still Proctor to deal with. Proctor was a small woman, with mousey brown hair she wore rather short and wore Laura Ashley type dresses. She was a twitterer, constantly fiddling with her hands. Sharon questioned her about a conversation she had had with Katrina, after Sharon had cast doubt on the abuse by me ever having taken place.

"Did you tell Katrina about Freud's story of the retraction of father /daughter abuse in Vienna, as an example of how pressure can sometimes force people to retract, when in fact the abuse did actually take place?" asked Sharon

"No," replied Proctor, "I told her about Freud just to educate her."

"And you just happened to pick on that topic, when there were so many other parts of Freud you could have mentioned?" Sharon asked.

Proctor sat and said nothing, fiddling with her hands.

"Did you tell Katrina it was her right to commit suicide?" asked Sharon.

"Yes," said Proctor.

"What possible reason did you have for telling someone as vulnerable as Katrina that she had a right to commit suicide?" I asked sharply. "Are you aware she tried to hang herself within twenty four hours of having that conversation?"

"Suicide is a regular feature of my discussions with Katrina and sometimes it is better to discuss these issues rather than ignore them." she replied and then stunned us completely when she volunteered the information,

"On one occasion I suggested to her that she write farewell letters to her family."

Philip and I looked at one another and we were both finding it difficult to keep our tempers. Looking at Yellowlees, I could not hide the contempt in my voice when I said quietly,

"And you had the gall to write to me, telling me that it was pressure from the family that provoked Katrina's attempt to hang herself."

Sharon decided to continue to push Proctor, who constantly fidgeted in her seat, fiddling with her hands and touching her hair. During an explanation of Dissociation, Proctor had mentioned "body memories", which was new to us, a term we had not heard until now.

Turning to Proctor, Sharon asked,

"What do you mean by body memories?"

Proctor seemed to settle, as if she was now in "her territory" her own comfort zone.

"Sometimes when a patient dissociates because of the nature of the trauma they are experiencing, such as rape, they will have no immediate memory of the trauma, but at some later date, their body will remember what happened and there will be a reaction, sometimes physical."

"Can you explain what that means?" asked Sharon, "because that does not tell us very much."

Proctor hesitated for a moment before explaining,

"A patient presented with recurrent chest pains which her doctors had been unable to explain. After therapy, it was discovered that her father had raped her as a child, and that the pain was her body's way of remembering that rape. It came from the pressure of her father leaning on her chest as he raped her."

"How old was she when she was raped?" asked Philip

"She was aged between two and three years old," answered Proctor.

"Did she actually remember the rape or was it similar to Katrina's memory, coming through flashbacks?" I asked.

"The memories came through flashbacks," answered Proctor.

"Therefore they might not have happened at all," I said.

Proctor said nothing.

"Are you telling us that a person's body can actually remember something which their memory or their mind can't, or has forgotten?" asked Philip

"Yes," answered Proctor.

Throughout this exchange Inwood had sat very stiffly in her seat, with her eyes downcast the whole time. I wondered what she would say about this meeting. There were a few other exchanges but it was clear we were not going to get many more "gems" from either Yellowlees or Proctor, both of whom seemed to realise they had said more than enough. It was agreed that Sharon, Philip and I would discuss the meeting with the rest of the family and that I would telephone Inwood to discuss how this contact could be taken further. When we had taken our leave and were outside of the hospital grounds, we could contain ourselves no longer. Sharon was the first one to express her outrage.

"Can you actually believe what we have just heard?" she asked. "Yellowlees cannot tell the truth about anything. He lied to you Dad and was forced to admit it but continued to lie about everything he has told us, despite both Philip and I challenging him."

"Thank God we were all there together this time," said Philip. "That has been the problem; all our meeting with Yellowlees have been on a one to one basis. But this time we were all there. The man is a cretin."

"And Proctor is nuts," I said. "That woman is definitely dangerous. And I hate the thought of her having anything to do with Katrina."

"What are we going to do now?" asked Sharon.

"I will telephone Inwood tomorrow and take it from there." I said.

When I called Inwood the following day, I ensured I was able to take notes of all that was said because I trusted her no more than I trusted any of the psychiatric team to give a true account of what was said. The family had agreed we should continue contact with the hospital in order to monitor Katrina's treatment but I also wanted to confirm that we were going to receive a report on the original complaint. I should have known it would not turn out like that.

"I think the meeting went well. Do you want me to arrange another?" asked Inwood.

"We wish to continue to have contact, but for the moment we would prefer to wait until we have received your report on the original complaint before agreeing to another meeting." I answered.

"I will write to confirm that what we agreed at the first meeting was that I should investigate the possibility of getting a second opinion, that Katrina does not want a second opinion, and in light of that, there is not much else I can do." said Inwood.

"We also agreed at the first meeting that you would get to the bottom of the alleged rape in the shower and the statement that was made to the police in Jenny's presence." I retorted, letting Inwood know immediately that I was not going to let Jenny Hogg's statement to the police drop out of sight.

"The agreement was that I should investigate a second opinion. I am not qualified to comment on a police inquiry. I have no proof a police inquiry took place, I have only your word for it." said Inwood. That statement immediately gave me warning that Inwood had no intention of investigating anything.

"You are not being asked to comment on the police inquiry. You are merely being asked to find out if a report was received by hospital staff immediately after an alleged rape in Sharon's shower. According to Katrina's police statement, she reported the alleged rape immediately on her return to the hospital. This was confirmed by Jenny. If you do find the report I want to know the date it was received as I have office diaries and files which can be cross-checked as to my whereabouts on that date." I retorted, managing – just – to keep my voice steady.

The conversation rambled on for several moments while it became more and more obvious that Inwood was going to be as difficult as she could be. At the end of one of a particularly irritating response to one of my questions, I said,

"I don't know if you are being deliberately obtuse or if you are simply not listening but...." Before I could finish Inwood interrupted,

"Oh I am listening Mr Fairlie, indeed I am listening or else I would not have picked up on the fact that you have files on this rape. When I asked you at the second meeting to give me a date when the rape took place you told me you did not know. Now you are telling me you have files on the rape, as well as diaries!"

I could not believe that Inwood was as stupid as she was making out. She may well have been but I gave her the benefit of the doubt and assumed she was playing the daft lassie.

"If you listen very carefully I will explain it again. The files and diaries I have relate to my business appointments with clients. If you find there is a report of an alleged rape, there is bound to be a date recorded. I can then check to see if on that date and at that time, I was with one of my clients, or if I was in the office. Either way, I will be able to show I was not raping my daughter. But I am perfectly sure you know perfectly well that no such report exists, hence the prevarication about having it produced or, alternatively, admitting it does not exist because that would prove that Jenny Hogg made a false statement to the police. You were supposed to be mounting an investigation but when Yellowlees was questioned about it yesterday, he did not have a clue what I was talking about." I finished.

"I was not asked to investigate any rape," said Inwood. "If you..." I did not let her get any further before interrupting,

"Your memory is as faulty as Yellowlees's. He can never remember anything he has agreed to or said either. Either that or he just lies."

"You have no right to accuse Dr Yellowlees of lying," Inwood said, obviously rattled.

"He admitted lying to me yesterday," I laughed.

After a few moments, Inwood said,

"He did not admit to lying, he explained why he had not told you the truth."

I could not believe the way this conversation was going. Now Inwood was talking to me as if I was stupid.

"Because I had intimidated him?" I laughed again. "What was his excuse for lying to Sharon and Philip? Did they also intimidate him?"

Inwood then accused me of speaking to her in an intimidating fashion and at that point, I decided the conversation had gone far enough. I broke off, telling Inwood I would wait for her report with interest.

On 10th May, Inwood wrote to tell me that she would be sending her report to Frank Brown, Chief Executive of the Health Trust by the end of that week. Brown's first correspondence, dated 17th May, arrived the following week. It ran true to form,

Dear Mr Fairlie,

The first issue which you asked to be considered was your concern about Katrina's care and treatment whilst a patient in Murray Royal. We have no reason to believe that the treatment that Karen has received and is receiving is anything other than entirely appropriate. Further, I understand that Katrina is currently content with her treatment and care and does not support the request for a second opinion. Without Katrina's consent we would not feel it appropriate to pursue this issue.

Mrs Inwood has advised me that at the most recent meeting with yourself, your daughter Sharon and your son Philip, Dr A J Yellowlees and Dr C Proctor many of the issues you have raised have been clarified.

I understand that there are a number of allegations for which you have requested further information and confirmation of dates that can only be found in Katrina's case notes. The Scottish Home and Health Department document "Confidentiality of Personal Health Information – Code of Practice" does not allow disclosure of information without the consent of the patient and information should only be disclosed in connection with the purposes of health care…

The offer of another informal meeting has been made…"

My reply to Brown, sent on May 20th, expressed my irritation that he could not even use Katrina's proper name throughout the length of the letter. It was petty and under other circumstances, I would have put it down to a typing error and left it at that, but we were getting the run around from the Mental Welfare Commission as well as the Social Work Department and I was in no mood to be given the same treatment by another bunch of bureaucrats. I was also putting down a marker to let Brown know I had no intention of letting anything go, no matter how small or insignificant. Katrina had refused to speak to Inwood, therefore her information that Katrina did not want a second opinion came from Yellowlees and Proctor, both of whom had a vested interest in making sure Katrina did not get a second opinion. Katrina had not expressed strong objections to the family, about getting a second opinion.

I emphasised my reluctance to meet Yellowlees on an informal basis was on account of the fact I did not trust him and that he had admitted to lying to me, although he continued to deny all the charges of doing likewise with Sharon, Andrew and Philip. He had made similar statements to the police, that Katrina's flashbacks were actual memories and that she had been physically and sexually abused from a very young age. I asked Brown if he was arguing that my entire family, as well as the police had all misunderstood Yellowlees, that they had all "got it wrong?"

My final paragraph could not have been more contemptuous of him and his team. I wrote,

You state, "We have no reason to believe that the treatment that Katrina has received and is receiving is anything other than appropriate." You may care to ponder on the fact that Katrina was sectioned on Monday 13th inst., that I sat with her for 30 minutes in order to calm her down while she begged me to allow her to kill herself. She almost succeeded in hanging herself on Thursday 16th inst. I received your one-page letter on Saturday 18th inst. Even the bureaucratic mind may find that ironic." (the details of this episode are in the following chapter)

The reply from Brown was written on 17th June and from its tone, he was becoming as irritated as I was. He wrote,

It is unfortunate that you have not found any re-assurance or clarification of your concerns following the recent meeting with Dr Proctor and Dr Yellowlees. For their part, both Dr Proctor and Dr Yellowlees found the meeting to be helpful and communication appeared to be very clear. It seems, however, that a lot of what was said has been misinterpreted by you. In response to the specific points you raise:

1. *On no occasion have Dr Yellowlees and Dr Proctor ever indicated a second opinion would be detrimental to Katrina's*

> *health Dr Yellowlees has offered a second opinion on many occasions which has been declined.*
> 2. *Your statement that Dr Yellowlees was lying is totally unacceptable. At no time has Dr Yellowlees ever indicated to you or your family or in fact the police that he believed that you had abused and raped your daughter. He has at no time given any formal statement to the police and that was made quite clear to you at the meeting.*
> 3. *According to Dr Yellowlees and Dr Proctor it was felt the issue of traumatic memory had been adequately clarified at the meeting…*
> 4. *Senior Charge nurse Jenny Hogg has not furnished the police with a statement incriminating you. She has never been approached by anyone to provide any such statement.*
> 5. *Katrina has made it clear that many of her episodes of self-harm were a direct response to the pressure from her family. Katrina's expressions of suicide have been taken very seriously and issues of her safety addressed.*

It was obvious also from the contents of the letter that Brown was being given a version of events which was skewed, to say the least. It was difficult to know whether he was being fed a parcel of lies or, whether he was simply providing a smokescreen behind which Yellowees and Proctor could hide. For that reason my reply to him of 26th June was both lengthy and detailed.

> *"We took extensive notes at the meeting with Mrs Inwood, Dr Proctor and Dr Yellowlees, precisely because we had no doubt the Health Trust would attempt to present a totally false picture of what actually took place.*
>
> *Before making specific comment I would like to make the general observation that no matter what point is raised anent discussions which Dr Yellowlees has had, at different times, with different members of the family and the police, or anent remarks made by Dr Yellowlees or his staff to more than one member of the family at the same time, Dr*

Yellowlees and his staff either, deny they ever made the remarks or, insist we have all misinterpreted what has been said.

That gives rise to a number of possibilities. Either, my family and I and the police are all telling lies about the conversations we have had with Dr Yellowlees (despite Dr Yellowlees admitting he lied to me on the telephone), or we all lack the intelligence to understand what Dr Yellowlees and his staff are telling us.

The alternatives are that Dr Yellowlees and his staff, have difficulties with their memories or, are so lacking in communication skills that they are incapable of explaining anything about the nature of Katrina's illness; to such an extent that Katrina's family, both individually and collectively, have inevitably come away from those discussions with Dr Yellowlees and his staff convinced they have been told one thing when, according to Dr Yellowlees, they have been told the exact opposite.

Of course, there is another possibility; which is that Dr Yellowlees and his staff take the view that as some of the conversations were held on a one-to-one basis, it is safe to deny what was said, or to claim that they have been misinterpreted, knowing full well that their superiors and their lawyers will provide them with ample protection."

I then went on to itemise the occasions on which Yellowlees had lied, again explained how Hogg had confirmed Katrina's statement to the police, something which had already been done on at least three separate occasions. Finally I raised the accusation that Katrina's suicide attempts were as a consequence of the pressure she felt from the family.

"Can you explain precisely what pressure Katrina's family are putting her under that would cause her to take her own life? She has been told by her family that the abuse she claims to have suffered at the hands of myself, her mother, her three brothers and all of the seventeen others accused, did not take place. It has been shown to her that it could not possibly have taken place. Is Dr Yellowlees saying that Katrina's accusations must not be challenged, that she should be allowed to

continue to believe that she suffered, and is continuing to suffer abuse that never happened?"

We were to find out, when the medical records arrived, that that is exactly what Dr Yellowlees meant; not only him but his "expert witness", who wrote that to "challenge Katrina's accusations would be to destroy the relationship with her." In other words, Yellowlees and his staff were prepared to encourage Katrina to believe in a lifetime of abuse that never took place, for the sake of their "therapeutic relationship" with her. They went even further when Katrina began to improve and seriously question what had happened; they tried to persuade her the abuse had actually happened by questioning her closely after I had left the hospital. After each of my visits, Katrina was asked, "Do you still fear your father? How do you feel when he puts his arms around you? Ar you sure you want to give him a kiss?" These were all written in the medical notes and it was only after my visits that Katrina was questioned in this way.

Our next meeting with Yellowlees was not until August and was called specifically because Katrina had had several psychotic episodes, for which she needed hospitalisation. The one that caused us greatest concern was when she called our house in Crieff, from her flat in Perth. (she had moved into the flat in April but had spent very little time there). When Kay answered the telephone, Katrina was on the other end, obviously very distressed.

"Mum, Dad has just left the flat after raping me." she said, trying hard to make herself understood through her tears.

Kay was astonished and immediately concerned because we had had so many of these occasions, she knew exactly what was happening.

"Katrina," she said, "calm down, your Dad couldn't have raped you he is here in the house and has been here all day."

"You're just covering up for him," sobbed Katrina.

"Sharon is here too and has been here all afternoon, she can confirm your Dad has not left the house," said Kay.

There was no response from Katrina, but Kay could hear her crying, obviously very distressed. Sharon took the telephone from Kay and spoke to Katrina for a time, after which she had managed to calm her down enough for Sharon to feel she would be alright until she, Sharon, could make it back into Perth. Katrina was hospitalised that night and immediately sectioned. Yellowlees agreed to meet us within the next few days and Sharon, Katrina and I, met with him and Proctor.

It had been originally intended that Sharon and Kay would attend the meeting with Katrina because my correspondence with Brown and the Health Trust was getting more and more acrimonious and we felt that Kay might be able to take a "softer" approach.

That is not to say that Kay was in any way less determined than I was, to ensure Katrina's care was given the attention it deserved, but we were also concerned that I had once again, been accused of rape and it would be better if I was not involved in appealing to the psychiatric team to explain to Katrina it could not have happened.

Unfortunately Kay was unwell that day and although she waited until the last possible moment to eventually decide she could not attend, with less than an hour to go before the meeting was to take place, she finally called off. We debated whether or not we should call the hospital and tell them that I was going to attend instead of Kay but we did not want to give them any excuse for calling off the meeting, given Katrina's state of mind. Proctor met us in the corridor and when we explained that Kay was unable to attend and that I had come in her place, she was obviously reluctant to allow me in, stating that my presence had not been agreed beforehand. Sharon made the point to her that Katrina's health had obviously not improved and that we were concerned about the new allegations that had been made. Proctor disappeared for a few moments into a nearby room, where, we assumed, she discussed the situation with Yellowlees. Eventually they both appeared and said they were content to allow the meeting to go ahead, as if they were doing us a great favour.

We explained what had happened and told them of our concern that Katrina was still not improving. Sharon pushed Yellowlees who finally blurted,

"Sharon you seem to want me to tell Katrina that the incident never took place, but I can't do that because I wasn't there!"

"We know perfectly well you were not there, but we are telling you it could not possibly have happened and my mother and I can testify to that. Katrina needs to be told it did not happen," Sharon said obviously irritated.

Yellowlees just looked at her and before he could say anything, Proctor interrupted with that small, twittering voice she had,

"The only two people who will know for certain what happened are your father and Katrina," she said.

Dealing with that level of idiocy, had its price, a very obvious price. I had often wondered what planet people like Proctor inhabited, what parallel universe spawned the likes of Yellowlees and her, because there was absolutely no doubt in my mind, they did not live in the same world as the rest of us mere mortals. As the family had gained confidence in their dealings with the psychiatric team and it became obvious that their theories and pontificating could be so easily dismantled under close questioning, they also could see them for what they were – a group of less than ordinary individuals who quite obviously did not have a clue what they were talking about. They were no more than self-appointed experts on their own highly suspect "professional opinion", professional opinions that deemed "evidence" as unnecessary, particularly if it exposed their own lack of logic.

Sharon and I were now faced with the two people most responsible for Katrina's care, one of whom found it impossible to tell Katrina that on the "evidence of two other independent witnesses, it is impossible for you to have been raped by your father" – because he "was not there". What went right over his head, was the obvious irony of his extreme willingness to testify to the fact that rape, sexual abuse and murder all took place, despite his absence from the scene of the crimes. His partner in crime – and in my opinion what they were doing bordered on the criminal – equally quick to dismiss any "evidence" that contradicted her own pet theories, could only fall back on that well worn mantra of the Recovered Memory therapist caught out like a rabbit in headlights, "the only people who can say etc. etc."

I looked across at Katrina, who sat with her head slightly bowed but listening closely nevertheless. The position being adopted by Yellowlees and Proctor was conveying exactly the same message to Katrina as was conveyed when she was given the pregnancy test, when she had the flashback of being raped in the shower. Both rapes *could* have happened, only her father and her really *knew* what happened and obviously her father would deny it.

"Are you saying that the word of both Katrina's mother and Sharon are worth nothing, that they should simply be dismissed? Are you seriously saying that despite the obvious fact that Katrina is not well, you are prepared to do nothing to allay her fears about an incident that to any rational person, quite obviously did not happen?" I asked.

Proctor simpered and Yellowlees stared but neither said a word to Katrina that the alleged rape did not happen. Sharon and I looked at each other in total frustration and Sharon said,

"Katrina has been over-dosing on her medication, not enough to cause her harm, but it is obvious she is not capable of controlling the drugs she is being given."

"I have written to her GPs on several occasions, explaining to them about the medication," said Yellowlees.

"Are you saying her GPs are over-prescribing?" I asked.

"Yes," Yellowlees answered, "I have written to them on more than one occasion."

"And what was their response?" I asked.

Yellowlees looked uncomfortable but finally said there was no response and after a few more pointless exchanges, the meeting came to a close. I was not prepared to let things end there however and Sharon and I agreed that I should write to Katrina's GPs to confirm that Yellowlees had actually written to them because there was no way I was prepared to accept the word of Yellowlees without question.

It came as no surprise therefore when, after contacting the GPs who had been dealing with Katrina in both Perth and Crieff, I received the reply that Yellowlees had contacted neither of them and that all drugs which had been administered by them to Katrina, had been prescribed by Murray Royal. I wrote to Yellowlees on August 8th asking for an explanation and wrote to Frank Brown at the Health Trust with the same information on the same day, adding the following comment, *"It looks as if we can now add Katrina's GPs to the ever-lengthening list of those who seem to find it difficult to understand Dr Yellowlees."*

On the 17th August I received a reply from a very irate Dr Yellowlees complaining bitterly that I had accused him of being "less than honest". He wrote,

"I take great exception to your defamatory comment indicating that you thought I had been less than truthful in my dealings with Katrina's family. I would totally refute this since I have spent a great deal of time trying to explain those complex matters, most recently in the lengthy meeting Dr Proctor and I had with you, Katrina and Sharon on the 31st July.

Let me now turn to the matter of Katrina's medication which you feel requires further explanation. I am puzzled that you contacted Katrina's General Practitioner in Perth and Crieff in the way that you did following our meeting with you, Katrina and Sharon. This was not part of Katrina's management strategy which we discussed at some length." I still find it hard to believe Yellowlees actually wrote that comment, as if I had done something underhand, which inadvertanly exposed him as lying once again. His letter continued,

"I expressed concern about the amount of oral psychotropic medication that Katrina was consuming. (No, Sharon raised the quantity of drugs Katrina was taking)

"My view was that she had developed a degree of psychological dependence on these medications. (A bit rich given that he had been prescribing them since Katrina had gone into his care twenty months previously). *I hold Katrina's GPs in high regard and have no doubt that they have been prescribing the SPECIFIC TYPES of drugs that the hospital has specified. What has been of concern to me is the AMOUNT of drugs that Katrina has been consuming, particularly at times of crisis in the community."*

The only drugs Katrina was taking were prescribed drugs, prescribed by him but his next paragraph continued,

"Sometimes she might have been advised to increase her medication at these times in an attempt to control her symptoms. This however is a matter for the individual doctor in dealing with a given situation..."

I have personally written to the General Practitioners on a number of occasions recently and expressed my concern. I also spoke with them following receipt of your letter. I do believe that everyone involved in Katrina's care is aware of the need to keep a close eye on the amount of medication that she is actually consuming."

Yellowlees sent copies of that letter to Frank Brown- Chief Executive, Caroline Inwood- Director of Nursing and Quality, Dr Peter Connelly -Clinical Director, Charlotte Proctor and Alan Sharp – lawyer at Central Legal Office. Significantly no copy was sent to the GPs Yellowlees was blaming for over-prescribing drugs for Katrina. He was also repeating his claim that he had contacted them on several occasions, despite their denial that he had done any such thing. I answered Yellowlees's letter on 19th August in the following terms,

"I am in receipt of your letter of 15th inst. and have to point out that to date, it is the quickest response I have had from anyone associated with the Health Trust. It cannot be because I accused you of lying; I first did that during our telephone conversation in December 1995. I accused

you again at the meeting of 2nd May 1996 at which you, Caroline Inwood, Dr Proctor, Sharon, Philip and I were present. At that meeting you expressed the same outrage, blustered a little but finally admitted it. You will no doubt have a copy of the letter I sent to Frank Brown on 26th June 1996, in which I give at least two further examples of your willingness to stray from the truth. Petulant expressions of outrage and persistant denial will not change the fact that you have lied to both me and my family, not once but several times.

The amount of time which you have spent, as you put it, "trying to explain complex matters to Katrina's family" is totally irrelevant as much of that time has been spent attempting to deny remarks you had made previously.

You repeat your claim that you have written to the "General Practitioners on a number of occasions recently and expressed my concern." Are we to understand it has been necessary to write "on a number of occasions" because the GPs ignored your first expressions of concern? No doubt their own records will confirm the number of times you have written.

It is of no concern to me that you take exception to my comments, nor that you find them defamatory. Defamation is actionable and you have a legal team at your disposal. Not only will I not withdraw my comments but I will continue to make them to anyone with a concern in this case, until this matter is resolved."

I next received a letter from Frank Brown, Chief Executive, dated 23rd August 1996 and in response to my letter of 16th July. In light of the similarities in the letters written by both Jackson on behalf of the Social Work Department of Perth & Kinross Council and Brown on behalf of the Health Trust, we could have been excused for believing there is a school for bureaucrats out there somewhere, where bureaucrats are taught bureaucrat-speak, the language of sophistry, how to dissemble, massage the truth, or better still ignore it altogether; all the while dragging the complainant ever deeper into the vortex of total frustration. Every letter was a repetition of the dross and pap to which we had already been subjected by Yellowlees, Inwood and Proctor, every lie was given validity by the Health Trust's Executive. The following is a verbatim copy of Brown's letter;

Dear Mr Fairlie,

Further to my recent letter of 16th July 1996 I have asked those identified in your letter for their comments and I am now in a position to respond to the issues raised. I apologise for the delay in responding to your letter.

Dr A J Yellowlees has confirmed that he has never been untruthful to you regarding your daughter's illness or her statements to him. Dr Yellowlees admitted at the meeting on 2nd May that he did deny, during a telephone conversation with you, that he had previously stated that he found you intimidating at imposing. He gave you a full explanation at the same meeting and has nothing to add on the matter.

Dr Yellowlees at no time has ever indicated to your family or to the police that he thought you were guilty of the alleged abuse.

At the meeting of 2nd May 1996 Dr Yellowlees gave you explanations in relation to your accusations against him. It is unfortunate that you have not found these explanations helpful.

In relation to Sister J Hogg, she did not make a statement to the police. Her involvement was to witness Katrina's statement only.

With regard to your comments to the pressure Katrina feels, it is clear that she experiences the situation differently from you and your family. Dr Yellowlees has offered Katrina a second opinion at almost every interview he has held with her. Dr Yellowlees has also discussed the issue of a second opinion with Katrina's general practitioner.

In relation to Katrina's level of observation by staff. The report relating to the recent incident you described in your letter, Katrina was on one to one observation when this incident occurred and was not at risk. She remained under one to one observation due to her agitation until the staff believed it was safe to reduce the level of observation.

Dr Yellowlees and Dr Proctor have offered you further meetings to discuss issues that continue to cause you concern. I understand that you had another meeting with Dr Yellowlees and Dr Proctor on 31st July

1996 when you have been able to discuss your concerns further. Dr Yellowlees and Dr Proctor felt the meeting was productive and were disappointed that you have not perceived the meeting the same way.

With regard to your most recent letter your comments about adding "Katrina's GPs to the ever lengthening list" are unacceptable. During the meeting Dr Yellowlees expressed his concern about Katrina's increasing psychological dependence on oral psychotropic medication. In hospital she has often pressurised staff in order to receive oral psychotropic medication and there has been some suggestion that her general practitioners are put in the position of recommending additional oral psychotropic medication for her, particularly when some crisis presents itself to them in the community. There is also evidence that Katrina self medicates on medication which has been prescribed by the general practitioners and takes excessive doses of this medication when she feels she needs it.

Dr Yellowlees has recently written personally to the general practitioners indicating his concerns about her dependence on oral medication on more than one occasion in recent months. It is the amount of oral psychotropic medication that has to be watched. The general practitioners are correctly prescribing the specific types of drugs recommended by the hospital.

I hope that this explanation reinforces the one already given to you by Dr Yellowlees.

Yours sincerely

Frank Brown
Chief Executive.

Kay and I had left for our annual holidays to France by the time Brown's letter arrived in Crieff, therefore I did not respond to it until 1st October. Again, I am quoting verbatim and at length from my reply so that the reader can be sure that Brown, as Chief Executive of the Health Trust, was never left in any doubt about the nature of our complaints against Yellowlees and Proctor. Nor was he in any doubt about how I felt about his replies and his attempts to confuse the issues at every opportunity.

Dear Mr Brown,

Dr Yellowlees has never been accused of lying about my daughter's illness, nor about the nature of her statements to him. What he is being accused of is the way in which he convinced my family that I was guilty of abuse, by presenting his diagnosis of Katrina's illness and his interpretation of her statements, in such a way as to contend there was no explanation for Katrina's condition, other than that she had suffered severe sexual and physical abuse at my hands.

I have made that plain to you on several occasions in previous correspondence and I can only conclude that you are setting out to be deliberately obtuse by attempting to introduce and then deny, an allegation which has never been made. No doubt Yellowlees will continue to deny and deny (in much the same way as abusers are often accused of doing) despite the evidence to the contrary, but he also took certain actions which can only be explained in terms of his believing that I was guilty of abuse.

According to the police, Sister Hogg CONFIRMED Katrina's statement to them. You are no doubt aware of the difference between confirming and witnessing another's statement. Is Sister Hogg maintaining that she sat in silence throughout Katrina's statement, which is all that would have been required to bear witness. Is she saying she was never asked if it was a true account of what had taken place, and that she made no comment whatsoever to the police?

At the meeting of 2nd May 1996, Dr Yellowlees gave no explanation in relation to the accusations I made against him, other than to finally admit that he had lied to me on the telephone in December 1995. What Dr Yellowlees did was simply deny all accusations, despite being confronted by two of the people to whom he had made his damaging statements.

As to his explanation of his lying to me on the telephone, Dr Yellowlees is perfectly at liberty to find me intimidating and imposing, but he offered that as an assessment of me to my daughter Sharon when she questioned him about Katrina's allegations about my violence. It is the context in which the statement was made that makes it so damaging. At the meeting of 2nd May after he had finally admitted to lying to me, Dr Yellowlees tried to brush it aside as being simply an observation. If that was true, why try to deny it?

It is not only astonishing but crass for you to claim Katrina was not at risk. How can someone who is on one to one observation almost succeed in hanging themselves and not be considered at risk?

It really is becoming rather tiresome to be told that Dr Yellowlees and Dr Proctor think meetings that have been held with members of the family were "productive" when they can have been left in no doubt that they were nothing of the kind. At the meeting of 31st July which was attended by Sharon, Katrina and I, it was made clear to Drs Yellowlees and Proctor that Katrina's latest allegations of sexual abuse could not possibly have taken place for the simple reason that I was nowhere near her flat at the alleged times, was in fact at home and had witnesses who could prove it.

On being pushed by Sharon, Dr Yellowlees stated, "You seem to want me to say it did not happen, but I can't say that because I was not there." Sharon insisted there was proof the alleged incident could not have happened, that even Katrina accepted that it could not have happened. Dr Yellowlees continued to protest that he "was not there" and was therefore unable to confirm to Katrina that the incidents could not have taken place. Dr Proctor went even further and suggested that the only two people who would know for certain whether or not anything had taken place were Katrina and me. You will no doubt appreciate what a competent QC will do with that kind of argument in court but you expect us to accept that the meeting was "productive".

As you also insist that Dr Yellowlees has written several times to Katrina's GPs I can only assume that you have seen copies of those letters and can confirm the dates on which they were sent. Will you confirm that you have seen them and on how many occasions the GPs were contacted? This is obviously important if we are to establish that the GPs have been ignoring Dr Yellowlees's instructions, as he has claimed they have.

Your "explanation" as you call it, is no more than a regurgitation of the evasions, denials, expressions of outrage and general pap I have already received from Dr Yellowlees. If it reinforces anything, it is the sense of relief I have that my daughter is now going to be treated in Edinburgh."

By this time we had managed to have Katrina referred to another "specialist" in eating disorders in Edinburgh, through the efforts of our own GP, the details of which will be covered in depth in the next section and our relief was to be very short-lived. I received one final piece of correspondence from Frank Brown on the 12th November 1996. We had been in correspondence for almost a full year, as the Health Trust conducted its internal inquiry. Brown's letter ran as follows,

"I have given the contents of your most recent letter considerable consideration. I have also considered all of our previous communications with you and we have endeavoured to respond in good faith to both your concerns and questions over a considerable period of time.

I note that my reponse to your letters are followed by the same or very similar questions being asked again. Given that we have already provided replies I would have to advise you that I have nothing further to add to my earlier correspondence.

I understand that a second opinion has been given by Dr Freeman, Consultant Psychiatrist of the Royal Edinburgh Hospital with regard to Katrina and that he is now involved in her care management.

In the meantime, Dr Yellowlees, Dr Proctor and Mrs Inwood will continue to make themselves available should you wish to meet to discuss any further concerns you have.

I again enclose a copy of the information leaflets which describe how you may progress your complain should you remain dis-satisfied.

Yours sincerely

Frank Brown
Chief Executive.

Thus ended the great internal inquiry by the Perth & Kinross Healthcare NHS Trust. Had anything been achieved? Had anything been established? Were we any further forward? The answer to all of those questions is a very qualified "Yes". We had been given the opportunity to provide details of our complaints about Yellowlees and his team, therefore there could be no possible doubt that the Health Trust had no idea of the nature of our complaint. The same details had been provided to the Mental Welfare Commission, therefore it could never be argued we had not tried every avenue open to us, short of the Ombudsman, to have our concerns addressed. The Central Legal Office were also aware of what had been going on, therefore the people most in a position to actually address our complaints had all been given an opportunity to deal with them and all of them had done no more than gone through the motions.

What had been established was that none of the bodies to which our concerns had been addressed had any intention of even acknowledging there were any grounds for complaint. Jackson, Director of Law and Administration with Perth & Kinross Council had simply removed from our list of complaints, the behaviour of the Director of Social Work, Betty Bridgeford, the person whose conduct had led to the most damaging accusation being made against me and led her Director of Child Protection, Napier, to the false conclusion that I had engaged contacts in the SNP to act on my behalf. This had in turn, given my family cause to believe there just might be something in the allegations of abuse which had been made against me. Jackson, despite acknowledging there were conflicting accounts of what took place, decided to accept the word of his staff, without any explanation of why their account was more believable than that of the family, and came to the conclusion that everyone had performed admirably. It was perfectly acceptable to have shredded all original notes, to claim falsely, there was no file on me, to have concocted a file that was a total fabrication in order to cover up their own mistakes and to pass on sensitive information as a matter of idle gossip.

The Mental Welfare Commission had shown they had no interest whatsoever in our complaint, far less the welfare of Katrina. The Health Trust believed that Katrina's entire family, including her parents, her three brothers and her sister, the police and Katrina's GPs, were all either lying or lacked the intelligence to understand a single, simple piece of information, such was their faith in the integrity and infallibility of Dr Yellowlees and Dr Proctor. We were forced to learn an entirely new vocabulary as meetings which ended in acrimony and frustration were described as "productive" and an admission of lying was to be no more than "an explanation of why the truth was not told." "Professional judgement" was all that was required for the most heinous crimes of sexual abuse, rape and murder to have taken place. But witness statements could just as easily be dismissed, particularly if they ran counter to "professional judgement", because the good Doctors "were not there".

We had also learned the very valuable lesson that the Health Trust, in the shape of its executive officers such as Inwood and Brown, would procrastinate, evade, distort and blatantly lie if to tell the truth would highlight their mistakes or show them in a bad light.

The most blatant example was the allegation of the rape in the shower. There was no report, there never had been a report but Hogg had told the police there was a report given to the hospital because that is what Katrina had said. It would have cost them nothing to admit as much; to admit they had made a mistake by telling the police that Katrina had reported the rape when she returned to the hospital. For whatever reason, they just continued to lie about it, leaving Katrina to believe that she had actually made a report of a rape when what had happened was she had had a flashback. More importantly, the police were led to believe a report had been made of a rape which had just taken place. Why they did not ask why they were not called immediately was never explained.

In terms of progress, we had shown the allegations of abuse, rape and murder to be baseless as well as stopping the Social Work Department in its tracks. After our contacts with the psychiatric team which was at the bottom of all the allegations, we were entitled to question the sanity of some of those most responsible for Katrina's care. The Clinical Director McGuinness had refused to say whether or not he believed in alien abduction, Yellowlees was an admitted liar, while some of the rest of the team such as Hogg were proven liars and Proctor believed in body memories. By the end of 1996 the credibility of the entire team at Murray Royal/Gilgal had been well and truly shot but our battle to have Katrina restored to health was far from being over. In fact it had done no more than entered another chapter, one which created its own heartache. We were only half way through the long haul.

CHAPTER SEVENTEEN

THE LONG HAUL
March 1996 – October 1997

When Katrina discharged herself from Murray Royal on March 6th 1996, she was far from being well but, as she said at the time, she was afraid that if she stayed there any longer, she might never be well enough to come home. She was told repeatedly, as were we, that she was a very badly damaged young woman, who had been subjected to the most violent physical and sexual abuse from a very young age. No amount of evidence that pointed to a childhood that was very different from the one the psychiatric team believed she had, made any difference as their "professional judgement" took precedence. It is worth emphasising again, that no physical or forensic evidence of this abuse existed or could exist. There was nothing and no one that could corroborrate the allegations which were made, nothing that is, other than Katrina's drug-induced flashbacks and nightmares, together with the all-important "professional judgement".

Kay and I were very sensitive to Katrina's mood swings and her reliance on her medication. When she came to live with us in Crieff, she was still subject to psychotic episodes and hallucinations and we had to watch her twenty-four hours a day, every day. This meant that one of us stayed with her at all times, night and day with Kay and I sleeping in two hour shifts through the night. Unfortunately for Kay, I could not be on my own with her and if she woke up during the night when it was my turn "on watch", I immediately woke Kay. There could be days on end when Kay was lucky to get more than a few hours sleep, and that never came in periods of more than a couple of hours at a time. Within a very short time we were both utterly exhausted because I still had a job to go to and therefore much of the time Kay had the sole responsibility for looking after Katrina. It caused us to smile wryly when later, in their defence, Murray Royal wrote that "Katrina posed a difficult management problem." So, tell us about it.

In the short time we had been in contact with the British False Memory Society (BFMS), they had been an enormous help to us. They provided us with the information we needed to question Yellowlees and his team with some authority and gave us the lifeline that what had happened to us had happened to hundreds of other families in the UK and thousands of families in the USA. Their AGM was due to take place in London, the second week in March and I badly wanted to go. Sharon had been highly sceptical of the BFMS when we had first made contact because there were those in the child protection industry who were suspicious of anyone or any group that questioned their absolute belief that child abuse was everywhere and every man was a potential rapist. Her scepticism had lessened when she saw some of the material we had been sent, but she was not convinced it was a good idea to attend their AGM. Her concerns influenced Kay for a short time but I was determined to go, even if it meant going on my own.

Kay agreed to come with me so arrangements were made for Katrina to stay with Sharon while we flew to London. We took an early flight from Dundee to London City on the Saturday of the meeting, which allowed us to make the beginning of the AGM with time to spare. We were able to get an evening flight back so that although we had a very long day, it was only one day and we were able to have Katrina back with us on the Sunday. Kay and Sharon shared the concern about the type of people we would meet. Sharon's contacts had been vitriolic about the US counterpart, the False Memory Syndrome Foundation, claiming they acted as a refuge and mouthpiece for paedophiles and rapists. I thought it only natural that, given the nature of the issue with which we were dealing, there should be concern but some of the claims being made were simply outageous as far as I was concerned. I had no intention of condemning a group of people who had gone through trauma which mirrored our own, because someone had spoken to someone, who had a friend, who had met a woman at the checkout in Tescos, who had it on good authority from someone who had read it on the back of a raffle ticket.

When we arrived and made ourselves known to Roger Scotford, he immediately introduced us to Tanya Hunter, whose story in the Mail on Sunday, had prompted us to contact the BFMS. Both Kay and I were immediately attracted to Tanya, who came across as a very intelligent and open person. We chatted about her willingness to tell her story and we thanked her for having had the courage to do so, because without that initial information I still have no idea how things would have progressed for us. Tanya's daughter Anna, had recovered and although she was not at the meeting, she was well discussed by those who were. Roger Scotford opened the meeting by welcoming us and one or two others who were there for the first time. Roger likes to tell the story of the very early days of the Society when, after they had held a few meetings in the same venue, the lady who was responsible for the meeting place, had commented to Roger about the people who attend the meetings. She offered the opinion that they seemed to be a particularly nice group of people and asked what qualifications were needed for membership of the club. I have heard Roger tell that story on a number of occasions since that first meeting and it always raises a very rueful laugh from the membership.

We all found we had several things in common. Obviously we were all of a certain age group because the accusers were more often than not, daughters or other female relatives who were in their late teens at least, before the allegations were made. Without exception, the claims were historical and the accuser had had no recollection of any abuse until entering therapy. The reasons for therapy were often complex but there was a common thread which included women suffering from post-natal depression, young adult women with various types of eating disorder, highly intelligent young women whose studies had caused stress, which led to counselling which led to allegations of sexual abuse. It was not long before Kay said to one woman who was accompanied by her husband and whose daughter was the same age as Katrina and had accused them, that we were all in a position to finish each other's sentences, so similar were the stories.

One of the other features which was very obvious, we were predominantly middle class and professionals, intelligent, articulate and perfectly capable of fighting our corner with authority. Unfortunately, for a number of different reasons, some were not prepared to take on authority, which meant they limited their ability to clear their names. Some simply lived in hope that some day, their daughter would finally realise the abuse had not taken place and would retract. Their doors remained open always but unfortunately for some, their daughters never did walk through until it was too late. At first I found it difficult to understand why they would not take the fight to the psychiatrists responsible for their agony, but I soon realised there is no right or wrong way to fight the curse of Recovered Memory therapists. People deal with the problem in their own way and no one has the right to tell them they are wrong because they have chosen a different course. For me, the only way to deal with Yellowees et al was to fight back, to give them absolutely no quarter, not an inch, and to question every single statement they made until they provided evidence as opposed to their so-called "professional opinion". Of course, no evidence was ever produced, despite the allegations that rape and incest were on-going, even when Katrina was a patient in hospital. The lack of evidence meant nothing to the psychiatric staff, who continued to believe I was guilty.

Despite the nature of the problems we all faced, we made friendships at that first meeting which have remained as strong as some which we have had since we were at school. As one of those friends said on one occasion, "We all have friends who have been close friends all our lives and they will remain close friends. But the friendships that have been forged through the BFMS have a different kind of closeness and strength because we all share that common experience that cannot be shared with anyone who has not gone through it." We left that first meeting exhausted but remarkably cheered by the contact with others who had shared that experience and who knew exactly what we were going through. It was good to know we always had that contact because the problems with Katrina continued.

Katrina had been forced to give up the flat she shared with Eileen shortly after the confrontation in October 1995, a year after her admission to Murray Royal. She had been made redundant from the Post Office at the same time and in any case, there was no prospect of her being able to work when she discharged herself from Murray Royal in March 1996. We knew however, it was important to find her a place of her own and we were lucky enough that the local authority had offered her a flat in Perth shortly after her discharge. Unfortunately she was rarely able to stay in it, particularly in the early months. Her depression and dissociative episodes continued and we were forced to ask for her re-admission to Murray Royal on April 12th. It was very much against our better judgement but neither Kay nor I were knowledgeable enough to care for Katrina, nor did we have the facilities to cope.

Her stay in Murray Royal lasted only a few days, during which time she settled very quickly back into their routine. She was no sooner back in Crieff than she suffered from flashbacks and nightmares, forcing Kay and I to sit with her sometimes for hours, until she settled enough for one or other of us to snatch a couple of hours sleep. It was not just a case of sitting with Katrina, her moods were so dark and the risk of her harming herself were so great, that we never allowed her to have her dressing gown cord with her at any time, nor was she ever allowed access to anything with which she could harm herself. This meant taking the cutlery drawer into our bedroom at night and making sure there were none of my tools or knives anywhere where she could have access to them. We were forced to ask for her re-admission again on April 24th, but again her stay lasted only long enough for her to be stabilised, after which she was allowed back to Crieff.

We tried to encourage her to stay in her own flat and when she was discharged from Murray Royal at the beginning of May, after only a couple of days in Crieff, she moved into her own flat in Perth. That did not mean our responsibilities were reduced because we were summoned at all hours of the day and night if Katrina had one of her psychotic episodes, where she saw fairies or felt the urge to harm herself. On Monday May 13th, I was in my office in Tay Street in Perth, when I received a telephone call from Murray Royal. A Dr Tait was on the line. He had treated Katrina on occasion but was not responsible for her treatment and Kay had had more contact with him than I had but I considered Dr Tait to be one of the "good guys".

"Mr Fairlie, we have Katrina up at the unit just now and I am very concerned about the nature of her conversation. Is it possible for you to come up to the hospital straight away?"

"What is Katrina doing up at the unit?" I asked, immediately concerned both at what Dr Tait had said and at the tone of his voice.

"She was up visiting one of her friends who is a patient here and is making ready to leave. I am very concerned about some of the conversation that has passed between her and the other girl and I don't think it would be safe to allow her to leave on her own. However, I am fully aware of the situation between you and the hospital and I don't want to do anything that might make matters worse. That is why I telephoned you." he said.

"I will be up straight away. Where will I get you?" I asked, getting up from my chair and walking round the desk in readiness to leave immediately.

"I will meet you at the front door of Gilgal," Tait said as he hung up.

I was at the hospital door in ten minutes flat and hurried inside to find Dr Tait waiting for me in the foyer.

"Where is Katrina?" I asked quickly, "you haven't allowed her to leave have you?"

"No, she is still with her friend. I told her you were coming up to see me about something entirely unconnected with her but she said she would see you before you left. I do need to speak to you before you see her," said Tait, ushering me into an interview room off the corridor leading to the main ward, where Katrina was speaking to her friend.

"What is the problem?" I asked, "What was she saying that made you so concerned?"

"Her whole conversation was about committing suicide and given her recent history, I don't think she should leave here. I want to section her but I want your approval first." said Tait.

"I know she is bad just now and you will know she has been back in here twice since she discharged herself in March. Kay and I are at the end of our tether to be quite honest," I said. I then told Dr Tait just how difficult things had been and how desperate we were to get Katrina help. I explained in detail how much she had to be watched, about her psychotic episodes and our fear of leaving her on her own. Dr Tait was well aware of Katrina's recent history and my account of our difficulties of dealing with her at home, merely confirmed his conviction that she should be re-admitted. I agreed it should be done but cautioned Dr Tait,

"Katrina is not going to be happy, but I am prepared to tell her if you want me to."

"No, it will be better if I tell her but I will have to get two of the nursing staff to take her to the ward and have her re-admitted. Will you wait here until I attend to that? I'll not be more than a few minutes."

Several minutes went by and I was beginning to wonder what had happened when I heard a piercing scream that I recognised straight away as coming from Katrina. Then her voice sounded, it seemed just outside the door.

"Dad! Dad they're hurting me. Dad."

As I rushed to the door, Tait came bursting in.

"Can you come out here?" he said breathlessly.

I pushed past him into the corridor and immediately took in what was happening. Two male nurses had Katrina pinned to the floor, her face pushed into the carpet. They each had an arm and were twisting the wrists in opposite directions. This was not a dream. Psychiatric staff euphemistically call this "restraining the patient" allegedly to stop them hurting themselves. Katrina by this time weighed no more than seven and a half to eight stone. She could have been easily held by one of them with one hand, but these two bastards looked as if they were enjoying their work

I didn't say a word I simply slapped a judo choke on the nurse nearest me and pushed his Adam's apple back into his throat. Had he held on to Katrina's wrist he would have been unconscious in seconds, but as I put pressure on his throat and my knee into his back to increase leverage, he immediately let go and frantically clawed at my arm to try to release the hold. I increased the pressure pulling him upwards at the same time, to make sure his wind was completely cut off before spinning him around and slamming him into the wall. The other nurse immediately got up from his knees and backed right off. Dr Tait looked horrified. I picked Katrina up from the floor and she clung to me in floods of tears. I looked at the nurses and I can only guess at the look on my face because they were giving me a very wide berth.

"If ever I see either of you lay a finger on her again I will BREAK your neck."

Tait came towards me, his hands outstretched, signing for me to calm down. He pointed to a door further down the hall, to my rear and away from the nurses, who stood still, staring at me, with the one I had almost strangled massaging his throat.

"You will get peace in here," said Tait, holding open the door of the interview room.

Katrina still clung to me, sobbing and trying to speak at the same time.

We sat down and I put my arms around Katrina, trying to get her to settle. It was impossible to make out what she was saying as she continued to sob bitterly, catching her breath as she tried to speak.

"Dad, I just want to die. Why did you come up? I just want to die. I can't go on any more, it's too hard."

I just held her for a few moments and let her speak, without making any attempt to answer her. It was like holding a child and in many ways, that was what Katrina had become. She was no longer capable of looking after herself. I sat and held her, stroking her hair as she pushed her face into my shoulder and sobbed. Eventually she had cried herself out and sat up, but avoided looking at me.

"I'm sorry Dad, but I just can't go on. I still have those filthy images in my mind. I can still see you abusing me and I know it's not true but the images are still there." Katrina said, breaking into tears again.

"Katrina, the fact you know its not true is a big step forward. Your Mum and I are not going to let you die. You mean far too much to us, to Sharon and the boys. You are not going to die."

"But I'm worthless Dad. The trouble I've caused you and Mum. How can you want me to live?" she said.

"You are just as precious to us now as you ever were. We are going to find out what happened but it was not your fault. You have to believe that Katrina. It was not your fault."

For the next thirty-five minutes I sat and held Katrina, comforting her, letting her talk. She made the same comments over and over about how useless she was and how much trouble she had caused; about how it would be better for everybody if she died. I countered with the same arguments over and over; of how precious she was to the family, pleading with her to accept it was not her fault, that she was not to blame. Tait looked in several times to check if things were all right and finally Katrina was so exhausted, all the fight had gone out of her. She agreed to go to the locked ward and I went with her and waited until she was ready to go to bed, heavily sedated in order to keep her calm and let her get some sleep. Dr Tait and I spoke for a short time and we agreed he would call us at home as soon as he had had the opportunity to speak with

Katrina. I was also exhausted as well as upset, dreading the thought of going home to tell Kay, who knew nothing about any of what had happened.

I called my office and told my secretary I would not be back until the next day, making the excuse I had to see a client out of town. All I wanted to do was get home to discuss with Kay what we were going to do. We had spoken to our own doctor, who was trying to find another specialist somewhere, anywhere, so long as it was not Murray Royal and Yellowlees. There was no traffic on the back road from Perth to Crieff, which was just as well because my mind was not on my driving. I had hated leaving Katrina there. The conduct of the two male nurses still infuriated me and I could not get the image out of my mind, of Katrina pinned with her face buried into the carpet, with them twisting her wrists. I was quite distraught at the state she had been in, pleading with me to allow her to kill herself and the feeling of helplessness that enveloped me, as I thought of the effort that Kay and I had put in, trying to find an alternative hospital to which we could take Katrina in times of crisis.

About five or six miles from Crieff, there is a long stretch of approximately three quarters of a mile, with a right hand bend at the end of it. Normally I took that bend travelling around fifty miles per hour. By the time I entered that long stretch, my thoughts were in turmoil, thinking of Katrina as a child, laughing, playing with the rest of the family, running around the garden with her friends; then the state she had been in when I left her, the frustration and helplessness I felt at having to leave her, to be looked after by people I had absolutely no faith in and for whom I had nothing but contempt. Without really being aware of it, I was in tears. I could feel them running down my face, soaking the neck of my shirt, blurring my vision.

Suddenly I was aware the bend at the end of the straight was approaching much faster than it should have been. I glanced at the speedometer and realised to my horror I was hitting almost ninety miles per hour. I had just enough time to hit the brakes as hard as I could but there was no way I was going to slow down quickly enough to take that bend. Although I was having difficulty holding the car in a straight line, I let go of the wheel with one hand and pulled on the handbrake, keeping my foot hard on the footbrake at the same time. The car slewed round the bend and I suddenly found myself on the other side of the road, facing in the direction I had just come. Fortunately there are two farm roads just on the Crieff side of that bend and I had spun the car around at the entrance to one of them, which is why I was not wrapped around the wire fence which ran parallel to the road. If there had been another car coming in the opposite direction, both cars would have been written off.

The engine had stalled and I sat with my forehead on the steering wheel, shaking like a leaf and saturated with sweat. My heart was hammering inside my chest and for a few moments I had to fight for breath, feeling as if I had just sprinted uphill. Reversing into the farm entrance, I turned the car round again so that it was back facing in the direction of Crieff – and home, but I switched the engine off again and sat until I had calmed down and stopped sweating. I now realised I had to speak to the doctor, but this time about myself. I had given myself a real fright and was aware I was beginning to come apart at the seams.

As soon as Kay saw me she knew something had happened and we spent most of the afternoon discussing what we could do. Our own GP was trying to find someone who could take over Katrina's treatment but our main concern was finding someplace we could take her when faced with the kind of crisis I had faced that day. The discharge sheet had said Katrina had an eating disorder, although that was not the only problem, but our own GP was looking for a specialist in that area. Unfortunately, Yellowlees was the recognised "expert" in eating disorders, in the Perthsire area. Kay and I had no idea if this was the best approach but we were still very much in the hands of the medical profession, prepared to take advice when we felt we had little or no alternative. Within a few days we were desperately trying to get an appointment to see him because Katrina had made another attempt on her life.

I had agreed with Tait that we would give Katrina a few days to settle before Kay and I went to Murray Royal to visit her but Kay had telephoned her both morning and evening for the two days she had been in and had agreed with Katrina we would visit her at the weekend. She had been sectioned on May 13th and on the 16th, Kay received a telephone call from the hospital, to say there had been "an incident". Attempted suicides were always "incidents"; that sounded much softer somehow and covered a multitude of sins. When Kay said we would come to the hospital that evening, she was told it had not been serious, that Katrina was sedated and quite settled and that it would be better if we waited until the next day or the day after. Kay said we would be at the hospital the following day and we would expect to see some senior staff member to discuss what had happened.

We were able to see Katrina the next day but she was so heavily sedated, it was difficult to get any conversation with her. A nurse accompanied her and sat at an adjoining table the whole time we were there, which was not long given the circumstances. Katrina said very little about what had happened, except to tell us she had attempted to hang herself in the toilets with the cord from her dressing gown; the nurse professed to know nothing about the incident and we were told there was no one of any seniority, able to see us at that time. As usual, we left the hospital seething with frustration and more concerned than ever, if that was possible.

This attempt on her life by Katrina had come less than a fortnight after our meeting with Inwood, Yellowlees and Proctor, all of whom were so self-satisfied with their treatment of Katrina that there should have been absolutely no possibility of anything like this ever happening, if the reality of Katrina's care had borne any resemblance to their account of the care she was given. Two days later, we received Brown's letter, in which he repeated the fantasy with which he was being fed by Yellowlees and his team. My next meeting with my own GP gave me the opportunity to relate all of this and to impress on him yet again, the urgency we felt about finding alternative care for Katrina. I left with his assurance that he was doing everything in his power to find that alternative, together with a prescription for anti-depressants for myself.

The pressure was definitely beginning to get to me. My work as a financial adviser was demanding, I wrote two columns for the local paper each week, I was going through the so-called internal inquiries with both the Perth & Kinross Council and the Health Trust, as well as trying to force the Mental Welfare Commission to take the interest in Katrina's welfare it insisted was part of its remit. On top of that, Kay and I had the constant stress of dealing with Katrina. We were never sure what the next day would bring. There had been numerous attempts on her life, some of which could be dismissed as attention grabbing but there were others which were certainly serious and might very easily have been final, had it not been for the hospital staff. Regular visits to the gym helped to get rid of some of the frustration and aggression that had begun to build up, but there was no getting rid of the anger, sometimes fury, that gripped me each time we were met with the bureaucratic indifference to what had been done to our lives. The feeling of complete helplessness was the most difficult to deal with.

I was a keen hill walker and when the anger was beginning to get the better of me, spending time on my own in the mountains, which were right on our doorstep, was one of the best antidotes. Kay did not like my going away on my own, particularly to places like Glencoe, one of my favourite areas, but there were times when the last thing I needed was company and the mountains provided the solitude I needed, as well as being physically demanding enough to satisfy the need to get rid of the aggression. Unfortunately the relief was only ever temporary, largely because there was always something new that had to be dealt with and which would start the cycle of frustration and aggression all over again.

Kay found the best solution of all by encouraging me to buy my own horse. I had ridden as a child, having had my own pony from the age of seven until my teens. The opportunities to continue riding regularly did not arise again until our own family had grown up and left the family home, which was when we moved to Crieff. I had spoken about getting my own horse before but Kay saw my need for my own company at times, being more easily satisfied by owning a horse, than by going into the hills on my own. She would also be far less concerned. I was lucky enough to soon find just what I was looking for, a seventeen one hand, chestnut, three quarter thoroughbred, cross Irish Draft. Ben, as he was called, was rising eight years when I bought him and soon became by best pal. For the next eight years I spent countless hours with him, riding in the hills around Perthshire and there is no doubt he gave me far greater peace of mind than either the gym or the mountains. He was the gentlest of animals, although lively enough when doing cross country, and I was able to teach my grandaughter Ilona to ride on him, despite her being only nine years old.

If anything, the situation was more difficult for Kay because she did not have the same physical outlets I had, to get rid of her frustration and anger which were just as great as my own. We often walked around Crieff but Kay did not accompany me on the serious hill walks. She also had far closer contact with Katrina because we both felt it was impossible for me to be on my own with her and we were soon to be put into a position where her contact with Katrina would become even closer and more demanding, both in terms of time and emotional effort. Kay also provided me with the support when I needed it, which was often, although we supported each other. Fortunately, when one of us felt things were getting on top of us, the other always had the strength of purpose and mind to pull the other through. It is often claimed that crises such as the one we went through, make a marriage stronger, although it is also true, that such a crisis has broken many a marriage. In our case, our survival was testimony to the strength of our marriage, a strength without which it would never have survived, such was the pressure to which we were subjected. We were soon to be set another test as Katrina's contact with Yellowlees and Murray Royal was finally broken for ever.

The episode in July 1996 was the final act in the long-running saga of association with Murray Royal and Yellowlees and his team.

It caused all of us, not least Katrina, major concerns about her health. To some extent it confirmed Yellowlees's verdict that Katrina was not fit to leave hospital but it also confirmed our own fears that she was institutionalised and that the reliance on the hospital regime had to be broken. The problem we faced was how to cope with the fall out of leaving a regime which was geared to provide twenty-four hour care and attention. With the best will in the world, we were not able to provide twenty-four hour care. We coped, as best we could, and frequently managed for two and three weeks at a time. But it exhausted Kay and I and Sharon and Neil had had more than enough. Both had full time jobs and two young children, while Philip and Alison had three children and Philip worked long hours in the prison service while Alison was in her final year at college studying to be a social worker. Andrew and Ashley lived in Glasgow and Jim and Anne had two young children and Jim worked as a shepherd with all the working hours that dealing with livestock entailed.

Each time Katrina had to go back into hospital, she settled very quickly while each time she came back to live in her flat, or to stay with us, the psychotic episodes and suicidal feelings returned. Perhaps what concerned us most about her claim that I had just raped her in her flat, was the shattering of our own belief that she knew none of the abuse had taken place. If she had been convinced of that, why would she have been so certain I had just raped her, so certain that she called her mother to tell her? What did that say about Katrina's state of mind? How long would it be before this cycle of recovered memories could be broken? Would it ever be truly broken?

There were a series of minor scares and very short stays in hospital but in September, our GP finally managed to find a specialist in eating disorders who was prepared to discuss Katrina's case. He had been given some of the basic details and agreed to see Katrina, as well as discuss the history of the case with us. His name was Dr Chris Freeman, who was a consultant at Edinburgh Royal Hospital and was the Principal of the Cullen Centre, a specialist unit dealing with eating disorders and attached to Edinburgh Royal. A meeting was arranged for early October.

CHAPTER EIGHTEEN

October 1996 – October 1997

Both Kay and I approached the meeting with Dr Freeman with a completely open mind, so keen were we to give an opportunity to anyone who was prepared to examine Katrina's case objectively. We came away from the first meeting with a new feeling of hope and a sense of relief that at last, we had found someone who not only understood our concerns but actually shared many of them. In many ways Freeman looked like every person's idea of the stereotypical psychiatrist. He was a large, loose limbed man with unruly hair, who wore his clothes carelessly. Our initial discussion was relaxed and informal, as he listened with interest to what Kay and I had to say about our complaints and concerns. After about thirty minutes or so, he asked to speak to Katrina on her own. They spoke for almost an hour, at the end of which Freeman had another short discussion with Kay and I. His summary of what he had gleaned from the discussions he had had with all three of us, was short and to the point.

"I have found the points you have made very interesting and the first thing I wish to emphasise is that I do not think Katrina should be treated as an inpatient," he said. "I don't think she should have been treated as an inpatient in the first place and to continue with that approach would be detrimental to Katrina, in my opinion."

"Why do you think being treated as an inpatient is a problem for Katrina?" asked Kay.

"Patients who are as vulnerable and suggestible as Katrina would appear to be, are better treated as outpatients because they have a tendency to copy the behaviour patterns of other patients in the ward if they are treated as inpatients," replied Freeman.

"Our son Philip, raised that question with Dr Yellowlees, who agreed that he had also noticed some similarities in Katrina's behaviour with that of other girls in the same ward," replied Kay. "What do you propose to do?"

"I think it would be better if Katrina attends the Cullen Centre here as an outpatient until she can be properly assessed," replied Freeman.

"What exactly, will you be treating her for?" I asked. "The discharge letter from Murray Royal mentioned several conditions, none of which Katrina had before she went into hospital."

"The Cullen Centre is the annex of the hospital here, which deals with eating disorders and we will address that problem first of all." said Freeman.

"But what about the allegations of abuse?" I asked, "Surely they will have to be addressed, because although Katrina has retracted all of the allegations and withdrew the police statement, there have been other occasions when she went back into hospital, that she made the same allegations again," I persisted.

Freeman did not answer the question directly but he did assure us that the treatment Katrina had received at Murray Royal /Gilgal would be nothing like the treatment she would receive with Maggie Gray, the Counsellor that would look after Katrina in the Cullen Centre. Gray was a specialist in treating eating disorders. He also said that as far as possible, there would be far less reliance on drugs and "medication on demand", which seemed to be a feature of Katrina's treatment at Murray Royal. We were greatly encouraged by this assurance but the statement which really stuck in our minds, was his reply to my complaint about the difficulty I had had getting any kind of response to the accusation that I had raped Katrina in the shower in Sharon's house. When he was told Katrina had been given a pregnancy test, he looked at us for a long time before he finally said,

"That was just another form of abuse."

At that point our time was up and we were obliged to leave, without meeting Maggie Gray or in fact, covering some of the more recent concerns about Katrina's apparent inability to tell the difference between events which had just happened and those which allegedly took place some time before. Her insistence that I had recently raped her in her flat was a case in point which we did not have time to cover in detail, nor to get Freeman's assessment of what might be wrong. Kay and I agreed that I should call Freeman the next day to try to get an appointment at some later date, but soon, so that we could have a longer discussion with him. Unfortunately he was not available and we never did manage to meet with him again, until it was decided that Katrina should be admitted to the Priory in Roehampton as an in-patient.

The first meeting with Maggie Gray was arranged for the following week and it did not go well. I took Kay and Katrina through by car so that we could both meet Maggie Gray before she started to counsel Katrina. We were determined that she was made fully aware of what had happened. Gray was not openly hostile at the beginning of the meeting, taking Katrina's particulars and outlining the nature of the relationship she hoped to develop. It was agreed there should be weekly meetings, each one lasting a little more than one hour and we impressed on Gray how difficult it would be for Kay and Katrina to get to the Cullen Centre. There was no direct bus service from Crieff to Edinburgh, therefore Kay and Katrina would have to get a bus from Crieff to Perth, from Perth to Edinburgh and then a taxi from the centre of Edinburgh to the Cullen Centre, which was about three miles out of the centre of the city. There were times when the round trip took almost twelve hours, at the end of which both Kay and Katrina were utterly exhausted.

When we had been with Gray approximately thirty minutes, the question of the type of therapy to which Katrina had been subjected was introduced to the conversation. Gray was obviously reluctant to discuss it and made her opposition very plain. Neither Kay nor I was in the mood to be fobbed off again.

"We need to discuss it," I said.

"Why? What good would it do you?" snapped Gray.

"It is not what good it would do us," said Kay equally sharply, "but we have to be certain Katrina is not going to be subjected to more of the same. If we thought for one minute that that was likely to happen, this would be the final meeting she would attend here."

Unfortunately that set the tone for the meeting, with Gray making her hostility to me in particular, quite plain. However, we did get a degree of satisfaction in that she was forced to give us some idea of the kind of approach she would use. We were not convinced Katrina's main problem was any kind of eating disorder. She had always been a healthy eater and her slim build was exactly the same kind of build that the entire family, including Kay and I had. She had always participated in several sports and had never had any kind of problem with food until the latter stages of her stay in Murray Royal. We told Gray about our concerns about the concentration on Katrina's supposed eating disorder but she had her instructions, she said, and there was nothing she could do about that. She did agree to let Freeman know about our concerns, although we have no idea whether or not they were ever passed on. Freeman never returned my call the day after our original meeting and we had no further contact with him in person, although we later found to our cost that he would play a very important part in the proceedings that were to follow.

Between October 16th 1996 and February 1997, Kay took Katrina through to the Cullen Centre every week by public transport. There were a total of fifteen meetings and several times, Katrina's mood and general health was anything but conducive to travelling back and forward to Edinburgh by public transport. On only one occasion did Gray make any effort to speak to Kay and that was under duress because Kay insisted. There was no attempt by either Freeman or Gray to contact us or to include us in any way in Katrina's treatment. We were never brought into their confidence and we were never given any information about Katrina's progress or otherwise. We did not need to be told she was not getting any better. She was still living with us and we still needed to watch her twenty-four hours a day. There were no serious attempts at suicide but her moods were very dark, her conversation was non-existant unless it was to discuss Murray Royal and Yellowlees.

We both made attempts to get her to discuss her therapy at the Cullen Centre but she was anything but communicative about that. It was as if the place did not exist. Katrina spent every day in our house, drinking copious amounts of tea and coffee, never washing the cup she used, no matter how long it had sat with the dregs of the previous contents, smoking up to sixty cigarettes a day and walking endlessly from the sitting room to the kitchen, to her bedroom and back to the sitting room. She never read even a newspaper and had no interest in TV. Her personal hygiene suffered badly and that was probably the single most important indicator of the depth of her depression. Growing up in a family where each and every one of us was sport mad, daily baths and showers, sometimes more than once a day, were a fact of life. We were all fastidious in our personal hygiene and Karina's room had been kept spotless with a place for everything and everything in its place.

That Katrina had disappeared. In her place we were living with some one who avoided washing unless told to do so, whose hair was combed only on the days she was taken to Edinburgh by Kay, who smelled constantly of tobacco smoke and who would never have changed her underwear, had not Kay made her do so on a daily basis. She had pride in neither her appearnace nor her surroundings and Kay fought a constant batttle to get her to wash and keep herself and her room tidy. Watching your daughter obviously suffering in this way, without being able to do a damn thing about it, eventually has a devastating affect on you. Kay had to put up with it for twenty-four hours of every day; trying to engage Katrina in conversation, following her as she wandered from room to room because we could not relax and leave her on her own for any length of time. She was given very little respite when I came home in the evenings because I still could not be on my own with Katrina. In any case, I was constantly involved in writing letters, taking our complaints to another level and attempting to find out as much as I could about Recovered Memory Therapy and the effect it had had on those on whom it had been used.

Whatever kind of mental prison in which Katrina was incarcerated, to all intents and pourposes, she shared it with Kay and I. We were trying to lead life as normally as we could but our own health was beginning to suffer from the sheer exhaustion of dealing with someone we could never be sure that, given the opportunity, would not take her own life. We had had no further contact with Yellowlees and his team and Murray Royal, and with the silence that emanated from Freeman and Gray, we felt totally on our own, dealing with something that neither of us had either the knowledge or the skill to allow us to cope. It was with a certain amount of relief therefore, that towards the end of January 1997, Freeman informed us he was attempting to have Katrina admitted as an in-patient to the Priory.

This was completely contrary to everything Freeman had told us when he first took over Katrina's care and, as we had little or no communication with either him or Maggie Gray during that period, we had no idea what either of them felt about the success or otherwise of their treatment. We saw little or no improvement in Katrina's state of mind and the weekly journeys to Edinburgh were definitely taking their toll on both Kay and Katrina.

At the end of one of the sessions, Gray told Kay that Freeman would like to speak to us both and could see us the following week, if that was possible for us. Expecting to be given an update on Katrina's care and general condition, Kay readily agreed and we both accompanied Katrina the following week. He came to speak to Kay and I while Katrina was having her weekly session with Gray.

When Freeman told us what he intended, we questioned him closely.

"Why are you suggesting Katrina should go back into hospital as an inpatient, when you told us it would not be in her best interest when we first came to see you?" Kay asked him.

"Katrina has not made the progress we had hoped for," replied Freeman, "therefore I think we have to look at the alternative. You must be aware of her continuing depression and her eating disorder is serious enough to require more attention than we can currently give her."

"Why can't she be admitted here, in Edinburgh?" I asked.

"We don't have the bed available just now and I feel she needs to be admitted as soon as possible. I have tried to have her admitted to the Priory in Nottingham but that was not possible, therefore if you and Katrina agree, it will have to be Roehampton," said Freeman.

"Roehampton?" we both exclaimed, looking at each other in astonishment. "But that is the South of England," I said.

"I am afraid it can't be helped," said Freeman. "If it were not necessary, I would not suggest it but Katrina needs the kind of treatment which they provide. Unfortunately they are one of the very few places in the whole of the UK that can provide it."

Neither Kay nor I knew the first thing about the Priory, other than that it was a private clinic, used by celebrities when they were in need of de-toxification – and that it was very exclusive and very, very expensive.

"There is no way we can afford treatment in the Priory," I exclaimed.

"It will cost you nothing as the cost is being borne by the Health Trust," said Freeman.

Kay and I looked at each other, knowing instinctively what the other was thinking.

"Have you discussed it with the Trust and what did they say?" Kay asked.

"They have agreed," said Freeman.

"But for how long?" I asked, "What will happen if they think the treatment has gone on too long and refuse to pay the fees? What will happen to Katrina then?"

"That won't happen," Freeman assured us. "The Trust will pay for Katrina's treatment for however long it takes."

Kay and I looked at each other again and both asked the next question at exactly the same time.

"What are the fees to stay there?" Kay then said, "I have seen reports of several thousand pounds a week. Are you sure the Health Trust is prepared to pay that kind of money for Katrina indefinitely?"

Freeman smiled and said, "Katrina's fees will not be in that category and you must just accept my assurances that the question of payment is not going to be an issue."

"Will Katrina have to be assessed again and how will that be carried out?" I asked.

"Yeees," said Freeman, looking at us both and dragging out the word to make it sound like several syllables. "She will and it will have to be done in Roehampton. I have spoken to Professor Lacey, who will be her consultant and he is prepared to see Katrina as soon as it can be arranged for you to go down."

"Have you spoken to Katrina about this?" Kay asked.

"Maggie Gray is speaking to her now," Freeman said.

"What if she does not want to go? She has not had a good experience of being an in-patient and I don't think we should try to persuade her against her wishes, as we did the last time," Kay said, directing this as much towards me as to Freeman.

"I agree," I said emphatically. "There is no way I am going to put pressure on Katrina to go down to the South of England, hundreds of miles from us, if anything goes wrong and she wants to come home. What happens if she absconds from the Priory, they way she did at Gilgal?"

Surprisingly, Katrina did not put up any serious objections when she came into the room with Gray, who had obviously covered the ground thoroughly with her. Before we left the Cullen Centre, Freeman had called the Priory and arranged for Katrina to go there to be assessed the following week.

Kay and I agreed it would be best if we could get down to Roehampton and back again on the same day, worried about an overnight stay in London with Katrina. She and Kay would have shared a room but we were too aware of what might happen if Katrina took one of her "turns" and were not prepared to take the chance. We took an early morning flight to Gatwick, the train to London and then to Roehampton, arriving about 12.30pm for an appointment at 2.00pm. Our return flight was at 6.00pm, which meant we would arrive home in Crieff, some time after 9.00pm. That was the plan but unfortunately, it did not work out like that. Professor Lacey spoke to all three of us together at the appointed time but when he was ready to speak to Katrina on her own, he was called away to attend to some emergency.

He was away for over an hour and by the time he had come back and interviewd Katrina, we were too late to make our flight back to Glasgow unless we took a taxi to Gatwick. Even then, because of traffic, we had to run through the airport, something that neither Kay nor Katrina were fit for. We arrived at the boarding gate to learn our flight was delayed by an hour. We had had nothing to eat since morning and welcomed the chance to have a meal. In the event the flight was delayed for almost two hours and we did not get home to Crieff until almost midnight, exhausted with neither the energy nor the inclination to discuss the day's events. We had been on the go for about 18 hours and the day had cost almost £800. It was a harbinger of things to come.

The following day, after we had all had a decent night's sleep, we talked at length about the consequences of Katrina's going to the Priory. That the Health Trust was prepared to foot the bill for this meant only one thing to Kay and I, it was an admission that Yellowlees and his team had made a big mistake in their treatment of Katrina. Why else would they agree? Other than it gave us an argument which could be presented to our legal team, as far as we were concerned, we were not in the least interested in what the final bill would be to the Health Trust. What interested us is what it was going to cost us, both in terms of money and time involved in keeping in touch with Katrina. The Priory was over 450 miles from our home in Crieff and we obviously could not afford to fly up and down to see Katrina, as often as she would expect us. Now that she was going to be treated in a way that would concentrate on returning her to health, or so we thought, we were prepared to give whatever it cost to help that process along.

Katrina was admitted to the Priory at Roehampton at the beginning of the second week of February 1997. We decided to drive down from Crieff because it was the only way we could think of being able to take everything that Katrina would need for what we expected would be a fairly lengthy stay. It was also much cheaper than flying down and a great deal more convenient than taking any other form of public transport. It allowed us the freedom to stop at any time if Katrina felt unwell.

There was very little ceremony when we arrived at the Priory. We were shown to Katrina's room without delay and allowed the time for her to get settled in and for us to be sure she would settle. The room was small, comfortable enough but the facilities were basic although it did have en-suite facilities, something which we expected, given the reputation of the Priory. We were introduced to two of the staff who would be dealing with Katrina and all three of us were shown around the main building, where Katrina would have her meals as well as the lounge and recreation areas. The surroundings were pleasant, including the grounds which included some lovely gardens. Kay and I had decided we would not wait too long that first day because we felt the longer we stayed, the more difficult it would be for Katrina when the time came for us to go home. We also had a very long journey home to Crieff to look forward to.

It did not take long for a pattern to emerge, where Katrina would telephone home every day, reversing the charges so that she did not have to spend her own money. Kay and I had agreed to that, until we received the first telephone bill from the Priory, of over £900. It transpired they charged hotel rates and, as Katrina frequently telephoned four times a day, we rapidly became very conscious of how much it was costing us to keep in contact with her. Much of the time she had little or nothing to say, she just needed to hear Kay's voice and to be assured we were still there. We knew what it must have felt like for her being so far away and we called her at least a couple of times every day. We always made sure we called her last thing at night.

Katrina's homesickness became a major problem for the first few weeks, until she began to feel more comfortable not only with the staff but with some of the other patients, most of whom were being treated for some form of eating disorder. Diet and regular meals were obviously of major importance and soon became a regular topic of conversation with Katrina. We had no idea what the staff were being told but we were always conscious of the consequences of what Katrina had said about us to the staff in Murray Royal/Gilgal. We were determined we would not allow a similar situation to develop again.

Kay and I drove down to the Priory on the Saturday of her first weekend there, arriving just after lunchtime. There had been prior agreement that she could come out with us and after she had had lunch, we drove to Richmond Park, where we spent a very pleasant couple of hours. We questioned Katrina closely about what was happening and what her treatment involved, learning that her sessions with staff seemed to be much more relaxed than they had been with their counterparts in Murray Royal/Gilgal. Katrina also seemed more relaxed and Kay and I left her back at the Priory, rather more content than we had been. Listening to her telephone calls during the course of the first week had given us the impression we were going to have serious problems getting Katrina to settle.

That feeling of contentment was not to last but, at the end of almost 24 hours without sleep, driving from Crieff to Roehampton and back and spending a few hours with Katrina, we were totally drained when we arrived home. It was a feeling we were to experience on a number of occasions over the next ten months, during which we drove down to the Priory at least twice a month but more often than not, three times a month. Sometimes, I would catch a couple of hours sleep in the car while Kay chatted to Katrina.

At others, we would both sleep at some motorway restaurant for a short spell and I was never so glad of my life-long ability to sleep on a knife-edge for thirty or forty minutes, waken quite refreshed and capable of carrying on whatever I was doing for the next several hours without rest. Kay did not have that knack but she certainly soon developed one for sleeping for long periods in a car travelling at high speed on the motorway. The regime changed little for the first two months, either for Katrina or us and, while we did not get the impression she was making much progress in terms of showing any great desire to come home, or in her general moods, neither did we feel she was getting worse. Keen to find out a bit more of what progress, if any, was being made, we arranged to speak to two of the senior staff the next weekend we were down.

Kay and I were introduced to two of the senior members of staff, one a female nursing sister, the other a male dietician, the latter taking charge of our discussion straight away. Katrina joined us while we were given a detailed presentation on the different types of eating disorders and their treatments. We went to some pains to state that Kay and I were not convinced Katrina's main problem had anything to do with eating disorders, as there had never been any evidence of her having the problem before going into Murray Royal/Gilgal.

"It is not uncommon for parents not to notice the eating habits of their children for years, before the problem becomes acute," said the dietician.

"We obviously cannot speak from experience when it comes to other families," said Kay, "but because Jim did not go to university until after our children were born and we were always short of money, diet was always something to which I paid a great deal of attention. As a nurse, I had always been interested in diet and when the children were young made sure they had a balanced diet from a very early age."

"I am sure you did," replied the dietician, "but could you always be sure the children continued with that diet as they got older?"

"We always ate as a family," replied Kay, "right up until the children left home. It was a family ritual that each evening, the family meal was when the seven of us sat around the table and talked about what had happened that day."

The two members of staff exchanged looks that spoke volumes about what they thought of that comment and the dietician rose from his seat and crossed to the flip chart he had used already, when he wished to emphasise a point. He drew a vertical and horizontal axis which intersected at point zero. (see fig.). On the vertical he marked units denoting weight and on the horizontal he marked age. Point zero denoted Katrina's date of birth and her birth weight, which was just under 7lbs. He then drew a curve, showing Katrina's increasing weight in line with her age.

"Now, what was the heaviest weight you ever recorded Katrina?" he asked, speaking directly to Katrina for the first time since the discussion started. After a moment's hesitation, she answered,

"Probably just over nine stones."

"And what age would you be when you reached what we will call your optimum weight?" he then asked.

"In my late teens," replied Katrina

This weight was marked on the curve and that became the apex. He then continued the curve as a straight line

"And what height are you ?" he asked.

"Just under five feet four inches." she replied.

He made a face as if to suggest that was rather light for her weight but made no comment. He then asked,

"What was the lightest weight recorded when you were in hospital?" he asked.

"Under seven stone," answered Katrina.

"And by this time you were twenty four years of age?" asked the dietician, as he drew the rest of the curve as a downward slope.

"And what age were you the last time you were under seven stone?" he asked, drawing a straight line from the right hand side of the curve, back to cut the left side of the curve at a spot which indicated Katrina would be twelve or thirteen years of age. He then turned and looked at Kay and I, a look of smug satisfaction on his face as he asked,

"What trauma hit Katrina at that age (stabbing the flip chart as he asked the question) to make her want to stop her emotional and physical development dead?"

Although as he had continued with his demonstration I could sense what was coming, as soon as he actually said the words, my stomach turned over as I thought, "Not again! Not another nutcase!" As I looked over to Kay I could tell by the look on her face that her thoughts were a mirror of my own. We did not have to say a word to each other. The dietician looked at the nurse, who nodded sagely, then looked at Kay and I in turn, before saying,

"Something happened to Katrina at that age to make her want to stop her physical development, to hold back her development at a period before the trauma, whatever it was, actually took place."

As I looked at him standing in front of his ludicrous diagram it took all of my control not to burst into laughter and exclaim,

"You are certifiable."

Instead, I looked at him for a short time before asking,

"And you think this is the reason Katrina has an eating disorder, despite all we have told you about our lifestyle at home and our insistence on family meals? Despite the fact that Katrina has never been bothered with any form of eating disorder in the past and, if she has one now, it only developed after she was admitted to Murray Royal/Gilgal? This is your diagnosis?"

"Yes, I don't accept Katrina has had no sign of an eating disorder before coming into hospital. We have met any number of parents who made the same claim but whose children had been suffering from some form of eating disorder for years before it was finally diagnosed." he replied.

The only thing I could think of saying that would not immediately convey my amusement, was, "Is it not a wee bit mechanistic?"

"Perhaps, but it works," he replied obviously beginning to warm to the task he anticipated was in front of him viz. persuading two sceptical parents of the beautiful simplicity and symmetry of his diagnosis.

From bitter experience, Kay and I knew there was absolutely no point in debating the issue. We did not need to discuss our next move between ourselves, it was instinctive; we simply allowed the dietician to ramble on, amplifying his theory. As far as he was concerned, Katrina had an eating disorder which caused her weight to plummet from over nine stone, before she had gone into hospital where she had undergone two abdominal operations and then spent well over a year as an inpatient in a psychiatric ward; to under seven stone. None of that was of any importance or even relevance to her loss of weight, the dietician said. His theory dictated that Katrina was deliberately holding back her physical and, more importantly her emotional development, to correspond with her physical and emotional condition "before the trauma took place".

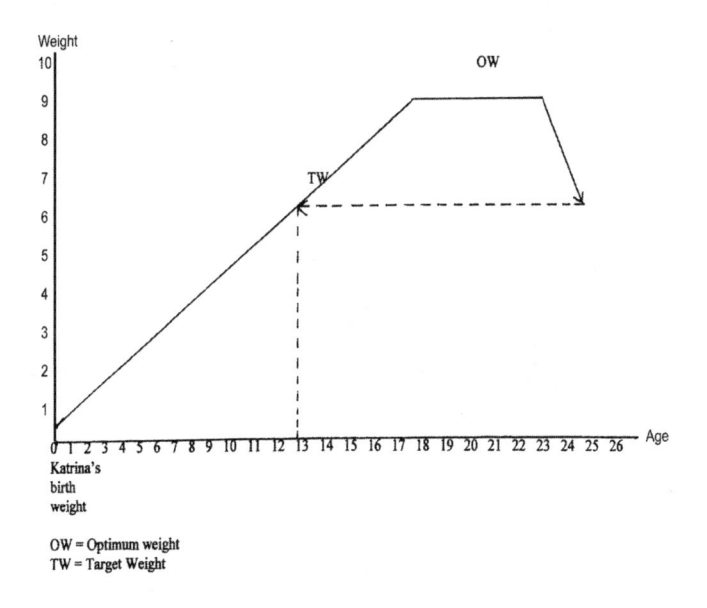

OW = Optimum weight
TW = Target Weight

This was the figure drawn by the dietician in the Priory, to explain Katrina's alleged anorexia.

"Will she be content if her weight stays at that level?" I asked.

"If it is the weight she wants to be, she will definitely be happier," he replied.

I didn't bother to ask about the repeated suicide attempts, the self-harming, the accusations of abuse and all the other bizarre behaviour of the previous two years. Kay had said almost nothing during all of this. Our account of our family dynamics and lifestyle had been dismissed by every "professional" involved in Katrina's care and at this late stage, Kay saw no point in attempting to change their minds. Fortunately, we were spared too much more of this nonsense because the dietician and nurse had other things to which they had to attend and we were left to take Katrina out for a meal. Kay and I decided not to pursue any discussion with Katrina, on the session we had just endured, and she obviously thought as little of it as we did because she made no mention of it during the rest of our day out. Kay and I did discuss it at length on the road home and while it caused us amusement, it also disturbed us that Katrina was again going to be under the care of people who believed in theories that we thought were such absolute nonsense.

We allowed another couple of months to go by before asking to speak to Professor Lacey, a meeting to which he readily agreed. There were a number of issues we felt we needed to discuss, mainly Katrina's apparent inability to understand what was being said to her during the course of our countless telephone conversations with her. It gave us concern because we could not help wondering what she was telling staff, when she seemed to misinterpret almost every conversation she had with us. We started the meeting with Lacey by telling him of our concerns, giving him several examples. He looked at us both, seeming to give his answer great thought, before saying,

"I really cannot comment on what was said during your telephone conversations with Katrina because I was not there".

Kay and I just looked at each other and shook our heads in dismay.

"I have never been to the North Pole, but I know it's cold," I replied. "It really is not helpful to be given this stock answer when we are desperately looking for help."

"What do you want me to say?" asked Lacey, "I cannot comment on what was said in a conversation that I did not overhear."

"We are not asking you to comment on what was said," answered Kay, "we are asking you to comment on the fact that Katrina seems to misinterpret a great deal she is told on the telephone. It leaves us in a position of not knowing if what she is telling us bears any resemblance to what is actually happening. Is this because of the medication she is on, because we have already experienced that when she was in Murray Royal/Gilgal, but we were under the impression her medication has been cut back substantially?"

Lacey again looked at us both for some time before repeating the mantra,

"I really don't know what to say that might help. I was not there therefore I cannot comment on what was said."

Our patience was being sorely tested and in complete frustration I said to Lacey,

"If you apply the "I was not there" test to every situation, how can you comment on any event which you did not personally witness?"

As Lacey looked at us and shrugged his shoulders, as if to dismiss the question, I continued,

"If you apply that test to every situation, the professional judgement you and the other psychiatrists we have encountered are so fond of quoting, must be totally meaningless. How can you form any kind of judgement, professional or otherwise, if you insist on witnessing each and every event before you can pass comment?"

Again, Lacey seemed to dismiss the question with another shrug, so I decided to push him further.

"So, are we to understand that if a patient in here approached you with the charge that a member of staff had sexually assaulted them, your only reaction would be to say, "I am sorry, I cannot comment because I was not there." Quite frankly, that does not give us much confidence for the safety of the patients here because if the "I was not there" test is applied, staff here are free to sexually assault patients with impunity, so long as they do it with no witnesses present. In fact, as far as you are concerned, eye witness accounts would simply be dismissed because you yourself, "were not there".

Lacey's response was still non-committal and our attempt to have a discussion about the abuse that Katrina actually did suffer and how and if that was being addressed was simply stonewalled. Despite the reservations we had about Katrina's treatment, she did seem to be making progress and whenever we went out for a meal, there was never any problem with getting her to eat and she seemed to enjoy her food. A measure of just how much she improved was evidence the following month, October, when she was given "time out" and travelled home for a long weekend. A few months earlier, the very thought of Katrina travelling alone from London to Crieff and back again, would have been inconceivable, therefore it was with some enthusiasm that Kay and I travelled down to see her the following week.

We had a lovely day out in Richmond Park, did a little shopping and when we returned to the Priory, we were all in good humour. We also had other news we wanted to discuss with Katrina. The anger Kay and I had felt at the failure of the internal inquiries by the Health Trust and Perth & Kinross Council, to find fault with the behaviour of any of those involved in Katrina's case, still burned as brightly as ever. I had already started legal proceedings and had talked to a QC, introduced by the legal firm for which I had worked for seven years. But what bothered us as much as anything was the fact that so many of those involved knew me either from my political activity or from the school where I had taught, when they had been there as pupils. This was especially true of both the police and the hospital. Given my high public profile, there was very little chance of what had happened ever remaining confidential, therefore we had taken the decision to go to the media but obviously had to speak to Katrina.

Her immediate reaction was one of shock and opposition but before we had had time to spend discussing it in detail, Katrina was called to speak to one of her carers. Left alone in her room, as we were told she would be only a few minutes, Kay started to idly rifle through some of the books which sat beside Katrina's bed. Suddenly she let out an exclamation which sounded as if she was in pain. I whirled around from where I had been looking out of the window, to find Kay sitting with her hand to her mouth, a look of absolute horror on her face. It took several attempts to get her to respond to my question, "What is it? What is wrong? Instead of answering, Kay held up what looked like a jotter with several pages of hand written notes. My heart missed a beat because I knew immediately it was another journal, the kind Katrina had been encouraged to keep at Murray Royal/Gilgal.

Kay was aghast as she started to read me extracts from the journal, stumbling over some of the words, shaking her head as she read, her voice faltering from time to time. She kept glancing at me to watch my reaction as she read the same accusations of abuse. It was as if nothing had changed, there had been no reconciliation, no retraction, no sitting through the rancorous meeting with Sharon, Yellowlees and Proctor. There was even an account of a day in Richmond Park with a nurse, to hold a short ceremony to commemorate the day her aborted child would have been born. Despite the fact we had gone over the previous treatment with Lacey on the day he assessed Katrina, it was obvious she was as immersed in her "recovered memories" as she had been in Murray Royal/Gilgal. It looked as if we were back to square one.

We heard the sound of voices and realised Katrina was on her way back to the room. Kay quickly stuffed the jotter back into the pile of books and stood up just as Katrina opened the door.

"We are going to have to get going or it is going to be very late before we get home," she said to Katrina. It was very, very difficult to act normally and to continue with what we now realised was a complete charade. It is impossible to describe the misery we felt on that journey home. Kay cried quietly for much of the 450 miles, interspersed with attempts to rationalise what we had just discovered. Would it ever end? Was there anything else we could do to combat the insidious effects of the treatment Yellowlees and his team had used on Katrina? The dietician's analysis of Katrina's eating disorder was as barking as Proctor's "body memories" and it was obvious Katrina was being allowed to drift back to the type of fantasy world in which she had lived in Murray Royal/Gilgal.

We had no intention of challenging Katrina about her journal at the Priory but we did question her a bit more closely about the staff and her conversations with them, in an effort to discover how her treatment was being handled. In early November she told us that one of her regular nurses had said to her on several occasions that as far as the "abuse" was concerned, the only two people who could say for certain what had happened, were her and me. We wanted that checked out but it was one of the stock mantra's of psychiatric staff dealing with those who claimed to have suffered earlier, historical abuse. No matter how often they made that statement, psychiatric staff never seemed to realise the stupidity of it. If they accepted that I could say "with certainty" what had happened and, I denied any abuse took place; did that mean there was no abuse? Obviously not, if they believed that Katrina could also say "with certainty" that abuse did take place. Independent eye witness accounts of circumstances that would show that abuse could not possibly have taken place, were simply dismissed as being of no account.

According to Katrina, the nurse had also told her that our decision to go public and speak to the media, was another form of abuse. If that was true, we intended to make an official complaint but we only had Katrina's word for it and the nurse may have said nothing of the kind. I wrote to Lacey on 4th November to express our concerns and to reiterate our disappointment with the outcome of the meeting we had had with him the previous month. His response of 11th November was a classic non-answer. It read as follows:-

Dear Mr Fairlie,

It is not the case that we avoid dealing with Katrina's alleged abuse. This is a core part of her current treatment, but this a matter that I must leave to Katrina to discuss with you, if she wants to. I did not enter into interpretations about the abuse when we met, firstly because I felt it would be premature and secondly it would only be meaningful if it was part of family therapy. Therefore, the examination of the past insofar as it is pertinent to the future, revolves around Katrina's own therapies. It may be it is pertinent for Katrina to share these with you, but that is her decision, not mine.

You will agree that my brief is to assist Katrina to get well. That is the most important matter, not for me to comment on conversations between Katrina and her therapist. If Katrina shares them with you, it is presumably for a reason, and this she should advise you of.

It was obvious we were going to be faced with the same obfuscation and evasion we had already endured in Perth and neither Kay nor I had any intention of embarking on another lengthy series of correspondence, where nothing would be achieved. Katrina had said on more than one occasion she wanted to come home and after Lacey's letter arrived and we had discussed the ramifications of Katrina's remaining in the Priory, being encouraged to repeat all that had gone before, Kay and I decided that the quicker she left the better it would be. It was obvious that she was better than she had been but she was still in need of help. But we felt that she could get it a lot nearer to home. We motored down to the Priory to collect Katrina and bring her home the following week.

CHAPTER NINETEEN

March 1996 – November 1997

I knew that I was not ready to leave Murray Royal/Gilgal when I discharged myself in March 1996, at least in terms of being well. But I had grown to hate the place so much and the relationship with the staff had deteriorated to such an extent, that I had to get out. Every day was a living nightmare of trying to cope with the effect of the drugs and the flashbacks. I convinced myself that if only I could get away and get back to a flat on my own, I would be fine. Yellowlees did his best to persuade me I was far from ready to leave and his discharge letter to my own doctor, emphasised I was leaving against his wishes and advice. He placed greatest emphasis on the number of times Dad still appeared in my flashbacks, which is not what I either wanted or needed to hear. That is what I wanted to get away from above everything else.

I didn't care what anyone said; I just needed to get away, but it was not to be as easy as I had hoped. I knew it would be hard, but I had hoped that spending time in my own flat, with Mum and Dad there if I needed them would eventually allow me to learn to cope on my own. I knew I had to do it sometime and as far as I was concerned, I was ready to try. The Post Office had made me redundant but they owed me money and pension benefits and one of the first things I did, was to pay them a visit. The staff were pleasant enough but not exactly helpful as everything had to be done by writing to Glasgow or to the Union, things I just did not have the energy to tackle right then. Mum and Dad had arranged a flat for me from the local authority, as I had had to vacate the one I shared with Eileen. Some of my old furniture was still there and Mum and Dad arranged to pick it up because it was something else I just could not face. In fact, it soon became very evident that there was not much I could face and within a few days of living in the flat on my own, I asked to go and stay with my parents in Crieff.

Unfortunately, there were too many bad memories associated with the house and try as I might, a few days at a time was as much as I could manage. I lived like a nomad for the next few weeks, moving between Perth and Crieff as the mood demanded. Coping with the medication continued to be a major problem, which involved regular visits to and from both my own GP in Perth and my parents' GP in Crieff, who had attended me for months before I was admitted to Murray Royal/Gilgal in the first place. Both doctors were very sympathetic and were actively looking to get me help away from Perth. Having lost touch with all of my previous friends and not sure of how they would react to me in any case, I made the mistake of keeping contact with some of the girls I had become friendly with in Murray Royal/Gilgal.

That was a big mistake because the topic of conversation inevitably returned to abuse, medication, suicide and the attitude of the staff. On the occasion I visited one of the girls with whom I had been particularly friendly, my mood was very low before I arrived at the hospital and unfortunately, my friend did not help. She had been sectioned for the whole of the previous week and wanted to speak about ending it and nothing else. Within minutes I felt my own mood getting even lower, therefore it was no surprise when Dr Tait told me that Dad had come to see me. I still feel bitterly ashamed that he became involved with the nursing staff the way he did that day, but looking back on what happened, I now realise I needed to pour my heart out the way I did and probably should have done it weeks before. Attempting to hang myself a few days later was an inevitable consequence of having waited too long to speak to someone about just how low I had sunk. When I later learned Dad had almost crashed the car on the way home and could have been killed, I began to realise the pressure I had put him under. I would never have forgiven myself had anything happened to him that day.

Some of my previous attempts at taking my own life had been pretty half-hearted, not becaue I did not intend to do it but because they were attempts driven by opportunity rather than planning. When I tried to hang myself behind the toilet door, there was nothing half-hearted about it and I had planned it. The night staff tended to watch us closely enough, especially in the unit which was a locked ward, but there were always going to be opportunities during any shift, when the staff would be involved with another patient or dealing with some unexpected event. All I had to do was stay alert for such an opportunity to arise. On the night in question, I felt particularly low and was longing for the opportunity to arise. When it did, I was ready.

I now know my Dad had given the doctors all the details of how difficult he and Mum had found looking after me, how they made sure I was never left with access to anything with which I could harm myself, such as a knife or the chord of my dressing gown. For that reason, the staff should have made sure they did the same. That night, I was left with the dressing gown chord and that is what I used to hang myself from the back of the toilet door. When I was found, I was unconscious and very near death. Charlotte Proctor, the psychologist interviewed me two days later and was interested to know if I had seen the white light, but my parents were told it was not a serious attempt. It was not until we saw the medical records that we discovered just how serious it had been.

It was obvious things could not go on as they were and although I hated the thought of having to see another doctor, to go over the same stories again, to re-live the nightmares of abuse, both real and imagined, I reluctantly agreed to speak to Dr Freeman in Edinburgh. I resented being told I had an eating disorder. From what I could understand of the nature of eating disorders, I did not look in the mirror and see someone who was fat, therefore I needed to lose weight. The shape of my body was of no interest to me. I stopped eating because I wanted to die and I had told Jenny Hogg that on several occasions, as well as other doctors at Murray Royal/Gilgal. It was a simple as that.

I was not interested in Freeman's theories, or Maggie Gray's theories. I attended the Cullen Centre because that is where I was told I would get help. Maggie Gray never said she believed me or did not believe me. Our sessions were always couched in terms of, "Let us suppose," or "If this or that happened." My feeling at the end of a weekly session was usually one of relief that it was over but that nothing very much had actually happened or been said. The travelling back and forward from Perth to Edinburgh and the length of the time spent on the journey, were a far greater problem than the weekly sessions were. Mum tried hard to get me to discuss what was said but I genuinely never felt that anything of note or worth had been said, therefore there was nothing I could tell Mum. I knew this annoyed her, given the demands I was making on her time, not just in travelling back and forward to Edinburgh, but during the course of the rest of the week, when her and Dad would be asked to come into Perth from Crieff in the middle of the night or every time I had a flashback or nightmare that frightened me.

It was as much of a surprise to me as it was to my parents when Freeman said he wanted me to go to the Priory in Roehampton. I felt the time spent at the Cullen Centre had been a complete waste and I did not see how spending time at the Priory would be an improvement, particularly if they continued to insist that I suffered from anorexia. I agreed to go because it was the line of least resistance. I hadn't been allowed to decide anything since the first operation to remove my appendix, or at least that is how it felt to me. I agreed to go to Gilgal, although I hated the very thought of it; I agreed to speak to psychiatrists and psychologists and the consequences had almost destroyed me and my family. I had accepted the sessions with Maggie Gray and the trips to Edinburgh every week; and again, I had agreed to go to the Priory but it was only because there appeared to be no alternatives. I just went where I was sent and did as I was instructed. I had long since lost any control over my life and I hated it.

For me, nothing changed at the Priory, except that every meal was monitored. I was given target weights for the end of each week and each month. There was emphasis on exercise and talks on healthy lifestyles, as well as private sessions with individual carers. My greatest problem was loneliness, the feeling of being totally cut off from my family and familiar surroundings. I could tell how much my telephone calls irritated my parents because more often than not, I had nothing to say because there was nothing *to* say. The staff were pleasant and attentive, encouraging me to talk and the pattern of discussions began to follow a very familiar course. Whatever I said was accepted; there were never any attempts to question me when I spoke about Dad abusing me. I still spoke to my carers about the abuse. I still claimed the allegations I had made in Gilgal were true, I even wrote them down in the journal. Nothing had changed.

Why did I make the same allegations, when I knew in my heart they were not true? I still had the images, which I could conjure up with no effort whatsoever. But why did I write down accusations about abuse I knew had not happened, why did I blacken my father's name again, knowing perfectly well that none of it had ever happened? I don't know; I just don't know. Was it a part of the illness? I don't know. Was I just seeking attention? I don't know. Why did no one ever just stop me and say, "You are lying. You know none of it happened." I don't know. By now I was well aware that some of the allegations I had made were bizarre in the extreme, but none of the psychiatric staff had ever questioned them. Maggie Gray never questioned them and the staff at the Priory were no different. Whatever I said was simply noted, sometimes commented upon but never contradicted or even questioned.

Would the outcome of my stay in Murray Royal/Gilgal have turned out any differently, had my original allegations been questioned? Bearing in mind the allegations started as a consequence of flashbacks, which the staff maintained were memories, in reality, they were not my allegations in the first place. They only became my allegations because I was encouraged to believe they were memories, but as they became embellished to the point where their very nature became more and more bizarre, would it have mattered to the outcome if they had been challenged at that point? I don't know.

There were never any marks on my body, despite my claims of having been severely beaten and raped in the hospital grounds. Those claims were made because of flashbacks but given the nature of the claims, that the attacks allegedly happened while I was a patient in the hospital, should some member of staff not noticed the physical marks of the alleged attacks? If I had been taken aside and told, "Look, there is absolutely no physical evidence that any of this took place!" would I have continued to believe it had happened? I just don't know. I have no idea what staff should have done in the circumstances of being faced with a patient making ever more unbelievable allegations. I only know that I was never questioned, never asked to think again.

I did not make the mistake at the Priory, that I had made at Murray Royal/Gilgal, of making friends with any of the other patients and taking on board their personal histories. Some of the other girls were there for only short periods and a number of them were lucky enough to go home every weekend. My lack of friends added to my loneliness but I preferred it like that. So detached was I from the rest of the patients, that when we were visited by Princess Di, who, from all accounts was a regular visitor, I did not join the rest of the girls in a group photograph and stayed in my room during the whole period of Di's visit.

When I look back on the time I spent in the Priory, I now believe I simply went through the motions. I kept to the rules, there were no attempts to abscond. There were no attempts on my life or even to self-harm. To all intents and purposes, I was an ideal patient. That I found the dietician's presentation on eating disorders and his analysis of the reasons for my alleged anorexia, as amusing and irritating as did my parents, did not persuade me to question it or to rail against it. It didn't seem worth it at the time. My main aim was to get out of there and go home and if I had to jump through a few hoops to do that, then so be it. By the time I was allowed to go home on my own, there is no doubt I had improved and it encouraged me to think I could get home permanently.

I thought that Mum and Dad obviously felt the same way and on their last visit to the Priory before I finally left to go home, we enjoyed a very pleasant day out, spoiled to some extent by the announcement that they intended to go the the press. I had been sheltered to a large extent from the battles they had had, particularly Dad, with the Health Trust and the local council but I knew how badly it had affected both of them. Dad had obviously suffered and he was frequently short tempered with me. His anger often erupted, particularly when the very name of Yellowlees came up in conversation and I honestly could not see how going to the press would help. My other concern was obviously for myself and the fact that everyone would know what had happened. Being so far away from the rest of the family did not help and although Sharon had called a couple of times on the telephone, I had seen her very briefly when I was home for the weekend but had neither seen nor heard from any of the boys since coming to the Priory.

I very quickly learned, although we did discuss it briefly, that Dad was determined to use the press, whatever I said. Mum told me that Philip and Andrew felt they had no right to object, given the part the whole family had played in accusing Dad. Jim had been furious, as had Sharon but he soon came round when he saw the reaction of other people. Mum sent me copies of the articles and assured me that the reaction had been only positive but I still hated the thought of other people knowing what had happened and that I would be blamed, whatever was said to my face. When I spoke to one of the nurses, Amanda, she considered it was another form of abuse and that Dad should never have done it as it showed little or no consideration for me. I agreed, but I did not have too much time to dwell on it because a couple of weeks later I decided to go home for good, encouraged by my parents. I only learned later, much later that Mum and Dad had written to Professor Lacey, about their concerns that I was drifting back into the same kind of regime I had left at Murray Royal/Gilgal. My health had improved but I was to find I still needed help. It was November 1997 and I had been in almost permanent psychiatric care for a full three years.

CHAPTER TWENTY

THE DECISION TO GO PUBLIC
October 1997

"Kay, I think we should use the media"

We were sitting watching TV, although my mind was on other things and the comment caught Kay completely unawares. She looked across at me and said, with a quizzical look on her face,

"What? What do you mean use the media?"

"I think we should go to the press with the story about the case," I replied. "We have just wasted almost two years jumping through their hoops and what have we ended up with? Nothing! As far as they are concerned none of them has done anything wrong, which means I am an abuser and the only reason I have not been prosecuted is because they don't have enough evidence. Look at what Bridgeford said in her letter, there was "*insufficient evidence*". I know we agreed at the start that we would go through the internal inquiry route, but it really sticks in my craw that the bastards are going to get away with it, unless the court case is successful."

"That is a big step Jim and we have the rest of the family to consider." Kay said as she turned off the TV. "Sharon won't be in favour, for one, and I don't see Katrina being keen," said Kay.

"I know, I know," I said, well aware that this would have to be discussed but I had been turning it over in my mind for some time. "What do you think about it?" I asked

Kay thought for a moment or two but finally said,

"We would have no control over what was said and you know a lot of folk will think, "*There is no smoke without fire*" What if your father's abuse comes out? How will you feel about that?"

"I would tell the press from the outset and take the sting out of it," I said.

"But what about Katrina?" How do you think she will feel if everyone knows?" Kay asked.

There was no doubt this was a major consideration and I had given it a lot of thought before speaking to Kay.

"Quite honestly, I don't give a toss what they think of the old man. I do have concerns about Katrina but I think there are more good reasons for going to the media than there are disadvantages, even taking Katrina's position into consideration," I said.

"For a start, this is not going to remain a secret for long. When you think of how many people already know and the number of staff who were ex-pupils of the High School, it is bound to be well aired by now. It is the fact that we are helping to try to keep it a secret that bothers me."

"There is a big difference between gossip among hospital staff and social workers and the whole world knowing Jim," said Kay. "What would the firm say?"

"Kay, I don't care what anybody else says. The people it concerns most – Katrina and the family, and us – they are the only ones I am concerned about," I replied. "The biggest weapon the likes of Yellowlees and the Social Work Department have, is silence. Yellowlees is banking on me saying nothing. Look at what he said to Philip, *'I would huff and puff for a short time but then I would just admit it. I have too much to lose by going to court'* I want to ram those words right down his throat."

I started to pace back and forward in the sitting room.

"I honestly think Katrina will be given a great deal of sympathy and given that she lost her job, her flat and the last three years of her life, I think people should know what happened to her. If the allegations against me start to filter through and we have tried to hide it, I think people who don't know me will be more likely to wonder if it is true. I couldn't take that. I couldn't stand the thought of people who have no idea what happened and who know me only by reputation, wondering if it is true and spreading the gossip as if it might be. The other thing to think about is if it hadn't been for people like the Hunters telling their story to the press, we would have been floundering for long enough. That alone is a good enough reason for going to the press but it is not the main reason I want to do it. I want to do it for our own sake."

"You have obviously made up your mind but you are going to have to be careful about the way you approach the family Jim," said Kay, "they do have some say in this. When are you going to approach them?"

"Now," I said, reaching for the telephone.

I called Sharon first and she left me in no doubt she was totally opposed to the press being involved in any way. Nothing I said made any impression and when the call ended, Kay who had been listening to my side of the conversation, shook her head and said,

"I knew you were not going to persuade Sharon, what are you going to do now?"

"Speak to the rest of them and even if they are all against it, I am still going to go ahead," I replied. The conversation with Sharon had angered me because I thought that she really had not looked at it at all from my point of view.

I knew Andrew would be in the middle of service (he was head chef at One Devonshire Gardens in Glasgow) therefore I next called Philip, who took the view that it was my decision. He was not sure I was doing the right thing and he expressed concern about his own children and the impact it might have on them, but he was prepared to leave it to me. Philip carried a great deal of guilt over what had happened and although he had tried to rationalise the actions of the family when they were first told, he felt he had no right to try to stop me doing whatever I thought might be of benefit in the fight to make the Health Trust and the Social Work Department accountable for what they had done.

No sooner had I replaced the receiver on the hook than the 'phone rang. It was Jim, in a state of some agitation.

"I hear you are going to the press," he said sharply.

"I take it Sharon has been speaking to you. It didn't take her long," I said, trying to keep the tone light.

"What the hell do you expect?" he said, his voice beginning to rise. "Do we not get any choice in this?"

It was the tone of his voice that irked me, as much as what he said, which really, was a perfectly reasonable question to ask. Had I been thinking a bit more clearly, and been more in control of my emotions, I know I would have reacted differently. But I wasn't – and I didn't.

"You mean like the choices you gave me Jim?" I replied, tension rising in every bone in my body. I was holding the telephone so hard, I almost left the imprint of my fingers on the handset.

"You bastard, this is our life…." That is as far as he got. I hung up and turned to Kay, my face white with fury. None of my family had ever used that kind of language to me, and very, very rarely in my company.

Kay put her hand on my arm as I replaced the receiver. She could see how angry I was and asked,

"What did he say, to make you so angry?"

Instead of telling her, I turned and said quietly,

"If he had been standing in front of me and spoken to me like that, I would have decked him."

Kay did not pursue it by asking again what had been said and before she could say anything else, the telephone rang. It was Jim. I walked away from the sitting room to the kitchen to get a drink and heard Kay say,

"I don't think that would be a good idea just now. Just leave it until your Dad cools down. He won't speak to you just now Jim. Just leave it."

Jim was angry that I had hung up on him and had wanted to pursue the conversation but Kay had known that in the state of mind I was in at that moment, things might have been said that could never have been mended. We had come a long way towards bringing the family back together and it looked as if I was in danger of re-opening the wounds. But I was convinced I was right and I intended to carry on, come what may. Andrew took the same view as Philip and Katrina had neither the energy nor will to put up much of an argument. She was still in the Priory and therefore saw nothing of the initial reaction, although Kay and I kept her as informed as much as we could, sending her some of the articles. What she did miss out on unfortunately, was the reaction of those who telephoned the house to give their support and to ask after her health. Had Katrina been able to experience that, I firmly believe she would have felt a great deal more comfortable much earlier. As it was, it took a bit of time for her to fully accept what I had done but as her participation in the BBC series showed, her contribution to the media was vital.

Having taken the decision to go to the press, I then had to decide how best to do it. I had learned from my years in politics that being honest with the media paid its own dividends and I had made a number of contacts over the years, some of whom I regarded as friends. I decided to call one of them to discuss the situation with him. He was initially shocked and then very angry at what had been done and after discussion, he thought it would be better if the story was handled by someone who did not know me, other than by reputation, so that there would be an element of objectivity in the writing. Obviously whoever covered the story, would want to speak to the other side, and to the family, particularly Katrina. That was to become the most important caveat in all the dealings with the media, that Katrina could be contacted only through Kay and I and we were determined she would be protected from the worst of the tabloids, although that problem never really arose.

I wanted to get as much publicity as possible, but did not want the story treated in the manner of the tabloid press. The issues at stake were too important to be reduced to a series of lurid headlines and very little else. The Daily Mail had covered the recovered memory issue in the past and its sister paper the Mail on Sunday had run the original article which had introduced us to the British False Memory Society (BFMS). My friend had worked for them and had contacts there, therefore I left it to him to brief one of their journalists before they contacted me. The journalist turned out to be Annie Brown, who came to see me at my office and the piece she wrote was not only sympathetic, it was written in such a way that none of the family could possibly take exception to the tone or the content. Annie was good enough to confirm that what she had written was acceptable, before the article went to print. Both Kay and I were concerned about the tone that would be adopted because we were well aware that once this was started, our family life would be public property, that the reputation of all of us, would come under the public microscope. I was taking a chance that I would be pilloried by those papers who had not been given the story, that my reputation would be trashed, whether or not it was justified.

The article appeared on Monday October 13th and I have to admit that although I had pushed for this to be done, I was nervous about the outcome. The telephone at home started to ring just after 8.00 am and it literally did not stop for days, both at home and at my office in Perth. Every broadsheet in the UK telephoned and journalists with whom I was in regular contact when I was active in the SNP called, frequently to express their support but often it was to introduce one of their colleagues who wanted to speak to me. The media interest was intense and within the first week I gave interviews to BBC, ITV and SKY TV as well as radio. Every news bulletin carried the story and I also did interviews with Jimmy Young, who introduced a psychiatrist who explained to the audience the problems that recoverd memory therapy had caused.

We were contacted at the end of the first week by the Richard & Judy show and it was agreed to do the programme the following week. Kay accompanied me and we were interviewed by Richard Madely and Karen Keating. The station received thousands of telephone calls in the aftermath of the programme, which had also included a contribution from Denise Robinson, the programme's resident agony aunt. She made the very pertinent point that Katrina had been abused by the system and told of a conversation she had had with some paediatrician involved in child protection, who had admitted to Denise, that she did not care if she got it wrong ten times, for everyone she got right, so long as she could save the life of one abused child. The destruction of the lives of those she got wrong, was of no concern to her and I made the point during the programme that not a single life of an abused child was saved by the thousands of lives that were destroyed because of false allegations.

One of the callers to the programme had left her number and asked me to call, saying it was quite important. When I returned the call, I discovered it was an ex-pupil of mine who was married with a young family, to another ex-pupil. She said she had been in tears when she saw the programme because she and her husband had such fond memories of being in my class at school. She had felt she just had to telephone and tell me that.

Kay and I did several radio and TV programmes together in the weeks and months following the appearance of the first article and on only one occasion was it evident that the programme host was unsympathetic. Libby Purvis made it fairly obvious that she had little or no sympathy with our position and at one point during the course of our contribution in a programme which had three other guests, she asked what we had hoped to achieve by going public with the accusations. Both her tone and the question was critical. Kay answered with her customary dignity whenever there was even a hint of criticism, which was very rare.

"While we were going through the internal inquiries and it was impressed on us the importance of "confidentiality" and how the Health Trust and the Social Work Department refused to answer on the grounds of "patient confidentiality", it was presented as if it was our dirty little secret. In actual fact they were the ones who were being protected. We did not have any dirty little secret to keep."

At that point John Hannah the well known actor, who was one of the other guests interrupted by saying,

"That is right. I have a friend who has just come back from Rwanda where they are trying to recover from the massacres that took place there. There is no doubt in anyone's mind that for there to be any kind of reconciliation in that country, justice will have to be seen to be done. I can well understand why Kay and Jim would want this made public."

That is the kind of response we became used to but what completely astonished me, as well as made me feel very humble, were the letters and cards that poured into our home and the telephone calls we received, from friends, acquaintances, old political colleagues and members of the SNP. The very first letter I received the day after the article appeared, came from Bill Walker. Bill had been the Conservative Party MP for the constituency in which we had lived and had been politically active all my life. We were never friends but we had shared many a political platform, biting lumps out of one another in political debate but there was a mutual respect in our relationship and his daughters had been pupils at the High School. Bill put that respect into words that left me deeply touched.

Some of the calls and letters came from people who knew me only by reputation and towards the end of the first week, I was walking down the street in Perth when I saw two young women approaching from the opposite direction. They were pushing baby carriages and were accompanied by an older woman. It became obvious as we came closer to one another that they knew who I was and I began to rack my brains trying to remember if I should know them. I gave them a half smile and suddenly the older woman walked right in front of me so that I had to stop. She clasped one of my hands in both of hers and said,

"Mr Fairlie, you don't know us, these are my daughters," gesturing to the two younger women, "they were at the High School when you taught there although you did not teach them. We have been reading what has happened to you and your family and we just want to say how sorry we are. We know you are a good man and we will pray for you." With that, she turned and the three of them hurried away, leaving me completely stunned and quite overcome.

Although the partners in the legal firm which employed me, had known from the day I was confronted, only two other members of staff knew about the allegations, therefore the article in the Daily Mail came as a tremendous shock to the rest, many of whom I had known for many years. The first of them put her head round the door at 9.15 and from then on there was a steady stream for the rest of the day. Many of them were in tears as they struggled to know what to say, some of them just giving me a hug before disappearing again. The one group that was totally absent from the stream of well-wishers, were the partners in the firm – my employers. Despite throughout the course of that week, I passed them regularly in the corridors and on the stairs and even on occasion, had to discuss mutual clients with some of them, none of them said a word. In fact, I did not leave that firm until March 2005 and during the ten years they had known about the allegations and the court case, there were three of the partners never once raised the topic, not even to ask how I was.

I had not told the partners I intended to go to the press, for reasons which had much to do with the attitude they had shown to the fact the allegations had been made. On the Friday of that first week, I waited until 4.00pm before deciding to take a file I had been working on, to the senior partner's office. He was a complete gentleman in every other way but he had avoided me the whole of that first week and when I placed the file on his desk, I had opened his room door and about to step into the corridor, before he said,

"Eh, your personal situation was discussed at the partners' meeting yesterday."

I turned to look at him and said,

"And?" having no intention of making it easier for him.

"The partners were very unhappy." he said, hesitatingly.

"And?" I said again.

"We have had some telephone calls from clients," he said.

"And?" I said for the third time.

"We had to consider the rest of the staff and their attitude but we told clients you would be continuing as usual."

"Good," was all I said as I turned and walked out.

The letters and calls I had had from clients were full of anger at what had been done to the family and sympathy for me. One morning I received a call from a client asking if she could come to discuss her investments. When she arrived, she immediately said,

"I did not come here to speak about business, the "Girls" (a group of my middle-aged female clients who were all friends and invariably referred to themselves as the "Girls") had a meeting and I was delegated to come and see if you are allright. And if there is anything we can do to help." The staff had shown enormous support and sympathy for me but had been questioned by the partners, who, for whatever reason, seemed to want to leave me with the impression that feelings among the staff were at best ambiguous. Shortly after my decision to go public, my secretary left to start a nursing course. She had been one of the two staff members who had known from the outset, as she fielded many of my telephone calls and occasionally photocopied some of my letters. She was not replaced and for the next four years, I was forced to deal with my own administration, adding greatly to the level of stress under which I was forced to operate.

When I decided to start court proceedings some months previously, I naturally went to the court partner for advice. His first action was to take personal statements from the family but it took six months and several reminders from me, before they were typed and sent to a QC the partner had suggested. He produced a very superficial and preliminary "opinion" which did not even begin to touch on what had happened. As a consequence of that he had a short meeting with the family and a further very short meeting with Kay and I. As the clock was ticking, if I wanted to pursue the case through the courts and I had no idea what, if any, case could be made, I pursued him for the next ten months trying to get him to give me an opinion that could be of some use. At the end of that time, a full eighteen months after I had first spoken to the court partner, we still had not received a scrape of a pen. I therefore decided to dispense with his services and at the same time, as my relationship with my employers had deteriorated substantially, I also dispensed with the court partner and spoke for the first time to the firm which represented me from that time until my case was thrown out in July 2004.

As the media intensity began to wane after the first two or three months, the family were able to appreciate the effects the publicity had had. Perhaps the greatest difference was in the attitude of Jim. We made up our differences within a short time of the telephone call which had gone so disastrously wrong but the most important aspect of the fallout from the media interest, was the overt sympathy Jim was shown by his friends and others who knew the family. When the boys were growing up and attending the judo club, our house was never empty of their friends and those friends were all young men now, some of them with families of their own. When the first articles hit the press, all of them contacted Jim, as well as Andrew and Philip, expressing their anger and support for the family. It made a great impression on Jim and he admitted after a few weeks that going public, was the best thing we could have done.

It also helped Katrina and when BBC's Frontline series asked us to take part in a documentary of our case in March 1998, Kay and I readily agreed, but we doubted whether Katrina would be prepared to take part to any great extent. The programme producers wanted to concentrate on Kay and I and Katrina if she was willing. Although she expressed some doubt initially, as soon as the filming started, Katrina surpassed everyone's hopes in terms of the nature of her contribution, which showed a level of self-confidence that she hadn't displayed for the past three years and more. Kay and I were delighted because it was the start of Katrina being able to speak to the media for herself and to relate in her own words what had happened to her. There were setbacks from time to time and she was not always willing to take part, but she had definitely turned another corner.

The BBC's programme was well received and started another round of media interest because it had also included a contribution from a journalist/researcher who was deeply involved in the Recovered Memory debate, but from the other side of the argument. She had called me to ask for a statement the previous month for an article she intended to submit to The Scotsman. She lied to me on the telephone claiming she worked for the legal department of The Scotsman and although her article was actually well written and reasonably balanced, I discovered after the article had been published, that she was very heavily involved with adult survivors of alleged childhood sexual abuse and was very much on the side of the people I was suing. She was surprised that I was prepared to say publicly that both the Health Trust and the Social Work Department had lied, challenging me to stand by my claims in public. In turn I challenged her to print the claims, which she did, pointing out that what I was claiming was indeed actionable. She was the only person who ever lied to me in order to get a statement.

Much to our surprise, Dr. Freeman from the Cullen Centre in Edinburgh, who had treated Katrina, also took part in the programme and it was the first time that Kay and I were able to see on which side of the argument he fell. Much of what he said during his contribution, completely contradicted what he had told us when we met him and he made a strong claim that it was highly unlikely that false allegations of abuse would be made in a family where the relationships between parents and children were stable. There would undoubtedly be underlying issues and the blame for the allegations could not be placed at the door of the therapist. He finished by concluding, "There is a lot of abuse out there that still has to be discovered." Obviously, if the abuse still has to be discovered, how does he know how much there is? But we were to find out that Freeman's claims about our family were to become even more outrageous, as he re-wrote the family history in order to protect Yellowlees.

Two days after the first article appeared, another article appeared in the Dundee Courier & Advertiser, in which a mother, whose identity was not divulged, claimed her daughter had been treated by Yellowlees and the same psychiatric team in Murray Royal/Gilgal and had accused her father of the same type of abuse that Katrina had alleged. Unfortunately the daughter had accosted her father with the allegations in the father's local pub, in front of his neighbours. The father had slapped the daughter and was convicted of assault. The girl had two other sisters, neither of whom gave her claims any credence. As a consequence of the press coverage, the Health Trust made a public statement, issued by Caroline Inwood, who had conducted our internal inquiry, and which said, "False Memory or Recovered Memory Therapy are not techniques that have ever been, or are currently being used by clinical staff working within Perth & Kinross Healthcare NHS Trust's mental health services. We would therefore like to make it clear that the therapeutic techniques used by professionals employed by the Trust are those agreed and approved as best psychiatric nursing and psychological practice by their professional organisations, which are in widespread use throughout the UK."

In the same article, I was quoted as saying, "Well, they would say that wouldn't they? In political circles they call it dissembling or 'being economical with the truth'. I think they are being very foolish in making that statement because thay have then got to explain how my daughter ended up in that condition." I cited the Brandon Committee's report which had condemned many of the practises and therapies to which Katrina had been subjected in a lengthy report to the Royal College of Psychiatrists. Referring to Inwood's statement I said, "If that is true, they should re-open the Brandon Committee and have a special investigation into Murray Royal because they must have been using another technique which has exactly the same effects."

This type of response from the Health Trust and the interest in the problem which the initial press article had created, was exactly what I had hoped for by going to the media in the first place. I firmly believed that silence was the greatest defence the authorities had and so long as people who were put into the same kind of position as we were, remained silent, psychiatrists and social workers would continue to wreck lives with impunity. I was determined that was not going to happen. At every opportunity, I publicly accused the Health Trust and the Social Work Department of lying and any number of friends and others who had followed the case, commented on the fact there was no reaction from either side to those accusations. That was to continue to be the situation right up to the final hearing in July 2004.

One other very important factor which arose from the public nature of our campaign, was the fact that so many other families who were in a situation similar to or exactly the same as our own, began to contact us. Frequently Kay would be at home during the day and on her own, when the call would come through from someone who had been falsely accused by a female relative, usually a daughter. Kay became expert at listening to these people who were desperate to have someone who understood their plight, without having to dot all the "I"s or cross all the "T"s. We found that simply being prepared to listen provided enormous comfort to many of them, but we were also able to offer practical help by giving them contact numbers of the BFMS or other organisations such as FACT (falsely accused carers and teachers).

Although the intensity of the media interest tended to wane, when my case was thrown out on a legal technicality in July 2004, the interest was immediately rekindled with legal debate conducted in the columns of the press as to the likely impact the decision would have. The ramifications of the decision to pursue the case through the courts will be covered in a following section but there was no doubt about the depth of interest that was generated. The same intensity of interest was experienced in October 2007, when Katrina's case was finally settled out of court. We were approached by two TV companies who wanted to do a docudrama but unfortunately neither had the money available at the time.

At the time of writing (July 2009) the debate surrounding Recovered Memory Therapy is far from over and vulnerable people are still being damaged by the same mistakes, mistakes that need to be brought into the public domain so that the public are more aware of the potential damage that can be done. This type of therapy is not, and never has been, the preserve of the therapist in private practise. Unfortunately many of the worst examples of the application of Recovered Memory Therapy have taken place during treatment of patients in the NHS. Although my decision to use the media was not welcomed unequivocally by the whole family, there is absolutely no doubt in my mind that it was a far better course of action than to attempt to hide "that dirty little secret". It has helped Katrina to grow in confidence and it let the public see what had been done in the name of psychiatry.

CHAPTER TWENTY ONE

THE MEDICAL RECORDS ARRIVE
November 1997 – November 2007

As soon as I began to think seriously, of taking legal action, which was as soon as we had discovered the existence of Recovered Memory Therapy (RMT) in December 1995, I realised we would have to have access to Katrina's medical records. I started to ask the Health Trust for copies of the records as soon as we had established regular contact with the Health Trust official, which was April 1996. I was stonewalled repeatedly throughout the period between April and December 1996, at which time, I asked the legal firm who employed me and, who at that time were still representing me, to start putting pressure on the Trust.

The first letter was sent to the Chief Administrator of the Trust on 10th December 1996, to which a reply was received on December 29th, telling me that they would take advice and get back to me. On January 14th 1997, I received notification that under the Access to Medical Records Act 1990, Section 5, I could not have access. Having checked the conditions of the Act, Katrina provided us with written permission to see the records and a further request was sent on January 21st. On the 30th January, I received another reply stating the matter was being considered. Having received no further contact by 24th February, another request was sent.

We received a reply on February 27th, stating that even with Katrina's permission, the Trust believed it "is likely to cause serious harm to Miss Fairlie's mental health as well as providing information relating to or provided by third parties who could be identified from that information." Obviously we then took advice from a medical expert who could not see how Katrina's health could be adversely affected, and wrote to the Trust on 2nd April, to that effect. It was also pointed out to them that under the Act, they could ask permission of "the third parties" and their failure to do so, would force me to raise a Court Petition to have access to the records. As we still had had no reply by May 22nd, a further request was submitted. We received a reply on 1st June, stating a meeting was being held on June 5th, at which our request would be discussed. By this time, more than a year had elapsed since I had made my first request.

On June 7th, we received a reply which stated that the Board had decided I could have partial access because they were still of the opinion it would be detrimental to Katrina's health and that they would inform me when the extracts were available and that I could view them at Murray Royal. On the 9th June, we sent a reply to say we would reserve our position, given that our advice was that there could be no conceivable threat to Katrina's health but that we would accept sight of the extracts, for the time being. By 8th July, there was still no contact as to when the extracts would be available, therefore another letter was sent to the Board, reminding them of the publication of the Brandon Commission in December 1997 and its severe criticism of RMT and its practitioners, something we believed was central to Katrina's care.

On July 9th we received a letter from the Central Legal Office, informing me that they were now handling my request and that I should appoint an appropriate medical adviser, who would liase with their medical adviser, "*with a view to agreeing or otherwise what material should be properly withheld in the interest of Miss Fairlie's health* in terms of the Act. Thus, after almost 18 months of stalling me, the Health Trust had finally reached the point where they would have to make the records available, therefore they turned the request over to their legal advisers at the Central Legal Office, so that the whole circus could begin again.

Fortunately, we had no need to get involved with the Central Legal Office because Katrina had started her own legal action and we decided to wait until she received her medical records, which had already been requested. They finally arrived at the beginning of November 1997 and they proved to be a veritable goldmine. Katrina had instructed her solicitor to inform me as soon as they arrived at his office. When I arrived, he was obviously excited and anxious to tell me something. He handed me a sheet of paper and said,

"Take a look at that".

"What is it?" I asked.

"Just read it," he smiled.

I discovered I was holding a Lab Report from PRI on Katrina's gall bladder, which had been removed the day before the report was written on 17th August 1994 and it noted the presence of a large gallstone and unequivocal evidence of "***chronic cholecystitis***". I could not believe it.

"She had a gall stone," I exclaimed. "She had a bloody gall stone and they have been telling us for three years there was nothing wrong with her."

"That is definitely going to make a great difference," said her solicitor.

"How the hell could they all have missed this?" I asked. "Katrina should never have been in a psychiatric ward in the first place. I must call her and Kay. They are going to be furious."

There were bundles of medical notes, divided into medical, psychiatric and psychology notes, but in no form of order and it was obvious there were pages where some things had been deleted. I couldn't wait to get them home and to start reading them. Katrina was with Kay when I called to tell them and they both burst into laughter when I told them about the lab report. But then the serious nature of what we had just discovered began to set in and the laughter turned to anger. Kay agreed to let the rest of the family know, getting the same reaction from all of them – excitement and then anger at the thought of what we had been put through because of medical stupidity and negligence. We were to find the stupidity was even worse than we had feared and that they were prepared to go to any lengths to cover it up.

We decided that the family should meet at our house in Crieff, to go over the medical records and to make notes about the treatment Katrina had received. The meeting was arranged for the Sunday and Sharon, Andrew, Philip and Alison, Jim, Katrina, Kay and I sat round our dining room table, with the bundles of notes spread out in front of us. It was the first time in almost four years that we had all sat together, round the table at which we had shared so many happy Sunday dinners and Christmas celebrations. I suggested that as we had all been involved with Yellowlees and his team at different times and for different reasons, we should divide the medical records so that each of us was reading the notes with which we were each associated or for which we could best identify the circumstances.

I had already read some of the notes and knew some of what they contained, therefore I thought it was important that I said,

"We are all going to read some things which will upset us. There are charges and allegations made about all of us that would make us angry under different circumstances but if we remember what it is we are reading and why the allegations were made, we can put them in context and simply concentrate on what it is we are here for – to identify the treatment that Katrina received and note where the staff, either told her what was in her nightmares, or indicated they believed I was an abuser. At the end of this there should be no recriminations directed at anyone."

There were nods of agreement all around the table and some half smiles as we divided the notes between us. In no time, each of us identified notes and comments by the nursing staff, the psychologists and Yellowlees, that fit the pattern of the material for which we were searching. It became very obvious that Katrina had not wanted to be there, refused point blank to do any disclosure work or discuss the abuse by her grandfather. Yellowlees later claimed Katrina initiated the disclosure work but all of the notes showed entry after entry, where she refused to work with Jenny Hogg at first and displayed open hostility to both her and Yellowlees. In fact the records showed that it took almost five months of medication and constant pressure to disclose, before they broke Katrina's resistance.

Each of us commented on the nature of the notes we had found, every time we unearthed another example of the pressure they had put on her. We also commented on the number of times they had spelt her name incorrectly, the general standard of grammar and spelling throughout the medical notes, causing us to wonder at the level of education of the staff who had been dealing with Katrina. Some of the entries caused us to laugh out loud and Sharon came across one entry of 28/7/95 where the nurse had written,

"*Katrina seems to have settled down since she started to take Prothieden and her sleep pattern has improved.* The following day there was an entry by the same nurse which said, "*Katrina made suicide attempt last night. Has not been taking Prothieden but saving it up and took overdoze last night.*" Under a heading **Action to be taken;** "*Stop giving Prothieden*". We all found this entry ridiculously funny, a measure of the tension we were feeling, but in the middle of the laughter, Katrina stood up and left the room.

I followed her into the sitting room where she was trying to light a cigarette and crying at the same time. I put my arm round her shoulder as she turned to me and said,

"It is all right for you all to laugh in there, but that was my life and I didn't find it funny. They almost destroyed me and nobody believed me when I told you what was going on. Do you believe me now?"

She was angry now and I tried to placate her by saying,

"We don't really find it funny either Katrina. It is just a release of tension when we are laughing."

"I can't go back in there, I can't read any more of that stuff. The last thing I want is to be reminded of what happened."

I returned to the dining room to explain what was happening and a short time later Kay also sat back and pushed the bundle of notes away from her.

"I'm sorry," she said, "I can't go on with this either. I can't stand reading their stupid comments and their stupid spelling mistakes, reading about what they were doing to her."

At that point I suggested we all take a break and relax for a short spell with a cup of tea or something. During the break we all discussed what we were finding and we could hardly believe what they had done. It was very obvious Yellowlees believed I was an abuser, as did the staff on his team. There was entry after entry which highlighted that. Almost every claim that Yellowlees and Proctor had made was contradicted by the notes – and we had only managed to scratch the surface.

After the break, Jim was the next one to call off, explaining that he had been involved so little with any of the staff, that he felt he could contribute very little to what we were doing. That was certainly true but the real reason was that Jim found it very difficult to deal with his guilt and this whole exercise was very upsetting for him. Those of us who were left, continued for another two hours but it became very clear we were not going to get anywhere near to the end of the notes that day. We therefore decided to divide them and Sharon, Philip and Alison and Andrew, agreed to take a bundle of notes home and work on them until we could meet again the following weekend.

It took us over three weeks to finish our review and to discuss the implications of what we had found. I summarised each section, highlighting the relevant points to note, some of which came as a shock, even to us. Jackson, Director of Law and Administration for Perth & Kinross Council had taken great exception to my opinion that there had been collusion between the Social Work Department and the psychiatric team, pointing out that my claims were defamatory. We were delighted therefore, to find among the medical notes copies of several letters I had sent to Jackson, outlining my complaints against the Social Work Department. I amused myself endlessly anticipating his face when he was asked to explain in court, their presence among the medical notes.

To my astonishment, I received notification there was a large box at the post office for me, a fortnight after we had received Katrina's records. Without ever having contacted the Central Legal Office, they had sent copies of Katrina's records to me, but a greatly sanitised version of the records, with great swathes missing. Significantly, as we worked through the version that Katrina had received, and I compared the two sets of notes, it became very obvious the Health Trust knew exactly what mistakes had been made and had removed the evidence. There was no Lab report, large sections which recorded the attempts on her life had been removed. The evidence which showed that staff watched my visits closely and questioned Katrina after every visit I made were also removed. It was important that in the notes Katrina had received, after she had retracted and I had started being allowed to visit again, we found the records of the staff questioning Katrina about how she felt about me and every time I touched Katrina, whether it was a cuddle, a pat on the back, holding her hand; all of it was recorded. None of that was in the bundle of notes given to me.

We obviously concentrated on the notes given to Katrina and found some of the psychology notes were particularly enlightening. On 10/7/95 one of the psychologists noted,

"*Yellowlees **told** me that Catrina had been forced into giving her father oral sex in one of the visiting rooms*". Not that Katrina had **claimed** I forced her; just a straightforward I had forced her. In another section the same psychologist noted that Katrina was afraid her mother would catch her with me, and then, the psychologist notes "*it seemed possible her mother had caught them before*".

Yet again, in a discussion with Jenny Hogg the psychologist notes that Hogg had told her about Katrina's latest "flashback" "*very violent and he has used tools and forced her to eat used sanitary towels.*"

In an internal memo from Yellowlees to Caroline Inwood, after it had been agreed there should be an internal inquiry Yellowlees writes,

"*Mr Fairlie should be given as little information as possible because he always misinterprets it then uses it to attack me.*"

Obviously it mattered little what I said or what the family said about the contents of Katrina's medical notes. Expert opinion was required and readers should ponder on the part played by "experts" in some of the most celebrated cases that have come into the public domain in the UK in recent years. Dr Meadows and Dr Southall are well known for their infamous interventions in the Angela Canning, Sally Clark and Trupti Patel cases and the tragedy of the false allegations and incarceration of Canning and Clark. Less well known but equally damaging was the part played by the pediatrician Dr San Lazaro in the notorious Shieldfield case, where the nursery nurses Dawn Reed and Christopher Lillie were falsely accused of child abuse. They successfully sued Newcastle Council and were awarded £200,000 each.

At the libel trial in 1998 Dr Camille San Lazaro had given evidence on behalf of Newcastle Council and had interviewed some of the children allegedly abused by the two young nurses. The Judge, Mr Justice Eady was so disturbed by the evidence given by San Lazaro he instructed that her conduct be examined by the GMC. He summed up her contribution thus, *"where physical findings were negative or equivocal, Dr Lazaro was prepared to make up the deficiencies by throwing objectivity and scientific rigour to the winds in a highly emotional misrepresentation of the facts."*

Dr Lazaro herself, admitted that some of her work was "inappropriate", irresponsible" and "unprofessional" and the GMC concluded they had sufficient grounds to find her guilty of serious professional misconduct. However they let her off after the intervention of a colleague who claimed Lazaro was "overworked" and "under stress".

When the decision of the GMC was published, the Daily Telegraph made the following comment,

"Such a decision is troubling for those facing charges of sexual or child abuse. Unreliable evidence from social workers and doctors often lies behind allegations that turn out to be false. Medical experts often give opinions in court without even having seen the child or carer, using inaccurate hospital records as the basis for conclusions that have a

shattering effect on the lives of the accused. Yet it appears that they cannot be held accountable if they plead tiredness and overwork – even if they are being paid large fees for their expert opinion."

That comment was brought home to us with a vengeance when we saw the reports provided by the Health Trust's experts.

We were fortunate that Professor Sydney Brandon, one of the most eminent people in his field and the author of the Brandon Report which had totally discredited Recovered Memory Therapy agreed to be our expert witness and examine Katrina's medical records.

It came as a great surprise to learn that Chris Freeman, who had treated Katrina in Edinburgh, was the expert for the Health Trust. Professor Brandon produced his initial report and then had a stroke, from which he never fully recovered and died a short time later. We were again fortunate that Dr Janet Boakes, who had been Professor Brandon's deputy on the Brandon committee that had produced the Brandon Report, agreed to take his place.

That there might be a difference of opinion or of emphasis in the reports from the "opposing" experts was to be expected but we were not only amazed but furious at the reports provided by Freeman, who completely re-wrote the history and dynamics of our family, without ever having met any of them. He produced his report in April 1998 and I was immediately angered by the attitude of Katrina's solicitor who called me to tell me the report was absolutely damning to our case and sent me the report, accompanied by a letter which said,

"*I am sending it to you rather than directly to Katrina as I do not wish her to read its contents without having some support available.*"

At this point it is useful to start with the reports from Professor Brandon and Janet Boakes where they outline general features of RMT and its practitioners, so that the report of Freeman can be given some context. Freeman provided a second report in September 2007, from which excerpts will also be taken for the sake of comparison. At the time of the Brandon Report, the memory wars had been raging for years, particularly in the USA, where the theory of Repression was given greatest credence and where the therapy of recovered memory had been developed.

The Brandon Report examined hundreds of cases and had come to the conclusion that Repression or dissociation, where a victim of trauma found the event so horrific that they "blocked" it from their minds completely, did not exist in the form that its proponents argued. Believers in the theory argued that although the conscious mind had "blocked" the memory, the subconscious mind had filed it away but in certain circumstances, known as triggers, the memory would resurface. The triggers could be therapy, where the therapist had recognised the "signs" of repressed memory from a number of physical signals that only proponents of RMT recognised.

Under therapy, the remembered trauma, which can frequently be very vague, begins to grow in detail as "flashbacks" become more frequent and detailed. The timesacle over which the trauma took place expands so that abuse, which lasted for perhaps only a few months will eventually extend for years. The recovered memories become increasingly elaborated, begin to draw in more and more people and become more and more horrific and bizarre. The most extreme are those which include memories of events in a past life or alien abduction. The problems arise when the stories stop just short of the impossible while still straining credulity.

Katrina's allegations showed every one of those traits. When Kay first found out about the abuse at the hands of my father, Katrina said it started when she was about six or seven and stopped before she left primary school at eleven. Her medical records have numerous entries at different times when the abuse started at age five, then three then two and "perhaps earlier" It allegedly went on until she was thirteen, fourteen, fifteen, eighteen and even into her twenties. The allegations of abuse in the hospital and in her flat were taking place when she was in her late twenties, but no one asked why if the abuse was happening currently, she had no memory of it and it only happened in flashbacks when she was under medication. Katrina's earliest allegation of abuse involved only me but eventually included seventeen different men, her mother and her brothers and an abortion where her uncle was the father. Her medical record shows Katrina was never pregnant. The abuse itself eventually included murder and savage beatings including the use of instruments and forcing her to eat used sanitary towels, although these were among some of the least bizarre and savage things that were supposed to have happened to her.

Both Brandon and Boakes highlight the use of certain jargon by RMT practitioners, who refer to "survivors" and needing "to be in a safe place." Freeman's first report contains a comment on her disclosures. Despite the fact the notes showed clearly how much Katrina objected to disclosure, something confirmed by both Brandon and Boakes, Freeman still manages to observe (Page 7. Para 8.1) "These begin to occur spontaneously. It is entirely predictable that such episodes should begin when Katrina was removed from her family and in a place where she felt **safe and secure."**

Mark Pendergast's book, "Victims of Memory" published 1997, is the result of three years of research into the RMT debate. He interviewed therapists on both sides of the debate as well as those who had been abused and who had alleged abuse. Pendergast writes, (P 197) *"I was particularly disturbed by the tendency of most therapists to absolve themselves of any responsibility. Almost all of them assert it doesn't matter whether the memories are literally true or not. The memories represent the 'internal truth' for the client and it isn't the therapist's job to search out the facts."* Compare that with Yellowlees's, *"It is not my job to get evidence".*

Pendergast also quotes two well known proponents of RMT in the USA, Barret and Scott who say, *"If parents insist that their child has been brainwashed by irresponsible therapists, they should consider what in that child's family experience has made her vulnerable to being brainwashed."* So, even if it can be shown that RMT has been used and that false memory has resulted, it is still the fault of the parents and not the therapists.

Compare that with the following quote from Freeman, on the BBC's Frontline programme recorded February 1998,

"I think the issue as far as false memory is concerned in sexual trauma is, can it be the case that a perfectly normal functioning healthy family, good relationships between mother, father, daughters, children etc. can be torn asunder by a completely false memory that is implanted in the context of therapy? My view is that it is extremely unlikely. That if you look at most of those families it doesn't mean that sexual abuse has occurred but there is some reason, some relationship which is not functioning well which has caused the accusation to be made, and you can't lay the blame entirely on a therapist implanting that seed there."

That view explains Freeman's determination to trash our family reputation, despite never having spoken to or meeting any of them. One of the main criticisms of Yellowlees, by both Brandon and Boakes, is that he did not speak to either Kay or I, nor did he attempt to get a family history before embarking on therapy with Katrina. Under the BMA's own guidelines, he had a duty to do so but one which he never fulfilled, together with his total failure to check her notes and find the lab report. Nevertheless, Freeman could come to some remarkable conclusions about the entire family. Remember this man is supposed to be an "expert" and as a consequence of the first report he wrote, Katrina's legal aid was stopped. I immediately wrote a detailed rebuttal and the legal aid was resumed but that is an indication of the willingness of the courts to accept "expert" opinion and the damage it can cause.

In his first report in April 1998 Freeman writes,

2.1 Katrina had a normal appendix and normal gall bladder removed. (By this time the existence of the Lab report and its contents was known by everyone associated with the case)

2.7 Katrina is blaming Murray Royal to some extent for her problems. It is recorded that this may be because her mother was repeatedly admitted to Murray Royal for periods of alcoholic detoxification and when Katrina had to stay with her grandfather and was repeatedly abused. (Did no one check the records? Kay had never been in Murray Royal for alcohol abuse)

7.2 "It seems agreed Katrina was seriously and repeatedly sexually abused by her grandfather.

7.3 This went on for a number of years (approximately six to thirteen).

7.4 Katrina's mother and father completely failed to protect her from this abuse, despite the fact that *I understand* that Mrs Fairlie was also abused, and *I think* I have heard Mr Fairlie say in a TV or press interview that he was also abused. (So much for a scientific approach)

7.6 Katrina's sister Sharon has also claimed that she has been abused by the same family members. (To whom?)

7.8 I could find no evidence that Katrina was wrongly or inappropriately diagnosed. (There were two diagnosis, one when Katrina was admitted to Murray Royal and one when she discharged herself. The second showed a massive deterioration in her mental health – see Boakes – If they were both correct, what was the cause of her deterioration under the care of Yellowlees?)

8.3 From the case records it would appear that the staff kept an open mind about the nature of subsequent revelations. They did suggest that she may have been influenced by her sister Sharon's reporting and it appears that it was after meetings with Sharon that the accusations about abuse by her father were made by Katrina. (So, now it was her sister's fault she made the allegations?)

8.6 Their (staff) prime concern had to be to maintain a supportive relationship with Katrina. *To have challenged her directly and said that these allegations were untrue, would almost certainly have damaged their relationship with Katrina.* (He later states they frequently challenged Katrina and Yellowlees also claimed they challenged her)

8.7 There was some discussion about whether other younger family members were currently at risk. *This discussion was*

>*entirely appropriate.* (Only if they believed I was guilty of abuse, which they claimed they did not)

8.8 Given that this family both in its nuclear and extended form has had such considerable problems and given that there was an extended history of abuse by family elders of mother and two sisters and perhaps other family members, it is entirely appropriate that the Clinical Team should seriously consider that Mr Fairlie may have been an abuser and that other family members might be at risk. When Katrina's brothers began to report that they had been abused and that they had witnessed Katrina being abused, this added further evidence in favour of these beliefs.

(Freeman really excels himself in this paragraph. He **ASSUMES** extended abuse of the family without any details or even speaking to any of them. He **ASSUMES** abuse of other family members but there is not a mention of that in the medical records. There is no mention in the medical records of the boys either being abused, or witnessing Katrina's abuse. These non-existent events are then used to apportion culpability in Freeman's own mind and held to be "evidence in favour of these beliefs". Thus in the space of a few lines, Freeman has transformed what was no more than a "consideration" of my guilt as an abuser, on the part of the Clinical Team, to "beliefs."

In his second report of September 2007, Freeman went even further, but this time, much of the report is given over to attempting to refute the report given by Dr Boakes. He is not even aware of the supreme irony of some of what he writes. For example, he attacks Dr Boakes for claiming that everything that Katrina disclosed was taken entirely literally and believed by members of staff, stating, "This does not accord with my reading of the notes."

He then claims to be puzzled by many of Dr Boakes's conclusions, although he makes no attempt to say why but continues,

> *"It is important to remember that in Katrina we have a young woman who comes from a very disturbed family, was abused over a long period by her grandfather and may have been abused by her uncle and who has a mother and father who have both been sexually abused. It seems remarkable that Dr Boakes is suggesting that this should not be taken into **account when formulating treatment plans for Katrina.**"*

What is remarkable is that this man who practises as a doctor, can be allowed to get away with creating a family history that did not exist in reality. In his first report he was still reporting that Katrina had had a normal appendix and gall bladder removed, despite the Lab report being noticed by both Brandon and Boakes and Katrina's entire family and being made known to the lawyers dealing with the case. In his second report, he chooses to ignore it because it is not within his sphere of expertise. In other words, he ignores the main source of the misdiagnosis of Katrina's illness and her reason for being in Murray Royal in the first place. Instead, he chooses to spend the rest of the report commenting on whether or not the use of Pethidine was the cause of Katrina's illness and unsurprisingly decides it is not. Or, he is defending Yellowlees and his team, unsuccessfully, against the criticisms in the report by Janet Boakes.

This man claims that Kay was taken into Murray Royal to be detoxified and that he thinks, then is sure that I was sexually abused. Where did that information come from?

He spoke to none of the family but can state unequivocally that they were abused, or were possible abusers or witnessed Katrina's abuse. He goes to great lengths to justify that Yellowlees and his team should think of me as an abuser, while they were doing their best to deny that they believed Katrina's allegations. It would have been easy enough to check whether or not Kay and been in hospital for detoxification or that I had been abused, but hey, these people are untouchable and if they are going to trash a family in order to protect a colleague, it is as well to make a job of it.

As far as Katrina's dysfunctional family is concerned, at the time of writing, Sharon her elder sister has spent over twenty years dealing with disturbed children, setting up and running a school in Central Scotland for the specific purpose of giving support to mainstream education for children with behavioural problems and is now deputy director of education in one of Scotland's local authorities. Andrew her eldest brother, is the most celebrated chef in Scotland with his own eponymous restaurant and the only two Michelin starred chef in the country. Philip is the vice chairman of his union, in regular discussion with government ministers on the direction of government policy and Jim the youngest brother, is a tenant farmer of five thousand acres running over three thousand sheep and was the architect and founder of the Farmers' Market movement in Scotland ten years ago, one of the most radical revolutions in Scottish agriculture for decades.

They all have grown up children and lead perfectly stable and happy lives. None of them has ever had any contact with psychiatric services, other than when we were fighting Katrina's case. If they were all abused, where is the evidence, where are the psychological scars that have been such a burden for Katrina? Why were none of them affected in the way Katrina was? The truth of course is that Katrina carried those scars only because of the intervention of Yellowlees and his team. It is recorded that Katrina was being abused as young as two but before Katrina went to school, she was constantly with Kay because Kay did not work until all the children went to school. For the two and a half years before she went to school, Katrina was never out of Kay's company, so when could the abuse have happened, unless Kay was a party to it?

It is also recorded that Katrina was kept at home by Kay to keep her company, that she regularly played truant from school and was frequently in trouble for insolence. Not only was all of this accepted as fact but comment was made about the nature of Kay's parenting. Had any of the idiots who swallowed all of this, including the so-called experts, spoken to either Kay or I they would then have had to work out how Katrina could be kept at home to keep Kay company when Kay, who went to work as soon as Katrina started school, was managing a shop in Perth for ten years, in other words throughout Katrina's entire school career, until the shop closed and she was made redundant. They would also have learned that I worked as a teacher for the whole of Katrina's school years, that I ran her and Jim to school each morning because they attened the same school at which I taught and I took them home in the afternoon, that if either of them missed a class, I was informed. As for insolence, none of the family were ever insolent with Kay and I and I certainly would not have tolerated their being insolent to my teacher colleagues, all and any of whom would have told me immediately if there had been any problems.

Freeman makes the following observation on page 25 of his second report,

"It may well be that Miss Fairlie's deterioration was related to her admission to Murray Royal Hospital in December 1994 through 1995 but as I have already concluded in my first report this is not because the treatment in Murray Royal was negligent or deficient."

This is the first and only reference Freeman makes, to the deterioration in Katrina's health during her stay in Murray Royal, in either of his two reports, and if it is not due to the negligent or deficient treatment she received, what is the cause? Freeman declines to offer an opinion. There are frequent references to Katrina's prolonged anorexia and her previous psychiatric problems before 1994. The only contact she had with psychiatric services prior to 1994 was her short contact with Powrie, the social worker in 1987, for a period of about three months. There was no further contact and there was never any evidence of anorexia.

Professor Brandon pointed out in his summary that Katrina's weight, even after her abdominal surgery and prolonged stay in hospital, was within the normal ranges that would be expected under the circumstances. He also comments that the belief among proponents of RMT that childhood sexual abuse often leads to anorexia or other eating disorders, led the staff to look for both anorexia and sexual abuse. He states in his conclusion,

"*It is clear the capacity for self deception is not confined to patients for the statements by Drs Yellowlees and Proctor to the effect that Miss Fairlie benfitted from her admission to Murray Royal and showed significant improvement with evident therapeutic progress is clearly at varience with the objective accounts of deterioration during and after her admission.*

Miss Fairlie was detained in a mental hospital for some fifteen months for no good psychiatric reasons. There is a strong probability that dependence, loss of confidence and self direction and regressed behaviour developed as a direct consequence of this.

The choice of Pethidine as analgesic is surprising. It is not particularly effective in long term use, is prone to create dependence and the manufacturers state that it should not be given to patients with severe liver disease or for pain following cholecystectomy, bilary colic or increased intracranial pressure. (APBI Data Sheet Compendium 1994-5 p.892)

There was some considerable debate between both sides about the use of Pethidine but Brandon and Boakes are the only two who offered definitive proof of the manufacturer's direction, as opposed to opinion, which is as far as those for the Health Trust could go.

In her summary Janet Bokes concluded,

"Over her year in Murray Royal, this young woman who on admission had no features of psychiatric illness, experienced an alarming deterioration in her mental health.

When admitted she had her own flat, was working in the Post Office, was slim but not underweight, had never self-harmed, had a history of one overdose in her teenage years but otherwise no formal psychiatric history and was not preoccupied with diet.

After ten months of continuous hospital admission she had given up her flat, had been made redundant by the Post Office and was receiving benefits, was thin to the point of gauntness, was worried about her weight, eating a poor diet and occasionally inducing vomiting, her face was scarred as a result of regular self-harming, she was suffering nightmares, dissociative episodes and flashbacks, was regarded as a very high suicidal risk and regularly experienced auditory, visual and tactile hallucinations."

One very important feature of the medical notes which Freeman ignores completely, is the content of Katrina's journals or diaries, a common feature of RMT. Janet Boakes gives a thorough account of the contents because they

9.1 "chart the evolution of her allegations and the deterioration in Katrina's health. They chart the erratic nature of the counselling with missed sessions, broken promises and sometimes economy with truthfulness on the part of the counsellor."

9.3 At the start of the diary she had no doubt that she had been abused by her paternal grandfather and had not been abused by anyone else.

9.4 15th March 1995 she has no actual memories apart from images which come to her in "flashbacks" and she struggles to decide if they are a product of her imagination or had really happened.

9.6 Katrina is increasingly distressed, seeing faces and hearing voices. It is not clear if she shared her doubts with her counsellor but there is *nothing to suggest that these doubts were explored by the professionals, or indeed if they harboured any doubts about her 'memories'. No one ever appears to have asked Katrina to think about the liklihood of her 'memories' or to compare them with what she knew about her family or to test them against the reality of other information available to her.*

9.12 She also appears to be under considerable pressure from members of staff to make a police statement, partly to support her sister.

9.14 The overwhelming conclusion from her diaries is that there is so much fantasy material contained within it that it is impossible to know what, if anything, is accurate. However, what comes across very strongly is her own sense of inner confusion, her constant tussle between belief and disbelief, and the lack of help given to her to resolve this."

Katrina's health problems did not disappear when she left the Priory to come home and for several years she attended the hospital in Dundee and a Professor Reid, became her consultant. The improvements were not immediate but they were progressive, to the point that it is now, at the time of writing, six years since she had to make use of psychiatric services of any description. There were frequent set-backs but the self harming gradually disappeared as did the attempts on her own life. The confusion was still there and even as late as 2007, when Katrina was given a psychiatric assessment by the legal team acting for the Health Trust, the accounts of her childhood, she gives to their "expert", are still wildly inaccurate but were accepted without question and his assessment based on an interview which lasted for just over one hour and the medical notes which are even more wildly inaccurate.

One of the most important features of RMT is highlighted by the Brandon Report under the heading, *THERAPEUTIC OUTCOMES OF MEMORY RECOVERY TREATMENT "*. *...the effects of distorted truth should not be overlooked. The damage done to families if the accusations are untrue is immense. Moreover, it is not only the families that are damaged by mistakes in this area. Patients who are mistakenly diagnosed as having been abused, frequently end as mental health casualties. (Loftus 1997) Where improvement is based upon a false belief, there seems a serious possibility of further mental distress.*

The psychiatrist who assessed Katrina for the court's final comment is,

"*Finally, and at a more speculative level, I cannot help wondering if this case (*her legal action against the Health Trust) *is currently having a stabilising influence on her. There does seem to be significant suggestions throughout the medical records that she has become somewhat* *fixated by it over a prolonged period of time, Unfortunately I have to confess that I do have some significant concerns that in the aftermath of the case, SHE IS LIKELY TO DECOMPENSATE AND HER MENTAL STATE MAY GO DOWNHILL AGAIN.* I think this would be irrespective of whether the claim is successful or unsuccessful, but rather as a response to heightened psychological tension of the whole affair. *I do think this is a period during which the pursuer could be at particularly high risk and I think it is important that her own legal team have given some consideration to how they might respond should she decompensate during the period of any Proof. In particular what they will do if she responds with threats of self harm or equally, threats made to Dr Yellowlees as have been made in the past. It would in my opinion, be adviseable that consideration is made as to how they would, for example liase with her current care networks and how it would be appropriate to act."*

The character assassination continued therefore, right up to the last gasp. Katrina's "fixation" with the court case "over a prolonged period" is seen as a sign of psychological instability. Had the Health Trust not spent tens of thousands of pounds of tax payers' money over thirteen years, in order to keep the case out of court, there would not have been a prolonged period during which Katrina would have been constantly asked by her own legal team, to deal with a mountain of correspondence. The snide "speculation" that she might be a threat to Yellowlees or that she might go to pieces once the case is over, speaks volumes about the kind of people we had to deal with and says a great deal more about them than it does about Katrina.

The final comment in this chapter should be left to the BMA, whose paper published in May 1999 had this to say about duty of care:-

"In many cases the clinician who accepts a duty of care is unsure of the diagnosis or the full facts of the situation. Part of the continuing duty of care involves taking appropriate steps – through history taking, examination, referral to specialist colleagues etc – to ensure that as accurate a diagnosis as possible is made… Good communication and clarity about what is established fact and what is hearsay or conjecture are essential. It is especially important that other professionals with a duty of care to the same patient are fully aware of areas of uncertainty so that mistakes are avoided and mixed messages are not given out… Doctors may be considered negligent if they imply – either verbally at a meeting such as a case conference or in writing – that they have verified facts or statements when they have not personally done so.

"The duty of care is primarily for the individual patient who is the centre of concern. Clearly however…a balance is sought between the needs of individuals and those of people *close to them and a duty of care may be owed to several people… Even where a doctor has not explicitly accepted a duty of care to several people, there is a general ethical obligation TO RESPECT THE RIGHTS OF NON-PATIENTS AND AVOID FORSEEABLE HARM TO THEM".*

"Where doctors become aware that an error may have occurred, they have an ethical obligation to take all reasonable steps to verify the facts as promptly as possible and acknowledge the mistake. WHERE PATIENTS OR THEIR FAMILIES SUFFER HARM AS A RESULT OF AN ERROR, THEY ARE ENTITLED TO APPROPRIATE COMPENSATION."

CHAPTER TWENTY TWO

LITIGATION AND THE CONSEQUENCES
November 1995 – November 2007

"It is indisputable that being labelled as a child abuser is one of the most loathsome labels in society and most often results in grave physical, emotional, professional and personal ramifications. This is particularly so where a parent has been identified as the perpetrator. Even when such an accusation has been proven to be false, it is unlikely that social stigma, damage to personal relationships, and emotional turmoil can be avoided. In fact, the harm caused by misdiagnosis often extends beyond the accused parent and devastates the entire family. Socity also suffers because false accusations cast doubt on true claims of abuse…" "No social utility can be derived from shielding therapists who make cavalier diagnoses that have profound effects on the lives of the accused and their family."

Those are not my words, they are the opinion of the Supreme Court of New Hampshire, USA, December 18th 1998 in the case of Joel Hungerford v Susan L. Jones. But they encapsulate beautifully, the impossible position in which an accused parent is placed when he or she (in the vast majority of cases the accused is the father) is the subject of false allegations of sexual abuse. In my particular case, I was far too well known both locally and nationally (within Scotland) for my daughter's allegations to remain secret for very long. In fact, Bruce Crawford, the SNP leader of the local city council already knew and he should never have been given any information in any way shape or form. The family had never expected any outcome in our favour from the internal inquiries from either the Health Trust or the Local Authority and, to accept their findings that "the staff had all acted appropriately" was tantamount to admitting the allegations were true.

The Social Work Department had issued an apology of sorts but couched in terms which stated *"there was insufficient evidence"* leaving the suggestion that there was **some** evidence, which was completely untrue. To this day (July 2009) fourteen years after I was confronted, the Health Trust has never even offered any kind of apology, choosing instead to attempt to destroy an entire family and its inter personal relationships, rather than admit a mistake was made. Those despicable people are beneath contempt, no matter how many apologists maintain they are well intended. Given the position taken by both the Local Authority and the Health Trust, litigation was the only option open to both Katrina and me, if there was ever to be any hope of some form of natural justice. Unfortunately, despite our best efforts it was not to be. Both the Health Trust and the Local Authority made bold statements at the very outset that **"they would defend the action vigorously"**. In the event, neither did anything of the kind, choosing instead to spend their energies and taxpayers money in successfully keeping the case out of court so that they had never any need to defend their actions; just deny, deny, deny and allow the legal system and their well-paid lawyers to the rest.

Although this is the final chapter in the saga, and the legal outcomes in the cases of both Katrina and myself, drew a line under the "official" battle, litigation and its consequences had been an ever-present part of my life from November 1995, the month following the first confrontation with the family, and July 2004, when Lord Kingarth "struck out" my claim, refusing me my day in court. Katrina had battled from November 1996 until her QC deserted her in October 2007 and she was forced to accept a derisory £20,000 in an out of court settlement from the Health Trust, for having had her life destroyed. As in theory, there could have been a conflict of interest, we were represented by different legal firms. In reality our cases were very similar, although Katrina did not pursue the Local Authority, and there was considerable co-operation between

Katrina's legal firm and me. As she became more able to act on her own behalf, Katrina took a greater and greater interest in what was being done and was far better able to question the actions of her legal team; but throughout her own campaign, right up to the end when my case had already been sidelined, we discussed every detail.

It is assumed by the court that when a pursuer makes averments (allegations) in a lawsuit, the pursuer is confident those allegations can be proved. It is horrendously expensive and no one in their right mind embarks on such a course lightly. I carried the expenses of my case for ten years, as well as the costs of the other side, which were awarded against me, therefore it is reasonable to ask the reader to assume that I believed my allegations could have been proved in court. It is also reasonable to ask the reader to assume my solicitor believed I could have proved my case, else he would have stopped me long before the case was thrown out. Katrina was eligible for legal aid, which was not given lightly and frequently had to be fought for at different stages of the long, tedious road. No one who has not experienced the kind of disappointment and anger both Katrina and I experienced, can appreciate fully just the depth of feeling we endured. The pain of disappointment was almost physical, it was so deep.

We had both longed for the opportunity to see Yellowlees, Proctor, Freeman et al on the stand, attempting to defend themselves and their ludicrous, junk science against forensic cross examination. Even my anger was no match for Katrina's, the day she was finally forced to accept their offer of £20,000, a figure that did not cover two year's salary, let alone the fourteen years she had lost, as well as the pension rights and other benefits to say nothing of the normal, happy life they had taken from her.

Kay and I discussed all the consequences of litigation before I approached the court partner in my firm because I could not have done it without Kay's support, which never once wavered, throughout all the pain and pressure of raising the money. The firm I worked for did little or nothing for me in the early stages, nor did the QC they had asked for a preliminary opinion, therefore their contribution is of no importance. It was not until I asked another local firm of solicitors to act for me, that things began to happen, although the QC they appointed at first proved to be an absolute disaster.

I discovered very quickly that a pursuer in a lawsuit such as the one I was pursuing, very quickly begins to resemble a money tree, at least in the eyes of the lawyers. The initial retainer was a paltrey £1,500 but that did not last long, by the time my solicitor had appointed an "Edinburgh Agent" who liased with the QC. The Edinburgh Agent, is just another firm of solicitors, who happens to be licensed to practise in the Court of Session, the highest civil court in Scotland, a privelege denied my solicitor who was based in Perth. If contact had to be made with the QC or the clerks of the court, my Perth solicitor would write a letter to the Edinburgh Agent, who would "peruse" it before passing it to the QC, who may or may not reply. If a reply was needed, it was sent in the first instance to the Edinburgh Agent, who "perused" it before passing it to my solicitor, who in turn would pass it to me, either with a covering letter or a request for a discussion. A simple, A4 sheet of paper, which required to be "perused" cost £60 a whack, so one letter and one reply cost me the perusal fees of three different people.

I had one consultation with the QC that was appointed for me and my first impressions were not encouraging. She had a very good reputation in legal circles in Scotland and was very highly thought of but she did not impress me, either in her approach to me, as a person, or in her approach to the case. She had been given the papers prior to our consultation, therefore did have some grasp of the complaints I had but she did not have a grasp of the case. Perhaps it was expecting too much of her to expect her to know the case as well as I did, or to have the same commitment to what I wanted done, but she immediately let me know that as far as she was concerned, she knew the case better than I did, although under my cross examination, she fell far short of the kind of knowledge I expected and required her to have. That was confirmed when I received her first set of pleadings.

I was taken aback when she suggested that instead of pursuing the Social Work Department, I should attempt to get "them on our side" in order to implicate Yellowlees. When she presented this as her preferred course of action, I immediately knew she had not read the papers thoroughly enough. I asked her how she thought we could do this, given that the Social Work Department had told us nothing but lies from the outset and for them to change horses midstream, would involve their admitting to their lies, which, I ventured was unlikely. When she offered the opinion that it did not matter they had lied, my heart sank.

When the first pleadings arrived, I was told they had been prepared by a junior council – a common practise – but checked of course by the senior. Between them they had managed to include five fairly serious errors, with the wrong doctor treating Katrina in the wrong hospital in the wrong time frame, among others. When I pointed this out, and made my displeasure known, the objections were ignored but not only were the errors ignored, every other issue which I though was important – such as Bridgeford's lies from the outset – were not even mentioned in the pleadings. I was well aware I was a complete novice at this and that I had no option but to rely on the "experts" in court procedure to present my case, but I could not understand how any proper case could be presented if some of the major incidents were ignored. During the two years I was involved with this QC, I found it impossible to get through to her the importance of Bridgeford's behaviour. She seemed to set her mind right from the outset, on refusing to make any kind of case against the Social Work Department, therefore it made no difference how much I stressed that if it had not been for Bridgeford's lies, Napier would **not** have assumed the SNP councillor was acting on my instructions, would **not** have told the family I was using my contacts and the family would **not** have been persuaded there was truth in the allegations.

Never having had any experience of dealing with the legal profession at this level, I had no idea what the procedures involved, in a case of this kind. For a start, I had to learn that the pleadings could go back and forth as both sides made their claims and counterclaims, making amendment after amendment, until both sides were satisfied that no further amendments could usefully be included. Although I had already been embroiled for over four years, I was amazed when my solicitor suggested we could be looking at another four years before getting the case into court, although he underestimated the time scale by another four years on top of that.

We had been used to the repeated denials by Yellowlees and his team but it still came as a shock to see the same denials, embellished even further, pop up in the Answers from the legal teams of both the Health Trust and the Local Authority. Fortunately, I was given the opportunity to check the Answers from the other side, and point out the evasions, the half-truths and out and out lies and it was finally brought home to me that there were no depths to which they would not sink, in order to cover their mistakes. To even acknowledge the existence of the Lab Report, which was now known to everyone involved, took until 5th January 2000, when the Health Trust's legal team finally admitted it to Katrina's counsel. There never was an admission to me since the Lab Report had been removed from the records I had been given. What that tells us about the legal system is difficult to guage.

In a detailed rebuttal of the pleadings from the other side on January 6th 2001, my frusatration boiled over. Freeman had done his best to blame Katrina's illness on her childhood and her dysfunctional family's history, albeit the history was a figment of his imagination. Yellowlees and his team denied everything, blaming Katrina and Sharon for not only the level of medication that Katrina received but the decision to involve the Social Work Department and the police. Freeman concluded that since the Clinical Team had decided to their own satisfaction I was an abuser, they were entitled to seek to defend the grandchildren. This is tantamount to saying that since the medieval witch finders had satisfied themselves their victims were witches, they were perfectly entitled to burn them.

I summarised my rebuttal thus;

"There is a clear implication here that not only did the Clinical Team, which I assume included Yellowlees, believe that I was an abuser, they were perfectly justified in holding to that belief. Nursing Notes Volume 1A, P28 contains notes anent Jenny Hogg. There are two pages of them and Hogg advises the family to tell their partners, then when the time is appropriate to tell their children. A member of the ClinicalTeam, recognised by everyone to be Katrina's main therapist, is telling the rest of my family to tell my Grandchildren that I have abused their aunt, without a shred of evidence or even having contacted me. Hogg also advises Sharon to contact Rhod Napier of the SWD. Are we to assume that Yellowlees allowed his staff to dictate policy, that he was not aware that Hogg held those views? According to the Answeres (to the Pleadings) with which we have been provided, Katrina seemed to exert an enormous degree of control over her own actions, despite the fact that for much of the time she was under strong medication, sectioned in a confined unit, suffering from PTSD, anorexia, borderline personality disorder, dissociative disorder, attempting suicide, running away, being raped, seeing fairies etc. etc. Despite all of this she and Sharon were responsible for calling in the SWD, informing the police and Katrina still had enough presence of mind to dictate the speed at which she would disclose, started journaling at her own initiative and recovered all of her memories all by herself. Can we conclude from all of this that the lunatics really had taken over the asylum?

My difficulties with the second QC were to have a major impact on the outcome of the case because of the time constraints that are imposed on anyone seeking redress through the court system. Anyone seeking to sue for damages is given three years to lodge their claim in court, otherwise, unless under very special circumstances, they will be ruled out of time. In the initial stages of the proceedings, it was vital that I make my intentions known to the court, after which the case could be "sisted" which means it is suspended until both sides are ready to proceed. My case was introduced with a set of pleadings which were far from complete or even accurate, and then sisted immediately. There was also debate with the QC about when the triennium, or the three year period I was given to make my case, would start to run. As no satisfactory conclusion could be reached, and it was important we did not breach the rules surrounding the triennium, a case was started which formed the base on which my third QC had to conduct the rest of my claim. He inherited a poor set of pleadings which he did his best to amend, being told by the judge on one occasion that he had strayed very close to the water line.

We did not have the medical records when the first pleadings were lodged in court and in hindsight, the case I should have made was one of defamation rather than one of negligence and breach of duty of care. Unfortunately the die was cast by the second QC and my third and final QC was forced to live with it. I was told that without the medical records, it would be difficult to prove malice on the part of Yellowlees et al, without which no case for defamation could be made. I had to accept that at the time, but again in retrospect and something that was realised shortly after, it was a wrong piece of advice. I was glad when we finally parted company because I not only had no confidnece in her, she made it perfectly obvious that she was not prepared to take on board any of the objections I made about her pleadings, nor to offer any kind of explanation for the way in which she presented the case. I found her whole attitude to be patronising in the extreme and when she wrote to my solicitor to complain about my questioning her and to withdraw her services, I was relieved as well as pleased. The final straw came when I insisted she re-examine the pleadings for the mistakes I claimed she had made and when they were returned, allegedly checked against the notes I had provided, with the mistakes still there. They were mistakes of fact, not of opinion therefore I initially refused to pay the fee of £250 but was told that if I did not pay the fee, I would be more or less blacklisted. The fee was paid and the relationship severed.

My third QC took an entirely different approach, being prepared to discuss my objections and point of view in meetings which on occasion ran for several hours. In order to keep my fees down, he dispensed with junior counsel. I was able to establish a rapport with this QC which had been totally absent from my relationship with his predecessor. He listened to my point of view and acted as Devil's Advocate as he questioned closely the arguments I advanced, to convince him that I had a case against both the Social Work Department and the Health Trust. My view was that even given the wide discretionary powers granted to Social Work Departments in their work in child protection, the law did not allow them to lie with impunity and Bridgeford had lied. My difficulty was in convincing him that her lies had had an enormous effect on our family and our relationships.

I had less difficulty convincing him I had a case against Yellowlees and the Health Trust and I spent countless hours looking at other stated cases in the USA, in England and later, in the Netherlands. Fortunately, there seemed to be a change in the attitude of the law in the UK, to the duty of care to third parties and I scoured the internet for the relevant cases. It was a much easier task in the USA because the majority of states had taken the view for several years that psychiatrists and therapists had no right to expect a general immunity if their conduct destroyed the lives of the families of their patients. The first successful case had been the Ramona case in Southern California, which set the precedent for other cases in the USA.

Despite the fact that Christopher Lillie and Dawn Reed, the nurses in the Shieldfield case in Newcastle, had sued Newcastle Council for defamation, I took great encouragement from the decision by Mr Justice Eady to award the nurses the maximum £200,000 each. I took even greater encouragement from the way he had dealt with the expert testimony of the witnesses for Newcastle Council. I took particular note of his ruling on the evidence of one of the four "experts" appointed by Newcastle Council to produce a report which would "prove" the nurses had committed child abuse. In his summing up of the evidence of Professor Barker, Justice Eady said,

*"It emerged early on in Professor Barker's testimony that he has fundamentally different attitude towards the weighing and analysis of evidence from that of a lawyer. At several points, it became apparent that he is rather dismissive of what he called 'a forensic approach'. He resorted from time to time to impressionistic mode, referring to his "profession judgement" and to discussion in academic and other published work. His colleagues were similarly minded. Yet the issue of whether any given individual has raped or assaulted a small child...**is not a matter of impression, theory, opinion or speculation. It should be a question of fact.**"*

His first presentation of my case in the Court of Session was a success, as was his second and third, as we crept ever closer to the point where there would be no further amendments and the judge would decide whether or not the case would be allowed to go to Proof. After the third appearance, I was feeling particularly pleased and when the QC and I met in Parliament Hall after leaving the side court, I congratulated him when he hit me with a real bombshell. He had decided to take a post with the Prosecution Service and join the "other side" as it were. As we still had some way to go I asked him where that left me, to which he said he had been given leave to "tidy up" his case load. This meant he would be able to take me on to the next stage but then I would have to find another QC.

We had reached a particularly important stage of the process of getting me into court and the QC had successfully changed the pleadings substantially but, there was still much to do. The judge's comments at the end of the session we had just completed, suggested we needed to offer another lengthy amendment – and to all intents and purposes, I did not have a QC. The case had already cost me tens of thousands and it had been relentless since I had started out in 1995. It was now March 2003 and I really did not feel like paying another QC to start all over again. I asked my solicitor how he would feel about me representing myself and his answer surprised me. He felt that no one knew more about the case than I did and he thought I was capable enough of making the case in court. He was only half right.

I had another major problem which was beginning to cause me serious concern. About fifteen years previously, while taking part in a judo championship bout, I had badly twisted my back. After months of physiotherapy, none of which made any improvement, I had to stop fighting although I continued to keep fit by running, weight training and horse riding. Unfortunately in the early months of 2002, I had developed serious pain at various places in my right side and after several examinations and suspicions of every ailment including cancer, it was discovered I had two old fractures in my vertebrae, which must have been done at the judo championship and gone undetected for over fifteen years. Completely unaware I was doing it, I had developed a method of walking which threw my body out of alignment, causing serious problems in my right hip. I had been offered a hip replacement and the waiting time was just about over, with the operation imminent.

Nevertheless, it was agreed I should submit the amendment, which was lengthy and complicated. My eldest grand daughter Stacey accompanied me to court that day. None of the family had been allowed to come to court during any of the other appearances, on the grounds that all of them might be called as witnesses if the case went to proof, but as I was going to represent myself, Stacey felt I should have some support and as she had been a child during the time of the allegations – she was now a young woman of nineteen – she was unlikely to be called as a witness. She was close to tears as she and my solicitor sat at the back of the court (my solicitor was not allowed to even sit beside me) watching me sit on my own, while the senior and junior QCs for both the Health Trust and Perth Council, accompanied by their clerks and piles of legal tomes, filed into the benches alongside me. There were seven of them in total and they made an impressive sight in their wigs and gowns.

My hip was very painful but as I had avoided taking pain killers to keep sharp, standing was causing me considerable discomfort. I started confidently enough, knowing exactly what I wanted to say but as objections started to be raised, I began to feel less and less comfortable. Had it been the proof and I was presenting my case and questioning witnesses, it would have been easier. I had often fantasised about getting Yellowlees and Freeman in the witness stand, but this was different. I was having to argue points of law and had neither the experience nor the intimate legal knowledge to allow me to do it with confidence. Nevertheless, I did mange to score several points and to my own surprise, Lord Kingarth allowed the amendment, which did improve the overall pleadings.

After he had given his judgement, he addressed me directly,

"Mr Fairlie, I believe you represented yourself because your QC was not available today?

"Yes, M'Lord, that is correct," I said.

Lord Kingarth, looked at me for a short time, probably noting the beads of sweat on my face as I struggled to stand comfortably.

"Do you feel comfortable enough to carry this on to the next diet?" he asked

I can help you as much as I can, but I am afraid I cannot make your case for you. You will be faced with some very complicated legal arguments which require detailed legal knowledge – and some experience," he finished.

"No M'Lord, I don't feel capable of taking this to the next diet. I know my limitations."

At that point there was an attempt to object from the other side but Lord Kingarth waived them quiet and said,

"Are you able to confirm that you will have a QC to represent you at the next diet if I set a date now?"

I had no idea if I would have a QC but I said I would, after glancing back to my solicitor, who nodded his agreement. While I had been preoccupied, he had found out that my QC had resigned from the Prosecution Service and would be available, if we asked him. It made sense, since he knew the case and had all his original notes. The date had been set for four months away, March 2004. I went into hospital on January 4th to have my hip replaced.

My QC agreed to pick up the case again, with one condition, he refused point blank to continue with the case against Perth Council, on the grounds that he was certain we could not win, that the Judge would rule in favour of the Council. I was angry because it meant that they had lied at every stage of the proceedings, lies that were so obvious that a child could have recognised them as lies and yet, had succeeded in avoiding having to answer in court. Unfortunately I had no choice and very reluctantly agreed to drop the case against Perth Council, which meant I was immediately liable for their expenses. I had no complaint about the case my QC made against the Health Trust, nor in the way he presented it. He was very forceful in the way he argued that Yellowlees had gone beyond the point at which it could be said he was protected by the discretions he enjoyed as a psychiatrist.

The court in New Hampshire had made the following decision,

"Accordingly…we hold that a therapist owes an accused parent a duty of care in the diagnosis and treatment of an adult patient for sexual abuse where the therapist or the patient, acting on the encouragement, recommendation, or instruction of the therapist, takes public action concerning the accusation. In such instances, the social utility of detecting and punishing sexual abusers and maintaining the breadth of treatment choices for patients is outweighed by the substantial risk of severe harm to falsely accused parents, the family unit and society."

This was the argument that was presented to Lord Kingarth and I thought we had a better than even chance of succeeding. In my discussions with the QC after the court rose, he was reasonably happy with the way in which the arguments had gone and I did get the impression he was rather hopeful that we would be allowed to go to Proof. It had taken ten years and five appearances in the Court of Session and my mortgage had increased to £130,000.

On the morning of July 8th, I was in the house with Kay when the telephone rang. It was a journalist from one of the broadsheets who said,

"How do you feel Jim, about Lord Kingarth's decision?"

"What decision?" I asked.

There was an audible intake of breath on the telephone before the journalist said,

"Have you not heard the decision Jim, have you not spoken to your solicitor?"

"No," I replied, "I have spoken to no one but I take it the decision is out. What is it?"

"I am afraid you have lost but I suggest you call your solicitor. Expect the media to be on to you because it was announced in open court this morning."

I had known nothing about it and when I replaced the receiver, Kay immediately asked what had happened, having heard snatches of the conversation.

"We lost," I said, as she threw her arms around me and burst into tears.

Lord Kingarth had produced thirty pages of closely argued legal argument before finally rejecting my plea to go to Proof on a technicality, stating at the end, "I stress as a matter of law because it goes without saying that if, as the pursuer claims, Dr Yellowlees made the diagnosis which it is said he did, and it was one reached carelessly and without proper investigation, the pursuer's concern to seek redress is wholly understandable. I am nevertheless required to decide this case within the boundaries of the law as it has recently developed." Earlier in his judgement, he had also stated, "Against that background it would, in my view, be wrong – as counsel for the defenders argued – to allow the pursuer to advance what is essentially a claim for defamation in the guise of a claim, of damages for losses caused by negligence."

As was pointed out by one legal expert in newspaper comments which followed over the next few days, I had fought the wrong case.

We had one chance left to get them into court. Katrina's case had still to be settled but that was not going well. Katrina had had four different QCs and not one of them had even had the courtesy to speak to her or to discuss the case with her in any way. Her

Edinburgh agent had ignored her from the outset and had it not been for the fact that her Perth solicitor kept me informed, only so that I could discuss things with Katrina, she would have been left completely in the dark. Her legal team were every bit as arrogant and contemptuous of her as her psychiatric team had been. Her case had been postponed several times for the most paltry reasons, usually because someone had mixed up the diary dates or someone else had called off at the last moment. Each time there had been a change of QC, the files had to be re-examined, thereby ensuring another delay.

In January 2005, Katrina learned there had been another delay, through the medium of the press but by this time, she was well enough to fight her own corner and she wrote to her Perth solicitor, telling him in no uncertain terms about how she felt. Not only did she learn from the press that her case had just been delayed for another year because some clerk had put the wrong name on the court papers, but she also learned that her Perth solicitor had decided to retire, which meant passing her papers to a young female solicitor with only a few years of experience. As if that was not bad enough, yet another QC had been appointed and he required to re-examine the papers. By the time Katrina was due back in court the following year, everyone claimed to be up to speed with the case and there had been no further changes of personnel. This was to be probably the final "day of debate" before going to Proof, assuming the court allowed Katrina's case to proceed to Proof. Before that final date was even reached, the legal team acting for the Health Trust, contacted Katrina's legal team to say they were now prepared to dispense with the "day of debate" and go straight to Proof, but the earliest date on which they could do that, would be a full year away.

By various pretexts, the Health Trust and their legal team had avoided having to appear in court for ten years. It seemed fairly obvious they were waiting to see what happened with my claim but since the Judge had ruled that I was owed no duty of care by the Health Trust, it did not help them very much. There was no question they owed Katrina a duty of care, she was their patient, and now they had decided to dispense with the day of debate, they would either have to defend themselves in court or, make an offer of an out-of-court settlement – and they had managed to negotiate themselves another year, before they had to make that decision. Despite their protestations to the contrary, we were confident they had no desire to defend themselves in open court and, that they would make an offer of some kind.

The final act of Katrina's solicitor was to take statements from members of staff at Murray Royal who had been present at the time of Katrina's presence there. She managed to take statements from five of them, some of whom had had more to do with Katrina's Care than others. Obviously the most important of them was Jenny Hogg. In his first report for the Health Trust, Freeman notes at the outset that Katrina had been given phsychotherapy and referred to the Clinical Psychology Department, but "*also starts seeing Jenny Hogg, Senior Charge Nurse on Gilgal Ward.*" Later, he notes a meeting at which " *Dr Yellowlees, Dr Howell, Charge Nurse Hogg and Clinical Psychologists Jackie McVey and Michelle McCann are present*". Significantly Nurse Hogg is the only member of the nursing staff mentioned by Freeman in his report.

In his report Professor Brandon notes that in December 1994 (Katrina went into hospital in November 1994) *"Katrina embarked on disclosure with S/C/N Jenny Hogg which she* **continues** *to find very traumatic and difficult,"* suggesting that this was not the first time disclosure work had been done. On 25/1/95 there is a note by Jackie McVey to the effect that *"K is progressing with her disclosure work with Jenny Hogg although she is still hostile at times."* Again on 15/2/95, *"K to remain on 10 minute observation following her sessions with Jenny Hogg."* On 23/2/95 it is recorded, *"K finds it difficult to trust her counsellor Jenny Hogg,"* and again on 8/3/95, *"K expressed to Jenny Hogg…"* On 14th March 1995 McVey notes, "***Jenny starts her first hospital diary***".

On 31/4/95 *"Continues her work with Jenny Hogg"*
On 14/6/95 *"Continues disclosure work with Jenny Hogg"*

On 26/7/95 Meeting with Dr Yellowlees, Dr Hull, SCN Hogg, Jackie McVey and Michelle McCann. Note all doctors except Hogg.

On 24/1/96 Review meeting with Dr Yellowlees, Cahrlotte Proctor and Jenny Hogg.

It is worth noting that whatever changes of personnel took place in Katrina's care team, the only two people who were always included were Dr Yellowlees and Jenny Hogg.

In her report Dr Janet Boakes recorded that Katrina's diaries *"chart the evolution of her allegations and her growing dependence on SCN Jenny Hogg."* Dr Boakes also notes that Jenny Hogg read Katrina's diaries and then lied to Katrina about it, although she subsequently apologised. Under the heading Disclosure Work, Dr Boakes notes,

11.8 *"K underwent disclosure work with SCN Jenny Hogg. There are no separate notes for this disclosure work though SCN Hogg regularly writes in the nursing records."*

11.11 *"It is not clear what was Jenny Hogg's experience or training for such psychotherapeutic work, nor whether she was having any supervision in the early stages."*

Despite her involvement with Katrina from the first week she was admitted to Murray Royal/Gilgal, right up to Katrina's last week there before discharging herself in March 1997 and even more importantly, despite Hogg's obvious senior position in the hierarchy of the clinical team in charge of Katrina's care, Hogg can remember little or nothing about Katrina's time in Murray Royal/Gilgal

In her statement to Katrina's solicitor on 1th October 2007, Hogg claimed to have no memory of anything other than the fact that Katrina was actually there. Her opening comment is,

"As regards the case I remember the circumstances as a whole. I have had access to the notes and without these I would not have remembered details."

I cannot remember if I was on duty when Katrina was admitted...

I do not know if I remember the reason for her admission....

I cannot remember anything about Katrina's initial presence in the ward...

I cannot remember our meeting for the first time...

I cannot remember if Pethidine had any significance on her admission...

I cannot remember when I became aware of the Pursuer's history of sexual abuse

I cannot remember if the symptoms Katrina displayed changed in any way when Psychotherapy commenced...

I do not have any specialist training in Psychotherapy. I did not do Psychotherapy with the Pursuer...

If the Pursuer was to say she did not want to participate in Psychotherapy, all I can say is that I cannot remember...

As regards the sessions I had individually with the Pursuer, they were not for Psychotherapy. My job was to speak to each patient, to support and reassure them...

I do not know if the Pursuer was experiencing flashbacks...

I cannot remember if the Pursuer's condition deteriorated when Psychotherapy started...

The statements from the other four nurse were all in the same vein. If such an attack of collective amnesia is common among nursing staff in the psychiatric services, it must be very worrying for the GMC and the medical authorities. They seem to have enormous difficulty remembering what happens from day to day and if they could forget totally, the circumstances of one of the most high profile cases in Scotland, a case that was in every newspaper in the country, had had widespread coverage on radio and TV and had been the subject of a BBC documentary, what hope was there of any of them ever remembering the more humdrum, ordinary cases, where patients, some of whom are very disturbed and need 24 hour attention, would need to have their cases reviewed from time to time?

Reading the statements from the nurses, it was perfectly obvious they had been coached and it was also perfectly obvious they had no expectation of ever having to appear in court. They obviously knew their protectors well. As the time approached for Katrina's day in court, which was earmarked for the third week in October 2007, we waited in expectation for the call from her solicitor. We were not disappointed and received the call about two weeks before the due date, asking Katrina to go to the Court of Session in Edinburgh, where a meeting had been arranged between Counsel for both sides. When her solicitor asked if she needed help with transport, Katrina said,

"My Dad will take me through. I want him to be there with me in any case."

Within minutes, there was another call from the solicitor, in a bit of a panic this time, to tell Katrina that under no circumstances should I accompany her to the Court. In fact she was told, it would be better if she was not even seen with me in Edinburgh because the media would be there. Obviously, I was regarded as some form of bogey man, and one which the legal team acting for Katrina certainly did not want to be seen with. We had no choice but to agree but Kay and I arranged to take Katrina through by car and to wait for her just round from the Court of Session. More importantly, we arranged to keep in contact by mobile 'phone so that we could discuss the offer with her before she agreed to anything and so that she knew we were just round the corner if she felt the pressure getting to her.

We did not need to worry because by this time Katrina's disgust with and contempt for the legal system was as great as my own and she was confident her own anger would keep her going during the meeting. Kay and I received the first telephone call within an hour and I could sense Katrina's shaking over the telephone, she was so angry.

"They have offered me £10,000 Dad!" "£10,000 and they were told where to put it,!" she shouted down the 'phone.

I had not expected a big offer to start with but this was an insult, it was derisory and even with the level of contempt I felt for them, even I did not expect her to be given an offer like that.

"What did your QC say?" I asked, fully expecting her to say he was as just angry as she was.

"That bastard told me I should take it because it was a good offer," she exclaimed.

I could not believe it and after we had discussed what was happening and being told she had been given ten minutes to discuss it with us, she returned to the meeting. When she turned down the offer, the Counsel for the Health Trust left the room for a short time and returned with an increased offer of £12,500, which her own QC again told her to accept, telling her it was the best offer she was likely to get. Katrina again refused, telling them that she had waited for over twelve years to get Yellowlees and his crowd into court and that she was determined she was going to get them there. Despite his best efforts to persuade Katrina to accept the offer, her QC finally accepted defeat and told the other side the answer was still no.

It was agreed to have another break for an hour and Katrina, Kay and I discussed what her next move should be. It was obvious she was going to get very little support from her own QC and we advised her to get the best deal she could get but not to allow herself to become too overwrought and stressed. When we received the next call just over an hour later, it was obvious that Katrina was very upset but she was even more angry than she was upset.

"They have made an offer of £20,000 Dad," she said and before she had time to say anything else, I asked her,

"Is that their final offer?"

"I have no idea because that bastard of a QC has walked out on me," she exclaimed.

"What the hell do you mean he has walked out on you?" I asked.

"I told them no, I was not going to accept it, that I wanted to go to court and he asked to see me outside," she replied, "He then told me that if I did not accept the £20,000 he would refuse to act for me. The bastard is deserting me."

I was so angry I could hardly speak. My opinion of the legal profession was not high at the best of times, although my own lawyer had always been an exception, but this was beneath contempt. There was no point in ranting and raving to Katrina, Kay and I could only imagine how she was feeling and what she needed was support and not some raving lunatic bellowing down the 'phone to her.

"That does not leave you much choice Katrina," I said quietly. "Make sure he means what he is saying and that he is determined to walk, if you refuse the £20,000. If you are sure he means it, just agree and get away from there as quickly as you can. Mum and I will pick you up outside the court where we dropped you off."

When we picked up Katrina, she was remarkably composed although she assured us she was raging inside. We all were and we headed for the nearest restaurant to get something to eat and calm down. Katrina filled us in on what had happened. She had determined her QC meant what he said before agreeing to the offer but with one caveat on which she refused to budge. There would be no gagging order and she gave them fair warning that we would be speaking to the media. There was no attempt to stop her. She had left the details of the arrangements for paying over the cash to her solicitor so that she could get away from them as quickly as possible.

Perhaps the most appropriate way of summing up the way in which Katrina's legal team had treated her, is to recount her next contact from the firm which had acted as her Edinburgh Agents throughout. When she had railed at the offer that had been made to her, her QC had had the cheek to remind her that the legal fees had to be paid. The insensitivity and stupidity of such a remark being made to someone who had had her life destroyed by the same kind of arrogance and stupidity was obviously lost on him. But they were not finished. The next piece of correspondence Katrina received was an offer from the Edinburgh lawyers, offering their services to manage her new found wealth, with a list of the fees they would charge.

They had approached her on the day the offer had been accepted, offering to set up a trust for her and trying to explain to her how that would best husband her capital. Obviously they did not tell her that to a lawyer, a trust is simply a dripping roast, from which they can have a regular flow of cash. She replied to the Edinburgh firm, informing them her father was a Financial Adviser and would handle her capital for her. Undaunted, they had held on to the cash and wrote to her again. A full six weeks after the agreement had been made, Katrina still had not received her compensation, not because it had not been paid by the Health Trust but because it was still sitting in the client account of her Edinburgh solicitor. I called one of the senior partners in the Perth firm which had acted for Katrina and told him that unless the money was in her hands within 48 hours, I would go to the Law Society. The cheque arrived the day after next and it was finally over.

AFTERMATH / EPILOGUE

"It is indisputable that being labeled a child abuser is one of the most loathsome labels in society and most often results in grave physical, emotional, professional and personal ramifications. This is particularly so where a parent has been identified as the perpetrator. Even when such an accusation is proven to be false, it is unlikely that social stigma, damage to personal relationships, and emotional turmoil can be avoided. In fact, the harm caused by misdiagnosis often extends beyond the accused parent and devastates the entire family. Society also suffers because false accusations cast doubt on true claims of abuse..." "No social utility can be derived from shielding therapists who make cavalier diagnoses that have profound effects on the lives of the accused and their family."

Supreme Court of New Hampshire, December 18 1998.
Joel Hungerford v Susan L Jones

Washington State in 1989, was the first to allow those who claimed to have been the victims of historical sexual abuse, to sue their alleged abusers. There then followed a deluge of law suits in which thousands of men – fathers, brothers, grandfathers etc – were sued by their accusers. Gary Ramona in 1994, was the first accused to successfully sue the therapist he held responsible for implanting false memories in his daughter's mind. Although he won his case, the price he paid was enormous as he lost his wife and daughters, his job and his house. Ramona nevertheless paved the way for other falsely accused men and a very few women, to follow on and the judgement from the New Hampshire Supreme Court in the Hungerford Case is fairly typical of the attitude in the majority of states in the USA, where psychiatrists and therapists are held to owe a duty of care to those who stand accused, by patients of the therapists, who had been subjected to Recovered Memory Therapy and who then claim to have "recovered" memories of abuse.

This is in stark contrast to the law in the UK, as confirmed by Lord Kingarth, when he stated the following:-

"I stress '**as a matter of law**' because it goes without saying that if, as the pursuer claims, Dr Yellowlees made the diagnosis which it is said he did, and it is one reached carelessly and without proper investigation, the pursuer's concern to seek redress is wholly understandable, I am nevertheless required to decide this case within the boundaries of the law as it has recently developed."

Lord Kingarth. Court of Session, 8th July 2004.
James M Fairlie v Tayside Health Trust

When Lord Kingarth "struck out" my attempt to seek redress from Tayside Health Trust on account of the behaviour of Dr Yellowlees, a psychiatrist in their employ, he expressed sympathy for my position but claimed to be bound by the law, as it currently stands. This book is an attempt to have the circumstances of my fight to clear my name of false allegations of murder and sexual abuse, brought by my daughter in October 1995, brought into the public domain. It also highlights the way in which Katrina was treated, first of all, by the medical profession on whom she was totally dependent, and secondly, by the legal profession who deserted her in a most despicable fashion.

Each year the British False Memory Society hopes that this is the year, its services will no longer be required and each year it is disappointed. The "memory wars", so-called, have been raging for almost three decades on both sides of the Atlantic, although the incidence of the use of Recovered Memory Therapy (RMT) is not so prevalent as it once was. Despite the toxic nature of the self-help book *The Courage to Heal*, the Scottish Executive's Labour Administration in 2007, gave its stamp of approval to a new scheme to educate those who might come into contact with people who may have been sexually abused. The individuals concerned, the "victims", may be currently being abused as children or, may be adult survivors of child sexual abuse. The target audience for the educational programme, health visitors, psychiatric nurses and so on, were given a reading list which included *The Courage to Heal*.

The whole approach to the educational programme was one which encouraged the hunt for sexual abuse, by use of the checklist system, so roundly condemned in the USA and in this country by the Brandon Commission. It continued to encourage the use of methods which have given rise to thousands of cases of false memory and false allegations of sexual abuse leading to the payment of hundreds of millions of US dollars in compensation and the striking off of those professionals in the field of psychiatry and psychology who use RMT. It took the intervention of myself, the BFMS, the equivalent organization in Australia and Canada as well as a number of other concerned professionals in the UK, to persuade a very reluctant Scottish Executive to have the booklet, which formed the base of the educational programme, withdrawn and revamped. The revamped version, reintroduced in April 2008 with no publicity and without any notice being given to those like myself and the BFMS, who had objected to the original, is now in circulation to government employees in the field. It is only slightly better than the original because the recommendation to use *The Courage To Heal* has been withdrawn, but despite the enormous controversy that still exists because of the use of checklists, and the very extensive library of literature which has condemned the use of checklists, not a single volume has been given as "recommended reading".

This book should act as both a warning and as an example. Katrina's courage should be an inspiration to other young women who have gone through the same treatment and suffered the same traumas. Until there is a successful court case in the UK, which holds accountable those who were responsible for damaging the health of vulnerable young women by the use of RMT, cases such as ours will be repeated, are being repeated. I now work with those who have been falsely accused of sexual crimes in particular, but also with those who have been falsely accused of other crimes and whose cases are being ignored.

Sexual crimes carry a particular stigma and those who are found guilty deserve to be punished to the fullest extent of the law. Sexual predators and paedophiles deserve no sympathy but it is the public's attitude to this type of crime that makes the fight to clear the names of those who have been falsely accused, so important if there is ever to be any kind of natural justice. It is only recently that women who have falsely accused men of rape, have been subject to prosecution. No one should forget the way in which the Hamiltons were treated by sections of the media, until they were proved innocent. The same is also true of Mathew Kelly but what of the many ordinary people who can neither afford to pay to defend themselves, not have the "celebrity" to have questions asked on their behalf?

The cases of Sally Clark, Trupti Patel and Angela Canning showed how badly so-called "experts" can get it wrong and how often the justice system allows it to happen. There is no doubt, however, that those tragic cases would have been allowed to disappear without trace had it not been for the determined efforts of a few well-educated, articulate people who cared enough to bring the details into the public domain. Without the publicity, would Meadows and Southall ever have been held accountable? My family's case has had widespread publicity in the UK and to a lesser extent in the USA. It has been the subject of a BBC documentary in their "Front Line" series but neither Katrina nor I had the satisfaction of seeing those responsible brought to account in the only way that matters in the eyes of the public. This book can provide a public record of what happened to a perfectly ordinary family, which was determined enough to fight back. Had we not had that determination the consequences, particularly for Katrina, do not bear thinking about.

It also highlights the difference in approach in law in the UK and the USA in particular, to the traumas created by the misuse of psychiatry. There is an on-going battle in the UK to bring to account those psychiatrist and psychologists who continue to believe in recovered memories and to make them take responsibility for the damage they have caused. Silence has been the greatest defence the RMT practitioners have had and the voices of their victims have gone unheard. Our family survived but we all paid a very high price. Katrina's siblings are all highly successful in their own fields and Katrina has been able to return to active participation in martial arts and horse riding and her tenacity and courage has allowed her to turn her life around. The young woman the self-styled "experts" claimed was so badly damaged that she would never fully recover, has proved all of them wrong.

Despite more than a decade of fighting the establishment, with all the stress and anguish that entailed, Kay and I have watched with pride, our family prosper and grow. We now have three great-grandchildren and while we are no longer called on to babysit or have to prepare to have a house full of happy, healthy children on regular "action weekends", we still enjoy their visits, when the discussions are about their plans for after collage or university, football and sometimes current affairs and politics. The family survived and to Kay and I that was all important.

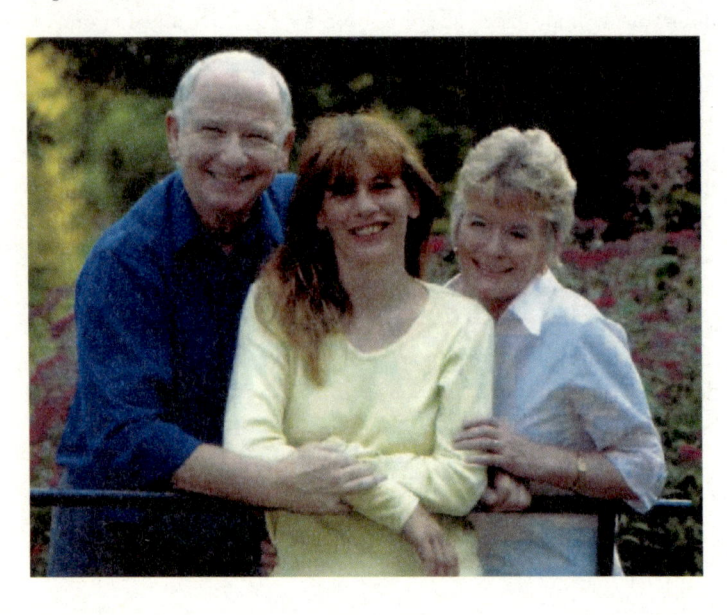

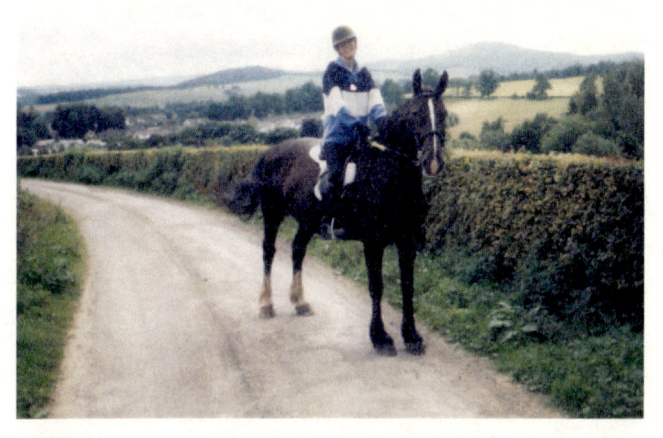

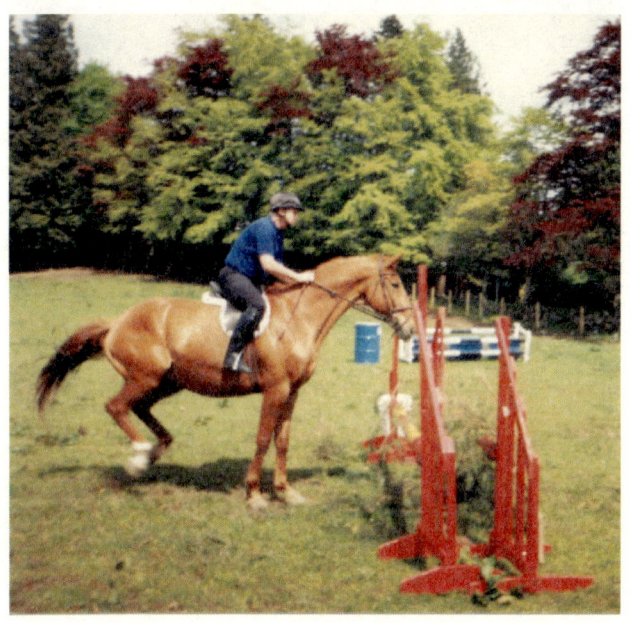